D1568731

THE HUMAN SKELETON

THE HUMAN SKELETON

Pat Shipman

Alan Walker

David Bichell

Harvard University Press
Cambridge, Massachusetts, and London, England

This book is printed on acid-free paper, and its binding materials have been chosen for strength and durability.

Library of Congress Cataloging in Publication Data

Shipman, Pat, 1949–
    The human skeleton.

    Bibliography: p.
    Includes index.
    1. Bones.   2. Human skeleton.   3. Anthropometry.   I. Walker, Alan,
1938–   .   II. Bichell, David.   III. Title.   [DNLM: 1. Bone and
Bones — anatomy & histology.   2. Bone and Bones — physiology.
WE 200 S557h]
QP88.2.S45   1985   612'.75   85-5497
ISBN 0-674-41610-4

The credits on pages 333–335 constitute an extension of the copyright page.

Contents

Illustrations

PART ONE
THE NATURE OF BONE

1
BASIC CONCEPTS

The subject is bone. But the word *bone* has two different meanings. Bone may be an organ, such as the humerus or upper arm bone, with a distinctive shape and function. Bone may also be a tissue or material with a particular capacity for growth, a distinctive chemical composition, and unique properties as a substance. As organs, the shape of bones reveals their functional constraints and illustrates the classic paradigm of whole organism biology that form reflects function. From the organization and structure of entire limbs down to the placement, frequency, and orientation of the microscopic canals that carry blood vessels to nourish bone tissues, bone form reflects the functional demands on bone for support and movement. The basic demands that carried over from the evolutionary heritage of an organism also come into play. Thus, the common heritage of all mammals dictates that they share mechanisms for bone growth, repair, and nourishment as well as identical microscopic components of bone. More specifically, the arrangement and shape of the wrist bones in humans carry concrete reminders of the time when our ancestors clung to branches with their hands.

In animals, the standard assortment of bones is known as the skeleton. In a human skeleton, normally there are 206 individual bones (Figure 1-1). Most of these come in pairs, such as the right and left humerus. Others are grouped into units. The backbone or vertebral column is made up of seven cervical, twelve thoracic, and five lumbar vertebrae. The ribs include twenty-four bones, twelve on each side of the thorax. The skull is comprised of eight major paired bones (the maxillae, palatines, nasals, inferior conchae, lacrimals, zygomatics, temporals, and parietals), three minor paired bones of the ear (the malleus, incus, and stapes), and six unpaired bones (the mandible, vomer, ethmoid, sphenoid, frontal, and occipital). The bones that provide the walls and roof of the cranial vault surrounding the brain (the frontal, parietals, temporals, and occipital) are sometimes referred to as vault bones. The hands and the feet are comprised of three groups of bones each. The hand has eight carpal or wrist bones (the scaphoid, lunate, triquetrum, pisiform, trapezium, trapezoid, capitate, and ha-

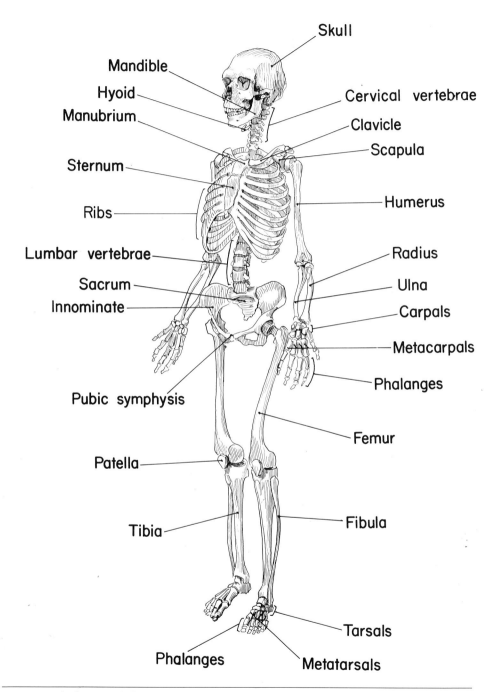

Figure 1-1

The human skeleton in anatomical position, showing the major bones or groups of bones.

mate), five metacarpal bones in the palmar region, and fourteen phalanges making up the fingers. The foot includes seven tarsal or ankle bones (the talus, calcaneus, navicular, cuboid, and first, second, and third cuneiforms), five metatarsals in the region of the sole, and fourteen phalanges in the toes, as in the fingers. In other mammals the number of bones is similar, although evolutionary specializations have often resulted in the loss or fusion of bones, such as the loss of toes in horses.

Study of the human skeleton in all its aspects — microscopic, gross, and functional — has a variety of uses. At a pragmatic level, fragmentary skeletal remains may need to be identified at archaeological, forensic, or paleontological sites. But much more than mere identification of the bones that are present can be revealed by studying skeletal materials. Relevant work is being carried out in a variety of fields, including embryology, cell biology, orthopedics, biomechanics, sports medicine, radiology, and anthropology. The results of many kinds of research on bone and bones are presented and synthesized here for the concerned student or professional who cannot hope to be a specialist in each of these fields.

ANATOMICAL RELATIONSHIPS

As a science, anatomy has developed its own vocabulary and language for the precise description of structures and parts of structures. Its most important concept, used in characterizing the relationships among the different parts of the human skeleton or body, assumes that the body is in the standard anatomical position: standing upright, with the arms at the side of the body, the hands palm forward, and the feet pointing straight ahead and parallel to each other (Figure 1-1). There are different conventions for describing anatomical relationships in quadrupedal mammals that do not habitually stand on two legs. The terms *right* and *left* as applied to parts of the human skeleton denote the sides of the body, not of the observer. Unless otherwise noted, all illustrations in this book show bones from the right side of the body.

There are six different sets of anatomical terms of direction in the human body: anterior or posterior; superior or inferior; medial or lateral; mesial or distal; buccal, labial, or lingual; and proximal or distal (Figure 1-2). Anterior and posterior refer to the front and back of the body or to planes parallel to the front and back of the body. Such planes lie perpendicular to the axis of symmetry, which divides the body into right and left halves. Anterior is toward the front, and posterior is

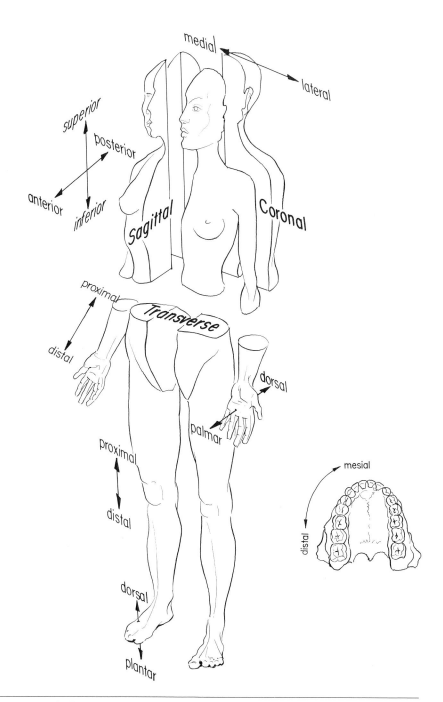

Figure 1-2

Anatomical planes and directions.

toward the back. These directions are relative. That is, a bone or other structure can be anterior to one structure and posterior to another. Thus, the external auditory meatus, the earhole on the skull, is posterior to the teeth but anterior to the back of the skull. In quadrupeds, *ventral*, meaning "toward the stomach," and *dorsal*, meaning "toward the back," are substituted for *anterior* and *posterior* when referring to the trunk. Structures in the limbs of quadrupeds are also referred to as having anterior and posterior aspects, although the standard anatomical position of their upper limb or forelimb differs from that of humans. In humans the hand is palm forward, or supinated. Since many quadrupeds supinate poorly, if at all, standard anatomical position for them is palm downward, or pronated.

Superior and inferior refer to the relative placement of structures along a vertical axis. Superior indicates a position closer to the head or the top of this axis; inferior, a position closer to the feet or the bottom of the axis. For example, the first cervical vertebra that holds up the skull is inferior to the skull but superior to the second vertebra lying directly beneath it. In quadrupeds, because of the different orientation of their body, superior is equivalent to dorsal, and inferior to ventral. A location that is closer to the head end of a quadruped is called cranial; its opposite direction, toward the tail, is called caudal.

Medial and lateral refer to a vertical plane that passes down through the head and body dividing it along the axis of symmetry. Medial is toward this plane; lateral is moving away from this plane. Thus, the shoulder joints are lateral to the sternum or breastbone.

Mesial and distal refer to the rows of teeth, called the dental arcade. Mesial is the direction moving forward around the dental arcade toward a vertical plane passing between the central incisors. Distal is the direction passing backward along the dental arcade from the central incisors. The third molars, often called wisdom teeth, are therefore distal to the second molars. Distal also refers to limb bones but has a different meaning in that context.

Buccal, labial, and lingual also refer to the teeth or the mouth. Buccal indicates the aspect of a structure closest to the cheeks. Labial is toward the lips, and lingual is toward the tongue. Thus, at least for the molars and premolars, buccal and lingual are perpendicular to mesial and distal. For incisors and canines, labial and lingual are perpendicular to mesial and distal.

Finally, proximal and distal refer to relationships among the bones or other structures of the limbs. Proximal is toward the trunk; distal is farther away from the trunk and closer to the digits. As with the other directions, proximal and distal are relative. For example, the distal end of the humerus or upper arm bone is proximal to the proximal end of the forearm bones, the radius and ulna, which it meets at the elbow.

All of these directions are relative and refer to a body in standard anatomical position. The importance of this is apparent in describing the bones of the limbs. For example, bending the elbow can bring the hand both closer to the trunk and higher from the ground than the elbow, but such an action can never make the hand either proximal to or superior to the elbow.

In addition to these six directions, the human body can be divided along three different planes or sections: the sagittal, coronal, and transverse. The sagittal plane bisects the body vertically along its plane of symmetry, dividing the right side from the left side. Thus, the sagittal plane runs in an anteroposterior direction. In Latin, *sagitta* means "arrow"; thus *sagittal* means "like an arrow" or "straight."

The coronal plane also divides the body vertically, but it runs medio-laterally or perpendicular to the sagittal plane. In other words, the coronal plane divides the anterior half of the body from the posterior half. The name of this section is derived from the Latin word for crown.

Finally, the transverse plane divides the body horizontally. This plane separates the body into superior and inferior parts. A transverse plane does not necessarily divide the body in half, however, and can be made at any level.

Bones themselves have a variety of features or structures. They have bumps or lumps, which in order of decreasing size are called processes, trochanters, tuberosities, protuberances, and finally tubercles. Bones also have elongated and narrow projections, called spines. A linear structure that is raised above the general level of the bone surface is a ridge or crest, and a depressed area is a groove or canal. Fossae or foveae are depressed areas that are less elongated in outline than grooves. A hole through a bone is a foramen (plural: foramina) or, if more tunnel-like in shape, a canal. The roughly spherical articular end of a bone is the head, and the narrower portion immediately adjacent to the head is often called the neck. The head of a bone is not necessarily the proximal end. The condyle is the vaguely knuckle-shaped, rounded articular portion of a bone. Both heads and condyles occur at freely mobile joints, where two bones meet, and they bear specialized articular surfaces to facilitate such movement. The main part of a bone, from which the various processes, condyles, heads, and so on protrude, is the body or shaft.

TYPES OF BONE

The skeleton as a whole has two major regions, the cranial and postcranial. Cranial elements are located in the head. They include the bones of the skull, the teeth, and usually the hyoid or bone that anchors the tongue muscles. All other elements are located in the postcrania, a term borrowed from mammalogy in which these parts of the body are typically posterior to the head, rather than being inferior to the head, as in humans. The postcrania are in turn subdivided into axial and appendicular regions. Axial bones are those of the trunk and thorax, such as the ribs, sternum, vertebrae, and sacrum, that part of the pelvis which articulates with the vertebral column. Appendicular bones are those in the limbs, including the bones of the shoulder girdle, upper and lower limbs, hands and feet, and innominates or hip bones.

The bones of the body also have four general shapes: long, short, flat, and irregular. Long bones are typically cylindrical; their length exceeds their breadth or thickness. Long bones include all of the major bones of the limbs, such as the humerus, radius, and ulna of the upper limb, and the femur, tibia, and fibula of the lower limb. The clavicle or collarbone, metacarpals, metatarsals and phalanges of the hands and feet are also long bones. Short bones are more nearly equal in length, breadth, and thickness than are long bones. Short bones are typically found in the hands and feet. They include the tarsals; the carpals; the sesamoids, which are specialized bones that grow within tendons, like the patella or knee cap; and various accessory bones that are sometimes formed by the unusual calcification of soft tissues, such as the cartilage that joins the ribs to the sternum. Flat bones are distinguished by the fact that their length and breadth far exceed their thickness. Flat bones include the sternum, ribs, innominates, scapulae or shoulder blades, and vault bones of the skull. Irregular bones are all other skeletal elements that do not fit any of these categories, such as the vertebrae, sacrum, and many cranial bones.

There are three gross types of bone tissue, based on morphology: compact or cortical, cancellous or spongy, and subchondral (Figure 1-3). Compact bone is the common type found on the external surface of skeletal elements. Nearly all of the bone in the shaft of any long bone is compact bone, so called because it looks dense and has few pores or spaces.

In contrast, cancellous bone is full of pores and spaces. Cancellous bone is made up of a network of small bars or plates called trabeculae. These trabeculae delineate marrow spaces that in life are filled with

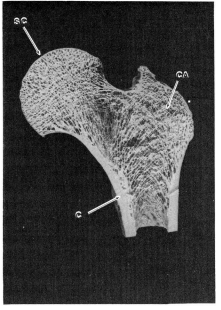

A

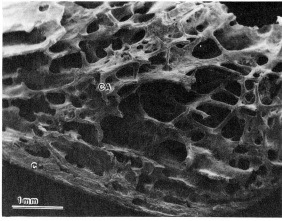

B

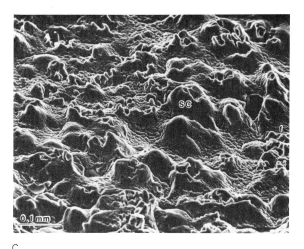

C

Figure 1-3

Types of bone based on gross appearance, *(a)* as found in a proximal femur. Compact *(C)*, cancellous *(CA)*, and subchondral *(SC)* bone. *(b)* Cancellous bone, made up of trabeculae, or small bony struts, and covered with a thin skin of cortical bone. *(c)* Subchondral bone, which underlies cartilage in life and is typically pierced by many small holes or canals for the blood vessels that help nourish the cartilage.

the hemopoietic tissues that produce red blood cells. Sometimes cancellous bone is also called coarse cancellous bone, to emphasize the large scale of these spaces. Cancellous bone is typically found in the ends of long bones, where it is covered with a thin protective layer of compact bone. In addition, cancellous bone is often found in flat bones, between two layers or tables of compact bone.

The third type of tissue, subchondral bone, occurs in the articular surfaces underlying the cartilage at particular types of joints. Articular surfaces differ from ordinary bone surfaces in having properties that facilitate movement. In life, articular surfaces are covered with a special tissue, hyaline cartilage, which is important in joint lubrication. Following death, the cartilage decays and disintegrates, exposing the subchondral bone, which is readily recognized as being unusually smooth and often slightly shiny. Subchondral bone is notable for the abundance of microscopic vascular canals piercing its surface. These canals carry the blood vessels that, in life, nourish the deeper parts of the hyaline cartilage.

FUNCTION OF BONE

In general, bone and bones perform four major functions in the body, having to do with its support, defense, movement, and supplies. First, the skeleton and its individual elements provide a framework or scaffolding that supports the soft tissues of the body and permits them to function without collapsing.

Second, the skeleton functions to protect the body. In one sense it acts as a sort of armor or hard, protective device to shield important soft tissues from damage arising from external sources. The ribs, for example, form a partial cage protecting the heart and lungs from blows or other injuries, and the skull acts as a bony box surrounding the fragile brain and special sense organs. In another sense, the joints and spongy bone tissue in the skeleton function as shock absorbers, modulating the impacts produced by locomotion and other movements so as to protect the soft tissues of the body.

Third, the bones of the body act as levers or struts, to be pulled upon by muscles, producing movement and locomotion. Although very small creatures, such as amoebae, are capable of slow movement without bones or other comparable organs, their method of movement is far from satisfactory if applied to creatures of human or even elephant size.

Finally, various cavities in the center of the major limb bones and in the cancellous layers of the skull, ribs, sternum, and innominates in adults serve as the loci of red blood cell or marrow production and storage. In addition, the bony tissues of the entire body are a huge warehouse of minerals to be tapped by the body in response to different physiological needs. For example, pregnant women with an insufficient intake of calcium will resorb part of their own bone tissue to supply the needs of the growing fetus.

Different regions of the skeleton are designed to meet particular needs. The four major functional areas of the skeleton are the head, trunk, upper limbs, and lower limbs.

There are twenty-eight bones in the skull or cranial region, plus thirty-two teeth in normal adults. By definition, a skull is comprised of a mandible and a cranium. A twenty-ninth bone, the hyoid, is usually grouped with the skull, although it is not properly part of the skull. The primary functional demands of the cranial region are associated with the brain, the senses, feeding, breathing, and noise making.

In terms of survival, the most important function carried out by the bones of the skull is protection and support of the brain. This function dictates much of the shape of the vault on many levels. The vault bones surround and protect the brain and bear the impression of the brain's external surface on their internal surface. In addition, the placement and size of the various foramina, canals, or other holes in the cranium, through which the nerves and blood vessels enter and exit, are finely controlled by the need for protection.

In addition to housing the brain itself, the skull houses four of the special sense organs for vision, smell, hearing, and taste, and it reflects their functional demands in its shape and structure. Vision and the visual apparatus are directly related to the size, shape, and placement of the orbits or eye sockets. In life, the bony orbits are lined with fat pads which form the actual sockets for the eyeballs, while the bony sockets provide stability and protection for these vulnerable tissues. The optic nerves that carry impulses from the eyes into the brain, where the information is processed, pass through special holes in the skull.

The olfactory apparatus, which is composed primarily of soft tissues, determines the size and complexity of the nasal conchae, delicate convoluted bones within the nose. In life, the nasal conchae are covered with tissues richly supplied by olfactory nerves. The importance of the sense of smell is also reflected in the cribriform plate, a part of the skull that lies below the olfactory lobes of the brain and above the nasal cavity and conchae. The cribriform plate is perforated with numerous holes through which pass all of the nerves associated with the sense of smell. The extent of the cribriform plate in an animal species directly reflects the extent of olfactory innervation and thus the importance of this sense to the animal.

Hearing is intimately associated with skull structure. The three tiny bones of each middle ear—the malleus, incus, and stapes—are all encapsulated within the temporal bone. The swelling of the large bony chamber within which these three small bones are found, as well as the shape and size of these bones, vary widely within mammalian species. Animals whose life may depend on hearing the low frequency noises made by their predators have greatly enlarged middle ear cavities, called tympanic bullae, which serve as resonating chambers.

The sense of taste is closely tied to mastication or chewing and processing of food. The masticatory apparatus is directly visible in the skull in the form, shape, and number of the teeth, in the shape and robustness of the maxilla or upper jaw and the mandible, and in the muscle markings on the cranial vault and zygomatics or cheekbones.

To some extent, the demands of breathing are reflected in the structure of the cranium. One major function of the nasal organ in humans is to warm and humidify air as it is breathed in. For example, in Eskimos living at lower temperatures the nasal conchae are elaborated and enlarged, at the expense of the maxillary sinuses, to provide a greater surface area for warming the air.

The postcranial skeleton has three functional units: the upper limb, the lower limb, and the trunk or axial portion. Each of these regions responds to different functional demands.

The upper limb and the lower limb are similar in general structure. The humerus of the upper arm is analogous to the femur of the thigh; the radius and ulna of the forearm are analogous to the tibia and fibula of the leg. Both foot and hand have five digits; phalanges, metatarsals, and metacarpals are arranged similarly. Despite these resemblances, the limbs are shaped by different functional demands that have resulted in structural modifications. In the upper limb, the major function is manipulation. The shoulder joint is extremely mobile, especially in comparison with the hip joint. The ball-and-socket joint at the shoulder is loose-fitting, and the cup of the scapula, the glenoid fossa, is shallow and only mildly concave. This arrangement allows free motion in a wide range of directions at the shoulder. The entire shoulder girdle is itself only weakly attached to the thorax or chest, both by a single bony connection between the sternum and the clavicle, which in turn articulates with the scapula, and by a complex series of muscles. The adaptations for manipulation are also visible in the freely pronating and supinating structure of the elbow, which permits the hand to be turned through at least 180°, and in the length and strength of the phalanges of the fingers. Finally, the long thumb has a specialized joint at its base to permit the thumb to be opposed to the other digits in a fingertip-to-fingertip position; this structure, which is lacking in the hallux or big toe, reflects the importance of the manipulative function to the upper limb.

The lower limb differs markedly in its attachment to the trunk, in the structure of its joints, and in the details of the foot. Support and loco-motion are the primary demands of the lower limb, although structural adaptations for efficient locomotion and support are compromised to facilitate childbearing, which requires different structural adapta-tions. In contrast to the shoulder joint, the hip joint is a highly con-gruent ball-and-socket joint with a much more restricted range of motion. The pelvic girdle as a whole is more tightly and inflexibly joined to the trunk. A ligament-reinforced joint links the lowest lumbar verte-bra and the sacrum, and strong sacroiliac joints link the sacrum with the ilia or blades of the innominates. The contrast persists in the more distal regions of the limb. The knee is built to have its major axis of motion in an anteroposterior direction; the joint between the femur and tibia is thus functionally similar to the joint between the humerus and ulna. However, in the elbow an additional pair of joints links the humerus with the radius and the radius with the ulna. These joints permit a second major axis of movement in the elbow. There is no joint at all between the fibula and femur, so that the knee is denied a compa-rable range of motion. Moreover, the joint surfaces of the knee are expanded, larger than those of the elbow, and cushioned by special fibrocartilaginous structures called menisci (singular: meniscus), which are additional weight-bearing features. In the foot, both the shortening of the toes and the restricted motion of the hallux reveal the supportive function played by this region. In humans, nearly all ability to grasp and manipulate with the toes has been sacrificed in favor of providing a broad, stable support for walking on a relatively flat and continuous substrate.

The third postcranial region, the trunk, plays the dual role of sup-porting and protecting the relatively delicate internal organs of the thorax and abdomen. Both movement, for breathing and speaking, and rigidity, for protection, are needed. The cage-like arrangement of the ribs over the heart and lungs is a protective device common to all mammals. The ribs also need to move, so as to increase the size of the thoracic cavity to facilitate expansion of the lungs in respiration. The movement of the ribs both outward and upward is permitted by the structure of the joint between the heads of the ribs and the vertebrae onto which they are anchored, which permits movement in two axes: superoinferior and mediolateral.

The vertebral column itself serves to protect the spinal cord, which passes through a bony ring, the vertebral arch, in each vertebra. In addition, the vertebral column serves to support the upper body. Finally, the vertebral column serves to support the skull and brain, and its structure is closely tied to this function.

The brain, though vital to life, is delicate, having the consistency of pudding. Yet it is balanced on top of the vertebral column inside the bony box of the skull. Such an arrangement would be doomed to failure without a cushioning device to shield the brain from the shocks of normal locomotion and movement. Two cushioning mechanisms are provided: the meninges and the S-shaped curve of the vertebral column.

The meninges (singular: meninx) are three membranes that surround the brain in layers. They anchor it within the skull, inhibit its movement, and buffer it against shocks with the cerebrospinal fluid that fills the spaces between the meninges and between the innermost meninx and the brain itself.

A major function of the cerebrospinal fluid is to impart buoyancy to the brain. The fluid literally supports the brain and greatly diminishes its effective weight. This buoyancy effect can be calculated simply. The weight of the brain and spinal cord in air is roughly 1500 grams; their effective weight when supported by cerebrospinal fluid reflects the weight of the displaced fluid:

$$\text{weight}_{\text{body}} = \text{weight}_{\text{air}} \times \left(1 - \frac{\text{fluid specific gravity}}{\text{tissue specific gravity}} \right)$$

$$= 1500 \text{ gms} \times \left(1 - \frac{1.007}{1.04} \right)$$

$$= 47.6 \text{ gms}$$

where weight$_{\text{body}}$ = effective weight of the brain in the body

weight$_{\text{air}}$ = effective weight of the brain in air

fluid specific gravity = weight of the cerebrospinal fluid per unit volume, relative to a standard

tissue specific gravity = weight of the brain tissue per unit volume, relative to a standard

Thus, the effective weight of the brain and spinal cord is reduced from

1500 grams to less than 50 grams, which substantially reduces the momentum of the brain in response to ordinary movements or forces.

The other cushioning mechanism, the double, S-shaped curve of the vertebral column, can be seen in lateral view. As a result of this shape, the entire column has the ability to flex and thus absorb shocks, like a spring.

At any region of the body or skeleton, a wide range of actions is possible, but few are of functional significance. Muscles function by contracting, not by pushing. Contraction produces a pull on the bone or object at the end of the muscle that is less firmly fixed or stabilized (unless neither end is fixed, as in weightlessness, when both ends may move). Thus, the same muscle can pull an object or an appendage toward the body, or it can pull the body toward the object or appendage. The determining factor is the relative mobility of each end of the system. For example, the muscles of the arm can be used both to move the hand relative to the stable body and to move the body relative to the stable hand, as in pushing off from a wall. Both directions of movement are equally possible as a result of arm muscle contractions. But in practice, the former is much more common than the latter. As a general rule, therefore, most muscle actions routinely operate in only one direction, which is the one that is functionally significant.

MOVEMENTS OF BONE

Contracting muscles anchored to bones, which in turn are articulated with other bones at joints, produces movement or action. Most muscles are attached to bones at two points. The origin of a muscle is the point of attachment that is more often fixed and immobile following contraction of the muscle. The origin is usually the more proximal or superior point. The insertion of a muscle is the point of attachment of the muscle that is most often moved by contraction of the muscle. Although these terms are to some extent arbitrary, since the bone at either end of a muscle is capable of moving, the distinction between origin and insertion is useful in considering the function of muscles.

Seven different actions can be produced by the movement of bones through muscle contractions: flexion, extension, abduction, adduction, rotation, gliding, or circumduction. These actions are either reciprocal, capable of occurring in two opposite directions, or else occur in a reciprocal pair with another action. For example, flexion and extension are a reciprocal pair of actions. Flexion decreases the angle at a joint or makes it more acute; extension is the opposite action of straightening out the joint or making it more obtuse. The muscles that habitually produce such actions are often collectively referred to respectively as flexors or extensors. Abduction and adduction are another reciprocal pair of actions. Abduction moves a bone or segment of a limb laterally or away from the sagittal plane at midline. Adduction moves a bone or segment of limb medially or toward the body's midline. Muscles producing such actions may be called abductors or adductors.

Rotation spins a bone or limb segment, usually about its long axis. Rotation occurs in two opposing directions, often medial or lateral. The muscles responsible are therefore referred to as lateral or medial rotators.

Gliding is the movement of one bone past another. It is an action typical of joints with planar or nearly planar surfaces. Gliding may occur in a variety of directions, according to the orientation of the joint at which it occurs, but is usually a movement of minor significance. Muscles producing gliding are not called gliders but instead are given other names derived from other aspects of their function.

Circumduction is an action in which a bone or limb segment is pivoted about a joint so that the distal end of the bone or limb segment describes the base of a cone, the apex of which is at the joint. Circumduction is such a complex action that it can be produced only by the cooperative actions of several muscles. These muscles are referred to by names reflecting their primary actions rather than the action of circumduction.

2
BONE STRUCTURE

The structure of bone as a tissue can be examined at three different levels: molecular, microscopic, and gross. But in reality each of these different aspects of bone structure is interrelated with the others.

MOLECULAR COMPOSITION

The molecular composition of bone is remarkably constant in all mammals. Regardless of species, bone is always a two-phase composite substance made up of two very different materials. Such substances are called anisotropic, meaning that they have two different sets of properties. The two major components of bone are the organic matrix, or osteoid, and the inorganic matrix. The organic matrix of bone is primarily collagen, a protein that occurs in long, flexible fibers made up of finer fibrils. The presence of collagen is not exclusive to bone; it occurs in connective tissues in various parts of the body, such as tendons, blood vessels, or the cornea of the eye. Collagen gives bone its elasticity, flexibility, and strength in tension or in response to pulling forces. The inorganic matrix of bone has the opposite characteristics. Various calcium salts, primarily hydroxyapatite $(Ca_{10}(PO_4)_6(OH)_2)$, are deposited in crystals within and between the long collagen fibrils. These inorganic crystals give bone its rigidity, hardness, and strength in compression.

GROSS TO MICROSCOPIC STRUCTURE

In addition to sharing the same molecular composition, bones share certain features of gross appearance. They are covered on their outer surface by a thick, tough membrane, called the periosteum where it overlies bone; it does not overlie articular cartilage but is continuous with the joint capsule. A similar tissue, the endosteum, lines the marrow cavities of the bones. In other respects the three gross types of bone—compact, cancellous, and subchondral—are distinguished by their appearance.

At the microscopic level, the differences between subchondral, compact, and cancellous bone blur. All types of bone have an identical microscopic structure at comparable stages of maturity of bone tissue.

The difference between them lies in the relationship of each to the blood supply. Cancellous bone is bony tissue surrounded by blood vessels; compact bone is blood vessels surrounded by bony tissue; and subchondral bone is more vascularized than compact bone and less vascularized than cancellous bone.

The microscopic structure of bone varies according to its maturity and the speed with which it must be laid down. There are three forms of immature or new bone: woven, laminar, and fine cancellous (Figure 2-1). Woven bone is deposited in the initial formation of bone in the fetus or where rapid repair of bone is needed. The surface texture of woven bone is characteristically coarse and fibrous in appearance, with many criss-crossing bundles of collagen fibers arranged in a disordered or random pattern. Many relatively large and tortuous channels for blood vessels wind through woven bone and across its surface. Eventually, woven bone is remodeled into mature bone, which has a more ordered structure.

In rapidly growing large animals, like humans, the remodeling process may be too slow to keep up with growth, so another type of immature bone is formed where greater strength is needed: laminar bone. Laminar bone is composed of sheets, or laminae, of bony tissue separated from each other by intervening networks of blood vessels. These blood vessels run primarily in the spaces between laminae and rarely traverse a lamina. As a result, laminar bone has a smaller volume of vascular canals than other types of bone and is probably stronger in some ways.

The third type of rapidly growing bone, fine cancellous bone, is found in places where transient reinforcement of the extant bone is needed. For example, fine cancellous bone may appear on the brow ridge of an animal when the stresses involved in chewing increase, as when a new tooth is erupting. Like coarse cancellous bone, fine cancellous bone appears grossly porous, although the pores are generally smaller. It also has a distinctive texture, since the surface is covered in tiny, meandering vascular canals separated by miniature ridges of new bone. In cross-section, these ridges appear to be shaped like mushrooms, separated from each other by blood vessels.

The differences between immature and mature bone lie mainly in the relationships between the vascular canals and the bony tissue. Mature or adult bone is called lamellar. Such bone is arranged in thin sheets or lamellae, which are roughly 3–7 microns thick (a micron equals 1/1000 of a millimeter). In each lamella, the bundles of collagen fibers are arranged parallel to one another, although the predominant

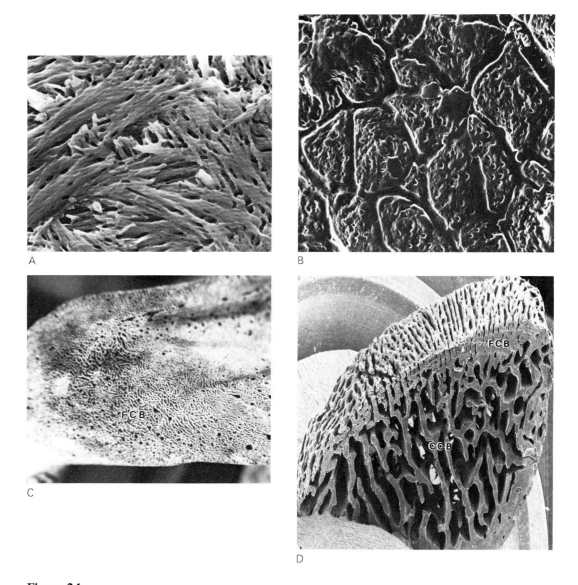

Figure 2-1

Types of bone based on microscopic appearance. *(a)* Woven bone has a coarse, fibrous texture that reflects its rapid growth. It is later remodeled into mature bone. *(b)* Laminar bone is also immature and rapidly laid down. It consists of sheets or laminae of bone separated by networks of blood vessels. *(c)* Fine cancellous bone characteristically has a surface covered by many ridges of new bone separated by vascular canals. *(d)* The prominent ridges of bone and vascular canals of fine cancellous bone, seen here in cross-section, distinguish it from coarse cancellous bone.

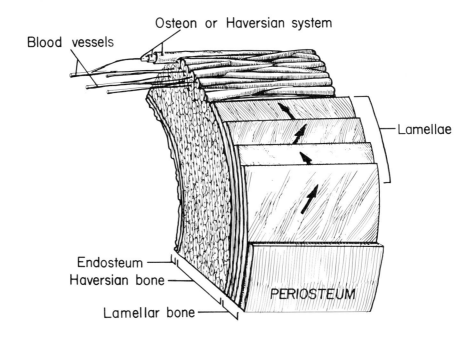

Blood vessels

Osteon or Haversian system

Lamellae

Endosteum
Haversian bone
Lamellar bone

PERIOSTEUM

Figure 2-2

Mature compact bone. The outer region is lamellar bone, made up of circumferential lamellae. Its predominant fiber orientation varies from lamella to lamella. The inner region is Haversian bone, in which blood vessels are surrounded by concentric tubes of bone tissue. Its basic unit is the osteon, a vascular canal plus its surrounding rings.

orientation may vary from lamella to lamella for strength (Figure 2-2). This arrangement gives lamellar bone a stratified or layered appearance in cross-section. Subchondral, compact, and coarse or fine cancellous bone may all be remodeled into lamellar bone.

A group of lamellae may be organized in one of two ways, depending upon its location within the whole bone. The basic unit of lamellar bone is the osteon, in which sets of 15–20 lamellae are arranged in concentric tubes around an opening for a blood vessel. The placement of vascular canals within these rings of bone differentiates mature from immature bone. Surrounding each osteon is a cement line, a dense ring that demarcates its boundaries and surrounds the outer lamella throughout the entire length of the osteon. Because osteons are formed by remodeling either immature bone or older mature bone, adjacent osteons may cut across each other, may touch each other at their cement lines, or may be separated by regions of less organized bone tissue. These intervening regions of bone, called interstitial bone, are irregular in shape. They may be remnants of woven or laminar bone, or they may be old, heavily reworked osteons.

The vascular canal at the center of each osteon is part of a network of canals, the Haversian system, which brings nourishment to the bone tissue. Within this system are two types of canals, Haversian and Volkmann's. Haversian canals are oriented more or less longitudinally within the bone. They are connected to each other, to the marrow cavity, and to the surface of the skeletal element by a complex system of oblique and transversely oriented canals, or Volkmann's canals. Volkmann's canals are not surrounded by concentric lamellae and in fact frequently cut through lamellae.

Not all mature bone is organized into osteons. Near both the inner and outer surfaces of long bones, this organization of bone tissue is replaced by several large-scale lamellae that encircle the entire perimeter of the shaft; these are called outer and inner circumferential lamellae. A comparable structure is found in the outer layers of other sorts of mature bones. Occasionally, coarse bundles of collagen fibers, called Sharpey's or perforating fibers, leave the periosteum adjacent to the outer circumferential lamellae and run perpendicularly into the circumferential lamellae and the underlying interstitial bone. Sharpey's fibers serve to anchor the periosteum firmly to the bone's external surface. They are particularly numerous at the attachment sites of various muscles and tendons and may in time partially ossify.

Although immature bone is a stronger substance than lamellar bone, it is nonetheless relentlessly remodeled into lamellar bone. One reason is that the greater vascularity of lamellar bone has a greater capacity for repair in response to stress, injury, or disease. Another reason is that remodeling permits a complete reorganization of the microscopic structure of a bone in order to meet radical changes in the daily stresses upon it, as when a sedentary individual takes up jogging.

BONE CELLS

Blood and bone are intimately related in terms of both development and function. Embryologically, blood cells, blood vessels, and bone tissue are all derived from mesenchyme, an embryonic connective tissue. A crucial step in the initial development of bone is the invasion of the bone's precursor by capillaries. The capillaries transport bone-forming cells into the precursor. These cells then begin to transform the precursor tissues into true bone. In adult life the vascular network continues to function as a transport system for bone cells, bringing bone-forming or bone-resorbing cells to sites where repair or remodeling is needed. In turn, bones serve as a repository for hemopoietic or blood-forming tissues. In adults, hemopoietic cells are present only within the marrow cavities of the different bones, while in children the liver also plays a role in blood formation.

Bone cells carry out two major functions, production of new bone and resorption or destruction of old bone, along with many minor functions. The microscopic features of the three different types of bone reflect the arrangement and activities of the different bone cells. Some of the most important features of bone cells are organelles, the membrane-bound components of the cell that carry out specific functions. The frequency and location of organelles reveals the overall functional capacities of each type of bone cell.

One of the main organelles is the Golgi apparatus. The Golgi apparatus is directly related to the high degree of secretory activity in a cell. Thus, it seems to have four major functions in any cell. First of all, the Golgi apparatus is thought to function in rearranging cell membranes so as to "wrap" or "unwrap" various products moving in and out of the cell. For example, it may wrap a secretory product in membrane, producing a vacuole that can move to the cell surface where the contents are discharged. The empty vacuole then returns to the Golgi apparatus, where the membrane is removed. Second, the Golgi apparatus may produce membrane-bound granules containing concentrated secretory products that are then stored in the cytoplasm for future use by the cell. Third, the Golgi apparatus processes various secretory products in the cell, which may end up being packaged in granules or vesicles. Finally, the Golgi apparatus is probably responsible for concentrating various digestive enzymes and wrapping them in membranes to form lysosomes, which are the digestive organelles of the cell.

The mitochondrion, another organelle, is the energy storehouse of the cells. It processes carbohydrates and other substances, releasing energy for various metabolic functions. As a result, the presence of many mitochondria shows that a cell is very active.

Another organelle is the endoplasmic reticulum, which contains many cisternae, or compartments, within which newly produced substances, such as proteins, can be segregated or processed further. One type of endoplasmic reticulum, known as the rough endoplasmic reticulum, has a surface studded with small, spherical structures called ribosomes. Encoded in the ribonucleic acid (RNA) within these ribosomes are instructions for synthesizing various products needed by the body. As proteins or other products are synthesized according to these instructions, they pass into the cisternae of the rough endoplasmic reticulum for storage or additional processing. From there, these products often move into the Golgi apparatus.

There are three major types of bone cell: osteoblasts, osteocytes, and osteoclasts (Figure 2-3). Osteoblasts are the major bone-forming cells. They are primarily responsible for producing large quantities of osteoid, the uncalcified organic matrix of bone. This collagen-rich substance is secreted from the nucleus-bearing end of the cell. Osteoblasts are derived from generalized cells, called osteoprogenitor cells, in the embryonic mesenchyme. Osteoprogenitor cells are present in the lining of the blood vessels on the periosteal surface and in Haversian canals. They are active both during initial bone production in the embryo and, after birth, at sites where bone injury is being repaired. As precursors, osteoprogenitor cells divide frequently and rapidly, but once they are transformed into osteoblasts, division is rare.

An active osteoblast is columnar in shape, having its nucleus at the end farthest from the bone surface. In an osteoblast, a well-developed Golgi apparatus lies between the nucleus and the cell base. At the far end of the cell, away from the nucleus, are rough endoplasmic reticulum and many mitochondria. The presence of these organelles reveals the active secretory function of the osteoblasts. Associated with the mitochondria are many dense granules that are believed to contain calcium and phosphate crystals, which are probably dissolved and released from the cell during calcification.

Osteocytes, the second major type of bone cell, are derived from osteoblasts that have become surrounded or trapped in matrix, regardless of whether calcification is complete or in progress, and have ceased to make osteoid. Instead, osteocytes seem to have a regulatory function, responding to the body's need for lower or higher circulating levels of the minerals contained in bone. There are three phases in the life of an osteocyte: formative, resorptive, and degenerative. In the formative phase, the new osteocyte resides in a space, called a lacuna, within either the osteoid or the bony tissue. It is losing its ability to manufacture osteoid but still has a large Golgi apparatus and endoplasmic reticulum. It is also well supplied with mitochondria but has few lysosomes. In this phase, the osteocyte develops long, dendritic processes, which reside in bony tubes, known as canaliculi. These processes act as a communication network between adjacent osteocytes.

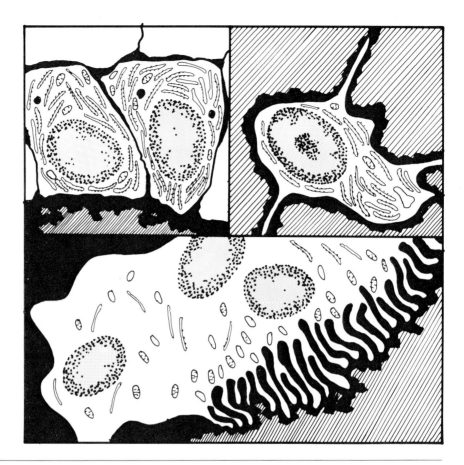

Figure 2-3

Bone cells. The diagonally shaded areas are bone. Within cells, the stippled structures are nuclei; short ovals are mitochondria; and elongate ovals are either rough endoplasmic reticulum *(studded perimeters)* or Golgi apparati *(plain perimeters)*. *(Top left)* Osteoblasts, responsible for secreting osteoid, are typically columnar in shape and have many mitochondria and much rough endoplasmic reticulum. *(Top right)* Osteocytes are osteoblasts trapped in lacunae in the osteoid. They communicate with other cells through long dendritic processes lying in canaliculi. *(Bottom)* Osteoclasts are large cells with many nuclei that are responsible for resorbing bone tissue. Resorption occurs at the ruffled border, at right, where digestive enzymes are released, creating a rounded depression or Howship's lacuna.

As the osteocyte matures, it enters the resorptive phase, in which it is surrounded with a pericellular sheath of osteoid-like material that lies between its edges and the lacuna wall. In this phase, the dendritic processes enable each osteocyte to pick up hormonal signals that indicate the need to resorb calcium or phosphate from the surrounding tissues. This resorption process is known as osteolysis. Because osteocytes can respond more rapidly to the body's needs than other resorptive mechanisms, osteolysis is crucial to maintaining appropriate circulating levels of calcium. By the time an osteocyte is in the resorptive phase, it is deeply embedded, its organelles have generally deteriorated, and the endoplasmic reticulum and Golgi apparatus are much less noticeable.

As osteocytes age further, they reach the final degenerative phase. At this point holes or vacuoles appear in the cytoplasm, mitochondria, and Golgi apparatus.

Osteoclasts, the third major type of bone cell, contrast with the other two types in being very large (20–100 microns in diameter), multinucleate, and involved actively in bone resorption rather than bone production. Osteoclasts were once thought to result from the fusion of the same osteoprogenitor cells that give rise to osteoblasts and osteocytes. Recent work suggests that osteoclasts are derived from the fusion of hemopoietic, not mesenchymal, cells with single nuclei in response to hormonal cues. These osteoclast progenitors are probably monocytes circulating in the blood stream.

In appearance, osteoclasts are distinctive for reasons other than their size and multiple nuclei. Actively resorbing osteoclasts are usually found in shallow depressions in bone tissue known as Howship's lacunae. These lacunae are probably formed by the osteoclasts themselves rather than being pre-existing concavities toward which the cells then gravitate. The resorptive surface of the cell, which creates the lacuna, is deeply infolded in what is called a ruffled border. This structure actively frees apatite crystals and collagen from the bone tissue. As osteoclasts resorb bone, large vacuoles filled with lysosomal enzymes move toward the ruffled border and apparently release the enzymes there to digest the bone tissue outside the cell. As apatite and collagen are digested from the bone tissue, these substances probably move into the deeply infolded areas of the ruffled border, which then pinch off to form vesicles. Such vesicles, filled with apatite crystals and collagen, have been observed in osteoclasts. The side of the osteoclast that is not in contact with the bone surface is smooth, and the abundant nuclei and mitochondria often occur near this outer surface of the osteoclast. Osteoclasts have many Golgi complexes and large vacuoles containing digestive enzymes. Finally, the endoplasmic reticulum is less abundant in osteoclasts than in osteoblasts.

Because of the bone's complex needs for nearly constant remodeling and growth, the three different types of bone cells often work simultaneously in adjacent areas of a bone. As woven bone is remodeled into mature, lamellar bone, osteoclasts work to resorb the young bone. At the same time, osteoblasts produce new osteoid, which in turn transforms the osteoblasts in osteocytes. Even at the cellular level, bone is a dynamic, responsive tissue.

3
COLLAGEN AND CALCIFICATION

Collagen, a fibrous protein, is the major organic constituent of bone as well as a major component in other body parts, such as hair, nails, tendon, and various connective tissues. It is also the most common protein in the body. Collagen is both elastic and flexible, able to deform and then recoil significantly without damage. It therefore contributes substantially to the strength of bone in tension or in torsion. Human collagen fibers can withstand a pulling force of several hundred kilograms per square centimeter without breaking or permanently elongating more than a small percentage of their original length.

COLLAGEN STRUCTURE AND FORMATION

The molecules making up collagen are distinguished by their large size, which is a function of their structure. Like all proteins, collagen's basic components are amino acids, linked together into peptides. Long chains of peptides, called polypeptides, form the basic units of collagen. Each polypeptide chain in collagen is a left-handed helix which then coils into a right-handed spiral or supercoil. Three polypeptide chains intertwined in this way form a large tropocollagen molecule (Figure 3-1). Each tropocollagen molecule is about 280 nanometers (nm) long and 1.36nm wide (a nanometer is 1/1,000,000 of a millimeter) and has a molecular weight of about 290,000.

In the body, collagen occurs as aggregations of tropocollagen molecules arranged in fibrils, which combine to form larger fibers. Different arrangements of peptides result in different polypeptide chains, and thus the exact composition of the tropocollagen molecule differs in different tissues. In birds and mammals, two of the three polypeptide chains found in bone, skin, and tendon are of a type called an $alpha_1$ chain, and the third is of a different type called an $alpha_2$ chain.

The process of aggregating the polypeptide chains into tropocollagen molecules is called polymerization. During polymerization, chemical bonds are formed, creating links not only among the three chains that make up a single tropocollagen molecule but also among the various molecules themselves. These bonds stabilize the collagen fi-

28

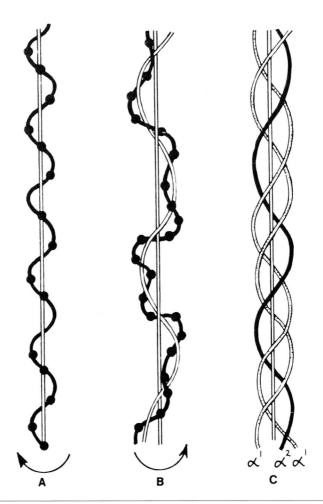

Figure 3-1

The tropocollagen molecule, comprised of three polypeptide chains wound together. *(a)* A single polypeptide chain *(black)* is coiled into a left-handed helix around an imaginary axis *(open)*. *(b)* The coiled chain is supercoiled in a right-handed helix around a second hypothetical axis. *(c)* Three such coiled and supercoiled chains are wound together to produce the tropocollagen molecule. Two of the chains are identical in structure (alpha$_1$ chains), and the third is biochemically different (alpha$_2$ chain).

brils and keep them from disassociating into their component molecules. Throughout the life of an individual, the number of these bonds within and among the tropocollagen molecules increases. This increase in bonding may account for the decreasing flexibility of bone with age.

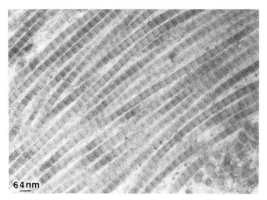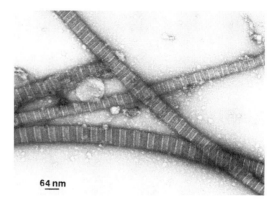

64nm   64 nm

Figure 3-2

Collagen fibers, showing characteristic dark bands at 64-nm intervals under different staining.

Apart from the typically large size and mass of the tropocollagen molecules, collagen in bone is readily recognizable because, when stained and magnified, its fibrils show characteristic dark bands at roughly 64nm intervals (Figure 3-2). Other forms of collagen show a different spacing of these bands. Only collagen with 64nm banding, however, becomes calcified into bone.

The precise arrangement of the tropocollagen molecules into fibrils and the cause of the banding are matters of debate. According to the most probable model, proposed by Hodge and co-workers, tropocollagen molecules are arranged in parallel lines, with holes between the head of one molecule and the tail of the molecule in front of it in the same line. However, the molecules in one line are staggered relative to those in the lateral line, so the holes are not aligned transversely across the fibril. Instead, the head of one molecule overlaps with the hole and part of the tail of the adjacent molecule (Figure 3-3). The dark bands that are visible at 64nm intervals are the holes between the heads and tails of subsequent tropocollagen molecules. Each of these holes is 26.5nm long and preferentially takes up the dark stain. The light bands interposed between the dark bands are areas of overlap between laterally adjacent molecules. These overlapping zones are 37.5nm long and appear light because they stain poorly.

The precursor of bone collagen is a molecule called procollagen, which is produced by osteoblasts. Other types of cells also produce procollagen that does not become bone. Chondroblasts, for example, make collagen for cartilage. Procollagen is even longer and heavier

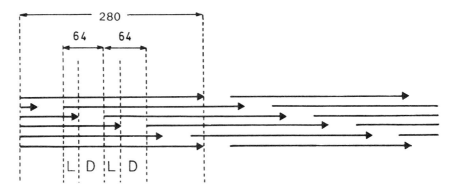

Figure 3-3

Model for the packing of tropocollagen molecules into fibrils (Hodge et al., 1965). The regularly spaced holes between the tail of one molecule and the head of the next *(D)* produce the dark bands seen in Figure 3-2. The holes appear dark because they absorb the stain. The zones of overlap between laterally adjacent molecules *(L)* show up in Figure 3-2 as light bands, where little stain has penetrated.

than the tropocollagen molecule, because it contains extra polypeptide chains at both its head and tail ends. These extra chains apparently prevent the premature assembly of the collagen fibril before the molecules leave the osteoblast.

The production of procollagen and its transformation to collagen are believed to occur in three stages. First, amino acids within the endoplasmic reticulum of the osteoblasts are assembled into unusually long polypeptide chains, which intertwine and become cross-linked into procollagen as they move through the endoplasmic reticulum and into the Golgi apparatus. Second, the Golgi apparatus wraps the procollagen in a membrane, creating a vacuole which is then sent to the cell surface, where the procollagen is excreted. Finally, once the procollagen is outside the cell, the extra polypeptides are removed by a special enzyme, procollagen peptidase, and the tropocollagen molecules assemble into typically banded, cross-linked collagen. Although the collagen is the major component of uncalcified organic bone matrix, it is not the only component. Other molecules secreted by bone cells are also found in osteoid.

CALCIFICATION

The calcification or mineralization of osteoid to form bone is a complex process. Calcium phosphate becomes crystallized into hydroxyapatite, or bone mineral, and is deposited in the collagen fibrils at specific sites, probably within the holes between the tropocollagen molecules. Precisely how this occurs is a matter of controversy. The calcification of osteoid into bone may be a process similar to the formation of ice crystals in water. This process is called nucleation, because the crystals start to grow from a nucleus or central core.

Three factors are important in inducing calcification by nucleation: the concentrations of calcium and phosphate ions must be high enough for the release of minerals, substances must be present either to trigger nucleation or to remove the barriers to nucleation, and a mechanism is needed for localizing nucleation to specific sites within the collagen fibrils. The first condition, adequate supply, is met with the help of the calcium phosphate that is stored as granules within or near mitochondria in the osteoblasts. As calcification begins, these granules may be either excreted directly from the cell or dissolved first, after which the ions are excreted. Other calcium and phosphate ions apparently come from the blood stream, because the different lamellae in osteons are calcified to different degrees, with the lamellae closest to the blood vessel being most heavily mineralized (Figure 3-4). If sites that are physically or biochemically suitable for calcification are lacking, or if a necessary mediator between the ions and the sites is absent, calcium phosphate may simply disperse, raising the calcium and phosphate concentration in the blood.

Different mechanisms are needed to trigger nucleation, depending on the kind of nucleation involved, homogeneous or heterogeneous. In homogeneous nucleation, molecules cluster together in a process called precipitation to form the fragments from which crystals grow. The precipitation is triggered by a temporary increase in the concentration of molecules. But homogeneous nucleation is an improbable mechanism for calcification, both because raising the circulating concentrations of calcium and phosphate ions in the blood stream to levels high enough for precipitation to occur does not always produce calcification, and because much of the collagen in the body remains uncalcified even when calcium and phosphate levels are high. Rather, the mechanism responsible for calcification must affect specific, local areas only.

The alternative pathway to calcification, heterogeneous nucleation, depends on the introduction of a foreign substance to the system which disrupts the equilibrium and causes the molecules to cluster. For example, ice is formed from water spontaneously and homogeneously at $-39°$ to $-41°C$ only if there is absolutely no dust or other foreign matter present. When silver iodide crystals are added, as in cloud seeding, ice

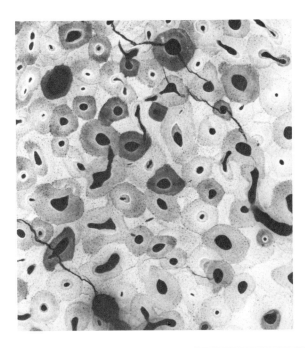

Figure 3-4

Mature compact bone, showing the lamellae of each osteon. In this microradiograph the inner lamellae of many osteons, which are closer to the blood vessel, are lighter than the outer lamellae, indicating that they are more heavily mineralized.

crystals begin to form on the surface of the silver iodide crystals at $-4°$ to $-6°$C. In bone, the foreign matter that triggers nucleation may be the appearance of tropocollagen molecules properly arranged into 64nm-banded collagen fibrils. The precise juxtaposition of particular components, such as the location of the holes in the fibrils, may serve to trigger heterogeneous nucleation. This arrangement would explain why collagen without 64nm banding does not calcify. Support for this view derives from the fact that in calcifying collagen fibrils, hydroxyapatite crystals are deposited at regular intervals that correspond to the holes' spacing.

Since collagen is widespread in the body as connective tissue and yet usually calcifies only in bone, there must be either an inhibitory mechanism preventing widespread calcification of collagen or a highly specific trigger mechanism, or both. The main candidates for the inhibiting agents are substances called pyrophosphates, found commonly in blood plasma. Pyrophosphates inhibit nucleation by making solutions containing calcium and phosphate ions more stable. The local concentration of pyrophosphates is regulated by an enzyme, alkaline phosphatase, which degrades pyrophosphates so that they are incapable of inhibiting nucleation. Significantly, alkaline phosphatase is always found at active nucleation sites where calcification is proceeding.

The final condition permitting appropriate nucleation and thus calcification to occur, the localization of calcification, is probably achieved by the action of a molecule that selectively binds to calcium and phosphate ions in one area and to the nucleation sites, or holes in the collagen fibrils, in another. It is easier to list the attributes of such a molecule than to identify exactly which molecule plays this role. The molecule would probably be manufactured by osteoblasts as one of the noncollagen constituents of osteoid, since such an origin would place the molecule in the appropriate region. Further, such a molecule must be able to bind only to collagen that will calcify and only at the nucleation sites within the fibrils. Finally, such a molecule must be able to bind simultaneously to those nucleation sites and to calcium and phosphate ions, while leaving the ions in a reactive state so that they can interact with each other to make crystalline hydroxyapatite. Several different proteins have been suggested to possess these attributes and would fulfill the localizer role. Among the more likely candidates are the protein osteonectin and a group of proteins, called phosphoproteins, which contain an amino acid, serine, bound to phosphate. Ongoing research should clarify which of these substances may function to initiate and localize calcification of osteoid.

BONE-BLOOD TRANSFER

Once collagen is calcified into bone, the tissue does not subside into inactivity. Bone remodels and resorbs nearly constantly in response either to the stresses and strains of daily activity or to the needs of the body for the calcium and phosphate minerals tied up in bone. The various parts of the body need a steady supply of calcium and, to a lesser extent, phosphate in order to carry out everyday functions. For example, even a fairly small drop in the circulating level of calcium causes the nerves and muscles to go into automatic discharge, producing spontaneous muscle spasms. Thus, mineral homeostasis must be maintained in the blood at all times, despite the temporary needs for the deposit, repair, or remodeling of bone in response to growth, injury, or disease. At the same time, sufficient calcium and other minerals must be maintained in the bones and kept available for growth or repair. For these reasons, there is a continuous

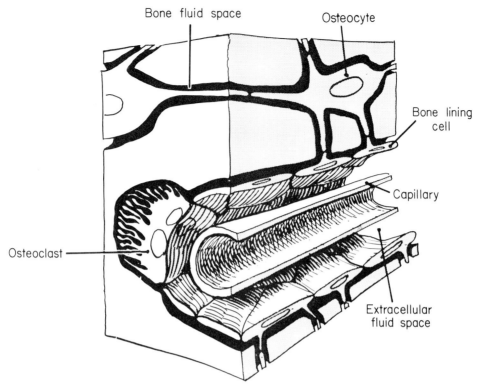

Bone fluid space

Osteocyte

Bone lining cell

Capillary

Osteoclast

Extracellular fluid space

Figure 3-5

Bone-blood transfer system. The extracellular fluid compartment contains nutrients, hormones, and other substances that have diffused out of the blood in the capillary. This compartment is lined with bone lining cells, which communicate to the embedded osteocytes the body's need to take up or release calcium and phosphate ions. This mode of mineral homeostasis responds rapidly to the circulating levels of parathyroid hormone or calcitonin.

exchange of calcium and phosphate ions between the bone tissue and the blood. This exchange is called the bone-blood transfer.

The bone-blood transfer is another example of the intimate association of bone and blood as tissues. It relies upon a precise arrangement of bone, bone cells, and blood (Figure 3-5). On the resting surfaces of bone, where neither resorption nor deposition is occurring, there is a special layer of flat cells, called bone lining cells, which resembles a membrane. These cells are either dormant osteoblasts or surface osteocytes. On one side they communicate with the embedded osteocytes via slender processes lying in canaliculi through the bone. Bone fluid bathes this surface of the bone lining cells, the processes, and the embedded osteocytes. On the other side of the bone lining cells is a compartment filled with extracellular fluid which is derived directly from blood plasma by diffusion out through the capillary walls. Thus, extracellular fluid both brings nutrients, hormones, and other substances to the cells by diffusion out of the capillaries and brings calcium or other substances back into the blood stream by diffusion back into the capillaries. Most of the regulation of mineral homeostasis occurs through the activities of osteocytes that take up or release calcium and phosphate ions in response to signals based on circulating levels of calcium in the blood plasma.

Regulation is accomplished through the activities of a pair of hormones secreted by the thyroid and parathyroid glands in the throat. These two hormones have opposite and antagonistic effects on the body. Parathyroid hormone increases the circulating level of calcium and phosphate ions. It stimulates osteocytes to initiate osteolysis, thus inducing resorption of bone mineral. Osteolysis results in the transfer of calcium and phosphate into the cytoplasm of the osteocyte, where normally it would be packaged into granules of calcium phosphate for storage in the mitochondria. However, parathyroid hormone also blocks the packaging of these minerals into granules. The result is a rapid build-up of calcium and phosphate in the cytoplasm. The response of the osteocyte is to pump the calcium and phosphate ions out of the cell into the bone fluid and, from there, via the bone lining cells, into the extracellular fluid. Once the ionic concentration is higher in the extracellular fluid than in the blood stream, the calcium and phosphate ions diffuse freely into the blood plasma, thereby raising the circulating levels. This response may occur in a matter of minutes.

The secretion of parathyroid hormone may also affect osteoclast activity, but osteoclasts are slower to respond to transient changes in parathyroid hormone concentration than are osteocytes. The effect of parathyroid hormone on osteoclast activity is more often a long-term function of maintaining appropriate mineral levels in the blood than a short-term response to the immediate needs of the body. Parathyroid hormone also facilitates the movement of calcium from the extracellular fluid into the cells of the gut and kidney. The circulating levels of calcium are not thereby lowered, however, because the extracellular fluid in turn derives much of its calcium from food that is being digested. Thus, parathyroid hormone increases the efficiency with which gut and kidney cells absorb dietary calcium and ultimately increases the total amount of calcium in the body.

Calcitonin, also called thyrocalcitonin, which is the hormone secreted by the thyroid gland, performs contrary actions to those of parathyroid hormone. That is, calcitonin serves in a number of ways to lower the circulating levels of calcium and phosphate in the blood stream. First, calcitonin reverses the flow of calcium and phosphate ions, moving them from the blood stream back into the extracellular fluid and then to the bone fluid. In addition, calcitonin blocks the resorptive activities of either osteoclasts or osteocytes, thus keeping calcium and phosphate ions locked up in bone tissue. Resorption by osteoclasts is inhibited by rendering the ruffled border of the osteoclasts inactive. Calcitonin visibly causes the ruffled border of osteoclasts to flatten and disappear, and it may cause the osteoclast to separate from the bone surface. Ruffled borders rapidly reappear if parathyroid hormone is released. Finally, calcitonin induces osteocytes to excrete their amorphous calcium phosphate granules into the adjacent osteoid, if there is any, to foster calcification.

These two hormones work in concert to control the interchange of minerals in the bone and blood. Both are constantly present in the blood of normal individuals, their concentrations fluctuating in response to the body's long-term and short-term needs.

4
BONE GROWTH

Bone growth involves a complex set of processes that occur once, in a particular sequence, in the life of an individual. These processes are coordinated with, but distinct from, the formation and calcification of bone tissue, which recurs throughout an individual's life. Bone growth begins prenatally, with the initial formation and ossification of the skeletal elements. Thereafter, growth continues in both prenatal and postnatal life, as the bones mature and increase in size, until skeletal maturity is reached and bone growth ceases.

During prenatal development, the bones of the body are laid down and ossified for the first time. At birth, the skeleton is immature, small, and imperfectly formed. All of the skeletal elements are present, but the proportions between them differ from those in adults. For example, an immature long bone typically shows three bony units with cartilage plates interposed between them (Figure 4-1). The middle portion of this bone, called the shaft or diaphysis, is a roughly cylindrical tube. In its center is a hollow, called the medullary or marrow cavity, which is filled with marrow-producing tissues and fat throughout life. At either end of the shaft is the metaphysis, the region in which most of the increase in length will occur with growth. The metaphyseal surface of the long bone is typically roughened, porous, and ridged. In fact, each metaphysis has a unique pattern of ridges or raised areas that distinguishes it from other metaphyses in the body. The articular ends of the long bone are separately ossified entities, called epiphyses. The epiphysis and metaphysis are joined together by a plate of epiphyseal cartilage, also called an epiphyseal plate, growth plate, or physis. When a long bone is almost skeletally mature, the epiphyseal plate is so reduced in superoinferior dimension that it is often called the epiphyseal line.

After the bone is formed, the second phase of growth commences, culminating in skeletal maturity. It has two major effects. One involves the epiphyseal plate and is reflected in its other name, physis, a word derived from a Greek verb meaning "to generate." Throughout the maturation process, bone tissue is generated at the interface of the metaphysis and the epiphyseal plate until all of the cartilage is replaced

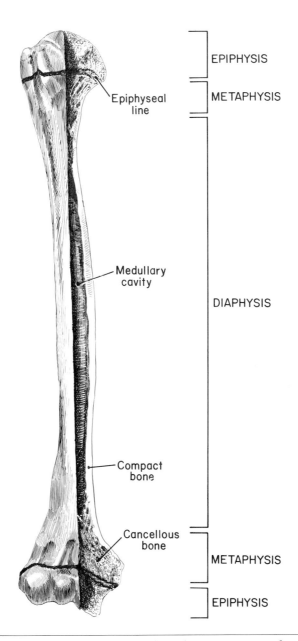

EPIPHYSIS

METAPHYSIS

Epiphyseal
line

Medullary
cavity

DIAPHYSIS

Compact
bone

Cancellous
bone

METAPHYSIS

EPIPHYSIS

Figure 4-1

Immature long bone. Both articular ends have their own centers of ossification, or epiphyses, which are joined to the diaphysis or shaft by an epiphyseal line or plate. The metaphysis is the actively growing region of the shaft next to the epiphyseal plate. In the center of the diaphysis is the medullary cavity, filled with marrow and hemopoietic tissues.

with bone. Skeletal maturity is reached when the epiphysis, meaning "over or on the physis," is firmly joined by bone to the metaphysis, meaning "after or beyond the physis," with no remaining trace of an epiphyseal line to indicate where the physis has been. Not all epiphyses in the body fuse simultaneously. For example, maturity of the distal humerus occurs just after puberty, but fusion at the proximal end is delayed until about 20 years of age. Many bones in the body that are not considered long bones also have epiphyses that fuse at maturity. The other major consequence of the second phase of bone growth is a tremendous increase in size and, often, minor changes in shape.

The second phase of bone growth is of special importance to many fields, because there is a fairly constant sequence and rate of skeletal maturation among different individuals. Therefore, the state of maturity of a complete or partial skeleton can be used to estimate the age of an individual at death.

PRENATAL BONE FORMATION

The sequence of bone formation begins with the fertilization of an egg or ovum by a single sperm, which forms a zygote (Figure 4-2). In the normal course of events, this single-celled zygote divides rapidly to form a ball of about sixteen cells, called a morula. By about the fifth day after fertilization, a cavity has appeared within the morula, transforming it into a blastocyst. The cells continue to divide and proliferate, but they are not evenly distributed around the cavity. Two different types of cells are present. On one side of the blastocyst is a dense clump of cells known as the inner cell mass; surrounding both this mass and the cavity is an even layer of different cells called trophoblasts. The embryo implants in the uterine wall at about the seventh day after fertilization. After this, the trophoblasts give rise to the placenta, and the inner cell mass begins forming the tissues of the embryo.

By the eighth or ninth day, the inner cell mass has differentiated into two cell layers. It is now called the bilaminar embryonic disc because it is a flattened structure of circular outline. The two layers are the ectoderm — which gives rise ultimately to such structures as the superficial layers of the skin, the hair and nails, some glands, and the central nervous system — and the endoderm — from which is derived such structures as the lining of the pulmonary and digestive systems, the tonsils, pharynx, and thyroid gland.

On or about day fifteen, a thickening, known as the primitive streak, appears along the midline of the ectoderm. Cells proliferate from the primitive streak and migrate laterally between the ectodermal and

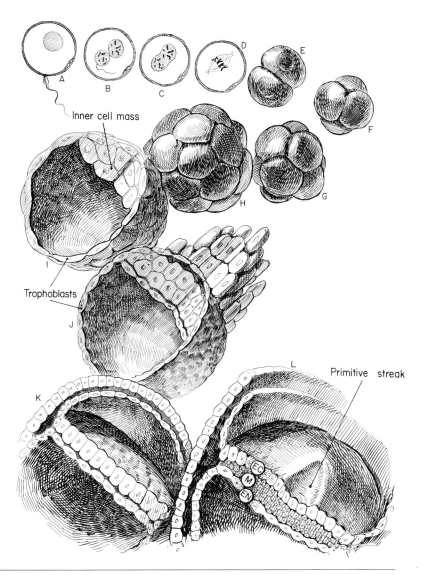

Figure 4-2

Development and early growth of an embryo. *(a)* The sperm penetrates the ovum or egg cell. *(b)* A fertilized, single-celled zygote results. *(c–h)* The zygote divides rapidly to form a 16-celled ball, the morula. *(i)* A cavity appears within the morula at about the fifth day after conception, transforming it into a blastocyst. *(j)* Blastocysts have two different types of cells, trophoblasts, which give rise to the placenta, and the inner cell mass. *(k)* By the eighth or ninth day the inner cell mass has differentiated into two layers, the ectoderm *(EC)* and endoderm *(EN)*, which comprise the bilaminar embryonic disc. *(l)* On the fifteenth and sixteenth days a thickening, the primitive streak, appears along the ectoderm; cells migrate from the primitive streak to form a loose connective tissue, the mesenchyme, which then gives rise to a third cell layer, the mesoderm *(M)*, lying between the ectoderm and the endoderm in the trilaminar embryo. The mesoderm gives rise to all of the skeletal elements.

endodermal layers, to form the loose, embryonic connective tissue known as mesenchyme, arranged around large, fluid-filled extracellular spaces. By the sixteenth day, the embryo is trilaminar, with a new cell layer, called mesoderm and derived from the mesenchyme, sandwiched between the ectoderm and endoderm. Ultimately, the mesoderm gives rise to all of the skeletal elements, the muscles of the body and viscera, the urogenital system, all connective tissues, and many other structures.

As the embryo and, after nine weeks, the fetus develop, the bones of the skeleton begin forming from the mesoderm by one of two modes: intramembranous or cartilaginous (also called endochondral) ossification. In both cases, bones develop through the transformation of previously existing tissues derived from the mesoderm. The major difference lies in whether those previously existing tissues are cartilage or mesenchyme.

Intramembranous ossification occurs when bone directly replaces mesenchyme. This mode of development occurs in the clavicle, the frontal, the parietals, the nasals, the maxillae, the vomer, the palatines, most of the mandible, and portions of the sphenoid, temporals, and occipital. Although many of the bones or parts of bones that undergo intramembranous ossification are flat, some flat elements, such as the scapulae and innominates, are not ossified in this way.

The center of ossification for bones that ossify intramembranously begins as a condensation and proliferation of mesenchyme to form a membrane, which then becomes highly vascularized. In the case of the cranial vault bones, this thickening of mesenchyme surrounds the developing brain tissues just as the future cranial vault will surround the mature brain. The mesenchyme cells serve as osteoprogenitor cells, which are transformed into osteoblasts. The blood vessels bring in the circulating monocytes that are the precursors of osteoclasts. Beginning in the third month after fertilization, these cells first ossify and then remodel the membranous tissue. As the condensed mesenchyme is replaced by bone tissue, a thick membrane is left surrounding the growing bone tissue. This membrane eventually becomes the periosteum.

By far the more common mode of ossification is cartilaginous. The limb bones, vertebrae, sternum, ribs, bones at the base of the skull, and parts of other bones all undergo a cartilaginous stage during embryonic or fetal development. Those parts of the cranium that are preformed in cartilage are called the chondrocranium. They include parts of the occipital, temporals, and sphenoid, and all of the ethmoid, malleus, incus, stapes, nasal cochae, lacrimals, and zygomatics. The occipital, temporals, and sphenoid are ossified in cartilage only in their denser regions, which contribute to the base of the cranium.

For such skeletal elements, the process of becoming a bone begins with chondrification, or the formation of a cartilage precursor or model, in the fourth or fifth week of fetal life. Mesenchyme cells condense and proliferate, as in intramembranous ossification, but instead of turning into osteoblasts, these cells become chondroblasts, or cartilage-forming cells. The chondroblasts turn themselves into mature chondrocytes, which are more rounded in outline, by secreting a matrix of collagenous fibrils that eventually surround and separate the cells from each other. Each chondrocyte is left within a primitive cartilage lacuna. In time, these cells produce a small, rudimentary model of the future bone out of hyaline cartilage.

These cartilage models are surrounded by a special, condensed mesenchymal tissue, the perichondrium. This tissue is essentially the same as that surrounding the intramembranous centers of ossification. In both cases, the tissue contains the osteoprogenitor cells that are ultimately responsible for making the bone tissue. The difference is one of timing. In intramembranous ossification, these osteoprogenitor cells are transformed into osteoblasts soon after the mesenchymal thickening appears; the osteoblasts then produce osteoid, which calcifies and becomes bone. In cartilaginous ossification, these osteoprogenitor cells remain dormant for a time, while the cartilage model is enlarged by the chondrocytes.

Long bones are good examples of bones that develop by cartilaginous ossification. Typically, long bones and vertebrae have three or more centers of cartilaginous ossification, one for the diaphysis and at least one each for the proximal and distal epiphyses (Figure 4-3). The cartilage model of a typical long bone is roughly dumbbell-shaped.

Growth of the cartilage model of a long bone occurs in both length and width (Figure 4-4). An increase in length is accomplished by interstitial growth, involving the multiplication of chondroblasts at the ends of the model. An increase in width occurs by appositional growth, in which new chondroblasts are contributed by the perichondrium. As the model grows in size, the cells at the center of the model mature and hypertrophy, or swell up; they also develop cavities in their cytoplasm. The matrix between chondrocytes thins and starts to disappear as those cells die, leaving empty, enlarged lacunae that are often confluent with each other. The remaining thin matrix walls calcify, but they are calcified cartilage and not bone. While the chondrocytes at the

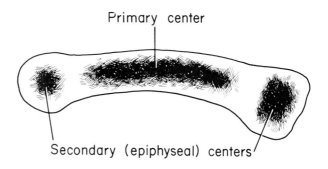

Primary center

Secondary (epiphyseal) centers

Figure 4-3

Typical long bone, with three separate centers of cartilaginous ossification.

center of the model are hypertrophying and dying, those at the perimeter remain normal.

Ossification begins at the primary center, within the shaft, as the perichondrium is invaded by numerous capillaries, which transform it into periosteum. The invasion by capillaries triggers the osteoprogenitor cells that have been lying dormant in this tissue. They turn into osteoblasts and begin producing osteoid in a thin sheet, called a periosteal collar, around the shaft of the model. The periosteal collar rapidly becomes calcified.

Nearly simultaneously, the central core of the model is invaded by capillaries carrying osteoblasts and osteoclasts. In a process called cavitation, these cells degrade the calcified cartilage, leaving a narrow cavity at the core. Within this cavity the osteoblasts lay down small struts and spicules of osteoid. These constitute the medullary center of ossification, which is often considered part of the primary, periosteal center. The struts rapidly calcify, filling in most of the cavity.

Calcification of the bone proceeds outward from the medullary center and inward from the periosteal center in a repetitive sequence. First the chondrocytes degenerate and die. The remaining lacunar walls calcify and are invaded by capillaries bringing in osteoclasts and osteoblasts. The osteoclasts resorb the calcified cartilage, and the osteoblasts produce osteoid. The osteoid calcifies and becomes true bone. The same repetitive sequence of events occurs in the epiphyseal centers of ossification, which are invaded by capillaries subsequent to invasion of the shaft. The epiphyseal centers are usually considered secondary centers of ossification.

As the cartilage model is replaced by bone, extensive remodeling occurs. First, the true medullary cavity is created and enlarged by resorption of the bony struts and spicules originally laid down in the

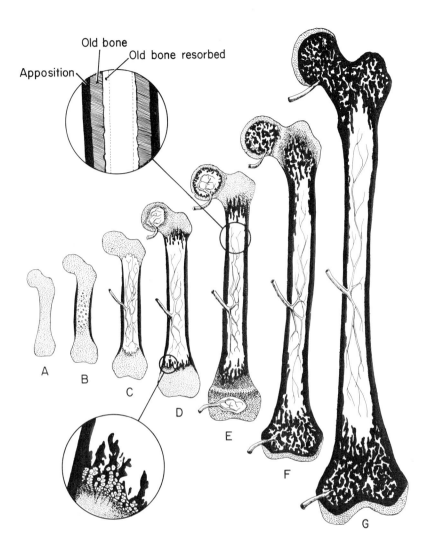

Figure 4-4

Growth of a long bone. *(a)* A long bone begins as a cartilaginous model, surrounded by perichondrium. *(b)* As the model grows, the cells at its center hypertrophy and start to die, leaving enlarged lacunae surrounded by thin matrix walls, which calcify. *(c)* The perichondrium is invaded by capillaries, transforming it into peri-osteum. *(d)* Osteoprogenitor cells in the periosteum become osteoblasts, which produce osteoid around the shaft. This periosteal collar is the primary center of ossification. The shaft ossifies and grows by resorption on its inner surface and apposition on its outer, as osteoclasts in its center degrade the calcified cartilage. *(e)* Secondary centers of ossification appear in the epiphyses. *(f)* As the bone approaches adult size, the diaphysis and epiphyses are fully ossified and separated from each other by epiphyseal plates of cartilage. *(g)* Eventually these plates are replaced by bone, whereupon skeletal maturity is attained.

medullary center. The newly formed medullary cavity comes to be lined with a highly vascular membrane, the endosteum, which — like the periosteum — is capable of providing osteoprogenitor cells for later remodeling. Second, the developing bone continues to enlarge by both interstitial and appositional growth, in a mode directly analogous to that used by the cartilage precursor to grow. The difference is that bone, not cartilage, is formed, so bone cells, not cartilage cells, proliferate or are recruited from the periosteum.

INCREASE IN SIZE   Once the shaft and epiphyses are ossified, leaving the cartilaginous epiphyseal plates between them, each skeletal element increases in size in a continuous process that ceases at skeletal maturity. Such growth in size involves both active resorption and active deposition of bony material, changing the bone's length and breadth. But while the overall diameter of the shaft wall increases with growth, so does the diameter of the medullary cavity. Osteoclasts for resorption are supplied by both periosteum and endosteum, as are osteoblasts for the production of new bone. Growth in size begins prenatally and continues postnatally.

The epiphyseal plates of long bones are cartilaginous at birth and remain so throughout many years of life. Many other bones are incompletely ossified at birth. Throughout the period of skeletal immaturity, the individual is constantly creating new bone by ossifying either cartilage or membrane. Resorption is also an integral part of the growth process.

At birth, ossification of the skull is incomplete. Much of the base of the skull is still cartilaginous, and the cranial vault bones, which ossify intramembranously, are separated from each other by six large membranous expanses, called fontanelles (Figure 4-5). The bregmatic or anterior fontanelle is located at midline where the two centers of ossification of the frontal bone meet the growing parietal bones. The homologous point on an adult is called bregma. The sphenoid or anterolateral fontanelles are located on either side of the skull where the sphenoid and temporal bones meet the inferior angle of each parietal. This point is known as pterion. The mastoid or posterolateral fontanelles are located on either side of the skull at the junction of the temporal, parietal, and occipital bones, at a point known as asterion. The lambdoid or posterior fontanelle, which is unpaired like the bregmatic fontanelle, occurs at the junction of the parietals and the occipital bone, at a point called lambda. These fontanelles are commonly known as the "soft spots" on babies' heads.

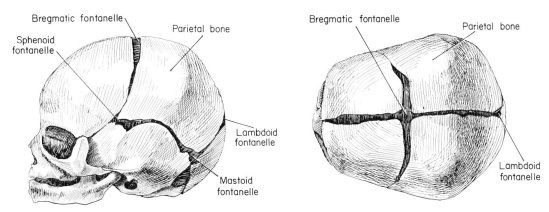

Figure 4-5

Neonatal skull, showing the six fontanelles between the ossifying vault bones. The bregmatic fontanelle lies at the junction of the growing frontal bone and the parietals. The two sphenoid fontanelles lie on each side at the anterolateral corner of the parietal, where it meets the temporal and frontal bones. The two mastoid fontanelles lie on each side at the junction of the temporal, parietal, and occipital bones. The lambdoid fontanelle occurs at the junction of the occipital and parietal bones.

The different fontanelles close by ossification at various times after birth. At 2–3 months the lambdoid and sphenoid fontanelles close; the mastoid fontanelles are closed by the end of the first year; and the bregmatic fontanelle closes between 18 months and two years after birth. The immaturity of the cranial vault at birth is an important feature. It allows a degree of malleability of the baby's skull, which facilitates passage through the birth canal. The skull's immaturity also permits the brain to grow after birth without being inhibited by the size of the skull, which in normal individuals increases to accommodate the enlarging brain.

Once the fontanelles are ossified, narrow, linear segments of membrane persist as sutures between adjacent vault bones. There are five major sutures in the cranium. Between the left and right halves of the frontal bone, which at birth are separate centers of ossification, is the metopic suture, which infrequently persists past early childhood. The coronal suture runs across the front of the skull, posterior to the frontal and anterior to the two parietals. The sagittal suture runs anteroposteriorly between the two parietals. The lambdoid suture, so called because it is shaped like the Greek letter lambda (Λ), joins the posterior parts of the parietals to the occipital bone. The coronal, sagittal, and lambdoid sutures all begin to ossify in the late teens, achieving closure in the thirties or later. The squamous sutures lie on either side of the skull between the inferior edge of the parietal and the superior edge of the temporal. Whereas the metopic, coronal, sagittal, and lambdoid sutures all are characterized by interdigitated fingers of skull bone separated by narrow strips of intervening membrane, the squamous suture is distinctively beveled, the superior edge of the temporal overriding the inferior edge of the parietal. The squamous or temporal sutures fuse later than the others, if at all, and they open and close slightly during breathing. The fifth suture is the basilar, which joins the body of the sphenoid to the adjacent basilar portion of the occipital bone. This suture generally closes in the late teens or early twenties. Many other sutures exist in the skull between pairs of adjacent bones. They are named for the bones they join, as in the zygomatico-maxillary suture.

Premature ossification of the fontanelles or closure of the sutures occasionally occurs as severe, congenital pathologies. Although closure of the cranial sutures generally begins at about age 17, proceeding from the interior of the vault outward, the rate and completeness of sutural closure are so variable from individual to individual that these are best used for age estimation in conjunction with other indicators.

REMODELING

Accompanying the appearance of new bone in any region of the skeleton is a continuous process of remodeling, which persists even once skeletal maturity is reached. This remodeling process is directly spurred by stresses and injuries incurred by the individual's actions and activities. Such remodeling transforms young, rapidly formed bone, with its primitive, disorganized vascular system, into highly organized, secondary lamellar bone with its mature Haversian system. This continuous remodeling process ensures a constant supply of newly formed osteons, which are more readily accessible than mature osteons as a source of the minerals needed for various metabolic functions.

Cancellous bone is also subject to nearly constant remodeling. Its remodeling follows Wolff's law that the organization of a bone reflects its function. For example, the orientation and arrangement of trabeculae reflect the trajectories of stress on cancellous bone. The corollary of Wolff's law is that changes in function or stress induce changes in structure. The mechanism whereby such changes occur has been investigated by Radin and co-workers studying the trabecular network of cancellous bone, which serves as a shock absorber for the joint. Ordinary stresses produce numerous microscopic fractures in the trabeculae. The repair of these fractures produces two measurable effects: a temporary increase in the density of the region, due to the formation of a callus, or new growth of woven bone, as part of the normal healing response; and a dynamic realigning and restructuring of the trabecular network so as better to absorb the stresses to which it is regularly exposed.

The complex interplay of the forces of bone growth and remodeling throughout an individual's life shows the dynamic nature of the skeleton. From the first formation of bones in the embryo to the final remodeling of Haversian bone near the time of death, both bone and bones are constantly changing. Various cellular and biochemical mechanisms work to fine-tune the structure, shape, size, density, and orientation of the bone tissue that makes up bones. Remarkably, the skeleton must change continuously so that it can maintain constant function in many different ways throughout life.

5
BONE AS
A MATERIAL

As a structure, the skeleton must function under an extraordinary set of circumstances. Throughout the life of an individual, the skeleton must change dramatically in size, resulting in changes in shape, and it must withstand an unusually varied set of functional demands, such as the many different types of motion and locomotion that are carried out even while the soft tissue mass, muscular strength, and mineral content of bones are undergoing change. One factor that allows bone to accomplish these operations efficiently and successfully is its ability to remodel and change biochemically in response to the body's demands. Another factor is its unique structural and mechanical properties.

MECHANICAL AND STRUCTURAL PROPERTIES

The mechanical properties of any material determine its response to different forces, such as tension, compression, and torsion. Both the forces and the properties are precisely defined. Tension is a pulling force, which tends to separate the atoms and molecules of the substance from each other. For example, tension is applied in the act of contracting a muscle which then pulls on the bone to which it is attached. The opposite of tension is compression, a force that tends to push an object or material into a diminished space, thus packing the constituent atoms and molecules more closely together. Compression is exerted by the body weight on the vertebral column, pelvic girdle, and bones of the leg and foot, even when the individual is standing passively. Running or jumping considerably increases the tensile and compressive force exerted on those bones; additional tensile force is created when muscles are used. Bending applies a combination of tension and compression to an object. Thus, both tension and compression are forces commonly applied to bones in everyday life. Torsion is a twisting force. It occurs more rarely but results more often in bone breakage. For example, in skiing accidents when the ski twists one way and the leg twists the other, one or more bones are fractured as the skier falls.

Bones are able to resist these three forces because of both the me-

50

chanical properties of their tissues and the design of their structure. Stress measures how hard external forces of compression or tension are pushing together or pulling apart the atoms and molecules of bone or any other substance. Mathematically, stress = load/area, where load, or force, is measured in terms of pounds or kilograms, and area is measured in terms of square inches or centimeters. Thus, the units in which stress is measured are either pounds per square inch (psi) or kilograms per square centimeter (kg/cm^2). Or in the international system based on the newton, which equals 0.102 kilograms or 0.225 pounds of force, stress is measured in meganewtons (one million newtons, or mn) per square meter (mn/m^2).

Strain measures how much the bonds between atoms or molecules are stretched by tension or compressed by compression during stress. Strain thus indicates how much effect a given stress has on the substance in question. In other words, unit strain = change in length/ original length, or the percentage increase or decrease of the original length. Since both the change in length and the original length of an object have identical units, such as inches, feet, centimeters, or meters, strain is expressed as a quantity, without using any units.

While stress is a measure of force on a substance and strain is a measure of the effect of force on the substance, strength is the amount of tensile or compressive force required to break the substance. Strength is often measured when the substance is under tension, because the ways in which a substance may fail or collapse under compression are more variable. Compression may cause deformation, buckling, or, with brittle materials, fragmentation.

Another major structural property of a substance is its elasticity, or relative stiffness or flexibility, as measured by Young's modulus of elasticity. This is an important quality in predicting how a substance will respond to stresses and strains. It is calculated from both of those values: Young's modulus = stress/strain. In other words, elasticity is a function of the force per unit area divided by the percentage change in length created by that force. Since, in deriving Young's modulus, the force per unit area is divided by a fraction, the resultant value (E) is expressed in the same units as stress, in either psi or mn/m^2.

Both stress and strain are variable, even for the same sample of the same substance; thus, Young's modulus can vary. However, the changing relationship of stress to strain is characteristic of a given material. Plotting stress against strain for a substance yields a curve that is distinctive for that substance (Figure 5-1). The slope of this curve roughly indicates the Young's modulus for the substance.

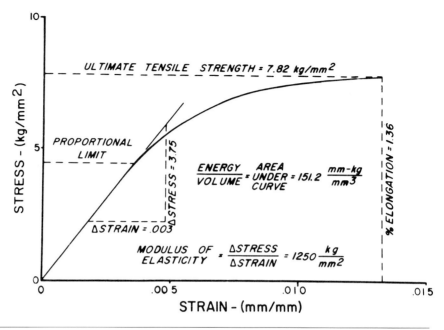

Figure 5-1

Stress/strain curve, demonstrating the material properties of a sample of cortical bone from the femur. The capacity of this sample for storing energy is shown by the area under the curve. Its ultimate tensile strength is a measure of the force required to break it.

The area beneath the curve on a stress-strain diagram reveals another important quality of the material, its potential for storing energy. Energy is a capacity for doing work, expressed as the movement of a load or force over a distance. It is measured either in foot-pounds (ft-lbs) or joules (.74 ft-lbs or 1 newton/meter). For example, when a 150-lb man jumps off of a step 2-ft high, he performs 300 ft-lbs (405 joules) of work. This energy is absorbed and dissipated by the ground, if the ground is relatively soft and flexible, but in some instances the energy can be stored and recaptured. The capacity of bone and, especially, tendon to store and potentially return energy is very important both in avoiding injury and in promoting efficient locomotion. For example, when a runner takes a step, the large Achilles tendon that attaches the gastrocnemius or major calf muscle to the calcaneus is stretched. This tendon stores the energy involved in creating strain or change in length, and it returns that energy by providing an automatic recoil which shortens the tendon again without expending additional muscular energy. Thus the energy stored in the tendon helps to push the foot off the ground again and increases locomotor efficiency. The stored strain energy in a particular volume of material is calculated directly from stress and strain: strain energy = (1/2)(stress × strain).

To summarize, stress is the force with which a material is pulled or pushed; strain is the degree to which this pushing or pulling changes the length of the object. Thus, the strain typically produced by a given stress is a major quality of any substance. This quality is its Young's modulus of elasticity, measured as an indicator of its stiffness or brittleness, based on the relationship of stress to strain. Strength, the stress at which the material fails, is an entirely different quality from stiffness or brittleness. Gordon (1968:43) provides clear examples: "A biscuit [cookie] is stiff [high E] but weak, steel is stiff and strong, nylon is flexible (low E) and strong, raspberry jelly is flexible (low E) and weak. The two properties together describe a solid about as well as you can reasonably expect to do." Finally, the ability to store energy, as indicated by a stress-strain curve, is an important quality of a material. All these qualities are relevant to bones and bone tissue.

PROPERTIES OF BONE

The properties of bone can be compared to those of other familiar substances, such as glass and steel (Figure 5-2). First of all, bone is unusual in that its tensile strength is high for a substance that is heavily mineralized. Measured with the pull oriented parallel to the long axis of the whole bone, the tensile strength of bone samples is about 16,000 psi (1128 kg/cm²); perpendicular to the long axis, the tensile strength is much lower, or about 10,000 psi (705 kg/cm²). By comparison, porcelain and other ceramics have tensile strengths ranging from about one-third to one-half that of bone. Predictably, because bone is comprised largely of hydroxyapatite, it is much stronger in compression than in tension, or roughly 21,000 psi (1480 kg/cm²) as compared to about 16,000 psi (1128 kg/cm²).

Torsional strength in a bone sample is lower than either its tensile or its compressive strength. The range of torsional strength is about 4,000–8,000 psi (282–564 kg/cm²), and the range of strain energy absorbed before failure is about 1.3–1.7 ft-lb (1.8–2.3 joules) in a 1-in² sample of cortical bone. Torsional strength, strain energy absorbed, and Young's modulus of elasticity all vary with the orientation of the sample. Some bones, notable humeri and tibiae, have obviously spiral alignments of their collagen fibers, presumably to help resist torsional forces such as commonly occur in those bones.

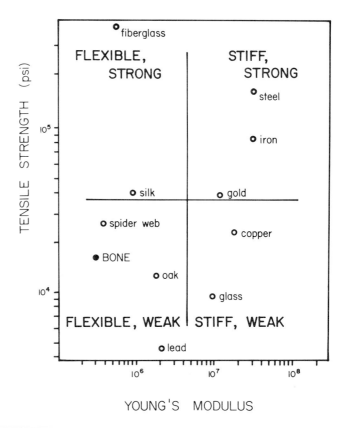

Figure 5-2

Properties of bone compared with other familiar substances.

Bone also has a fairly low Young's modulus of about 3,000,000 psi, slightly higher than that of wood, which is about 2,000,000 psi, and roughly one-third that of glass. Many biological materials, such as tendon and cartilage, have much lower Young's moduli. However, these other substances do not fulfill a major weight-bearing role, as bone does. The bones of infants have a lower Young's modulus of elasticity than do those of children or adults, which suggests that walking may be physically impossible until the bones become appropriately stiff.

Since bone is a two-phase substance, made up of flexible collagen and brittle hydroxyapatite, the collagen component might be assumed to take up the tensile stresses, and the mineralized component to withstand the compressive forces and impart stiffness. However, normal, intact bone is stronger than either hydroxyapatite or collagen by itself. Empirical studies of the properties of bone matrix, which is mostly hydroxyapatite, and bone protein, which is mostly collagen, isolated from whole bones reveal that collagen is stronger than matrix in tension but much weaker in compression (Table 5-1). Both collagen and hydroxyapatite are much weaker in either tension or compression than is whole bone, which has a higher Young's modulus of elasticity than either component.

The quality of bone that the whole is stronger than the sum of its parts characterizes various compound substances as well. Currey has drawn the analogy between bone and fiberglass, which is comprised of fine glass fibers embedded in epoxy resin, a type of plastic. Brittle substances fail under tension when minute cracks appear, because of either pre-existing defects or a slipping or dislocation of parts of the crystal structure. Once such cracks appear, they concentrate the stress locally and quickly spread throughout the material, inducing failure. In fiberglass, cracks in the brittle epoxy are stopped when they encounter the deformable glass fibers.

While collagen fibers in bone are also deformable, there are two additional reasons that bone is so strong and cracks are so difficult to propagate in it. First, in bone, hydroxyapatite occurs in tiny crystallites rather than in large units, with the result that cracks are likely to stop at the junction between units, where the bonding is weaker, instead of continuing to spread (Figure 5-3). The energy of the crack is thus dissipated in a direction perpendicular to the orientation of the force. Second, both osteocyte lacunae and the cementum rings surrounding osteons may serve as crack stoppers in bone.

The tendency of bones to decrease in strength and increase in brittleness with age is explained by four factors. First, the number of

Table 5-1	Properties of Organic and Inorganic Components of Bone		
Bone Component	Ultimate Strength		Young's Modulus of Elasticity (E)
	lbs/in²	kg/cm²	
	Compression		
Whole bone	21,400	1,509	1,480,000
Bone matrix (mostly apatite)	6,820	481	970,000
Bone protein (mostly collagen)	17	1.2	37
	Tension		
Whole bone	14,300	1,008	3,250,000
Bone matrix (mostly apatite)	845	60	2,490,000
Bone protein (mostly collagen)	1,010	71	30,700

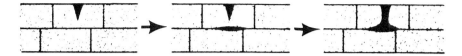

Figure 5-3

Effect of structure on crack-stopping. *(Left to right)* A crack is generated within a structural unit of the substance. Another crack opens between adjoining units. These two cracks intersect, forming a T-shaped crack that is much less likely to spread further.

chemical bonds within and among tropocollagen molecules increases with age, and this increased bonding may result in a loss of flexibility in collagen fibrils that decreases the strength of bones. Second, the bonds between the collagen and hydroxyapatite components of bones may weaken with age, thereby making the crack-stopping function of bone structure less efficient. Third, since remodeling proceeds throughout life, the frequency of osteons increases with age. The effect over time is that the volume of the bone occupied by "holes" increases and the volume of actual bone tissue decreases. This development may be compounded by osteoporosis, a common disorder of old age in which as much as 50 percent of the calcium in the bones is resorbed into the blood stream. Both of these factors act to reduce the strength of whole bones. Finally, the bonds between the inorganic and organic components of bone may weaken with age, thereby making crack propagation easier. Weaker bonds between the collagen and bone mineral may also explain the tendency towards osteoporotic bone loss with age.

STRUCTURAL DESIGN AND GROWTH

In light of the need for nearly continuous growth and remodeling, bones might appear to be inefficiently shaped to deal with ordinary stresses. For example, long bones would seem to work better if they were prestressed rods, like trees, rather than hollow tubes. Yet since the medullary cavity is not present in the initial stages of long bone formation in the embryo, it must be deliberately formed for some functional reason.

One reason that bones are not prestressed rods is the difference between the stresses to which they are subjected and those to which trees are subjected. Trees must be strong both in constant compression, so that they do not collapse under their own weight, and in bending, which for the most part occurs infrequently and in one predominant direction. Trees are virtually never subjected to tension ex-

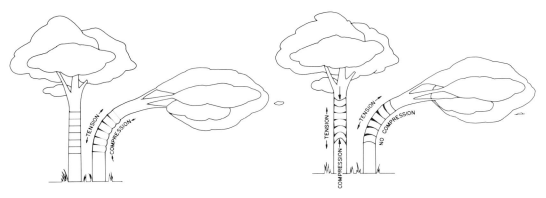

Figure 5-4

Effect of prestressing on bending strength. *(Left)* A tree is subjected to compression by its own weight and to tension by being bent. *(Right)* A tree is therefore prestressed, since it is built to withstand tension at its circumference and to withstand compression in its center. When the wind blows strongly, a prestressed tree can bend much farther than a tree that is not prestressed without breaking, because the prestressing counteracts most of the tension.

cept in the context of bending (Figure 5-4). Thus, they are built to be strong in tension around their circumference, where tension may occur during bending, and strong in compression at the center, where tension rarely occurs. Bones, on the other hand, are subjected to a variety of compressive, tensile or stretching, and torsional or twisting forces, during both stationary postures and locomotion. Further, the activities and hence the daily stresses of human bones change markedly throughout life. Thus, it would be difficult to prestress bones, because the forces to which a bone is subjected cannot be predicted.

Bones could also be shaped as solid rods instead of tubes, but that structure would be less efficient, for reasons of weight. Statically, bones can resist stresses, particularly the compressive ones to which they are most commonly exposed, only by the strength of bone tissue itself, although dynamically they can resist stresses by constant microfracture, repair, and remodeling. The strength of a bone may change as it increases in size.

In a long bone, for example, the increase in size is correlated with an increase in length, for the weight of a structure increases proportionately to the cube of any dimension of that structure. In contrast, the compressive strength of a long bone, measured as the cross-sectional area of the shaft, increases proportionately to only the square of any dimension. In other words, as a bone grows, it gets longer faster than it gets stronger, if it maintains its original proportion of length to shaft diameter. The net effect is a loss in strength, which gets more pronounced as the growth increases. To maintain comparable strength, then, a bone must become disproportionately thicker relative to its length as it grows. Having a hollow center is simply a means of saving weight without sacrificing strength.

This apparently simple relationship is complicated by the fact that bones are subjected to dynamic stresses in addition to static weight-bearing. In fact, it is rare for bones to be subjected to such high compressive forces traveling longitudinally down them that they break. Fractures are more commonly the result of tensile forces, arising through sudden bending, or torsional forces, such as are frequently applied in skiing or other sports where the hand or foot is twisted relative to the body or where the body is twisted relative to a fixed hand or foot. Thus, the cross-sectional area of a tubular bone is neither the only relevant measure of its strength nor the most important one. Bones are more commonly subjected to torsion and bending in addition to compression. Whenever an object is twisted, one part of it is subjected to compression and the other to tension. However, an axis through that object, called the neutral axis, is subjected to neither force. In cylinders, this neutral axis runs longitudinally through the center. It is therefore economical and functional to eliminate material along this neutral axis, thereby creating a tube, since to have material where it is not useful provides no structural benefit. Even in bending, the highest stresses are in the outer fibers of the bone. In short, a tube is stronger in resisting torsion or bending per unit of material, or per unit of energy expended to build that material, than is a solid cylinder of the same dimensions.

This aspect of strength, called the second moment of area or the second moment of inertia, can be measured or calculated mathematically. The second moment of area is the sum of the areas of bone or other tissue multiplied by the square of the distance of that tissue from the neutral axis. As a bone grows, its second moment of inertia stays proportional to a linear dimension, such as length, to the fourth power if functional equivalence, or comparable strength, is maintained. During life, the amount of bone tissue and its distribution around the medullary cavity are adjusted to compensate for regularly occurring stresses. An ideal compromise between strength and weight is achieved when the hollow center of the tube has the maximum diameter that leaves sufficient material to resist stresses. Of course, in life the center of the tube is in fact filled with marrow, fat, and other soft tissues; it is hollow only in structural terms.

EFFECTS OF HEATING

Predictable changes occur in bones and bony tissues with heating. These effects are important to anthropologists and forensic scientists, enabling them to determine whether skeletal remains have been subjected to fire, as in cremations, accidental death by fire, or cooking.

An obvious change with heating occurs in bone color. Heating causes a predictable sequence of color changes in bones and teeth:

Temperature range	Predominant colors
20°–<285°C	Neutral white, pale yellow, yellow
285°–<525°C	Reddish brown, very dark gray-brown, neutral dark gray, reddish-yellow
525°–<645°C	Neutral black with medium blue and reddish-yellow
645°–<940°C	Neutral white with light blue-gray and light gray
940°C+	Neutral white with medium gray and reddish-yellow

In addition, the heating of bones and teeth dehydrates and denatures collagen and produces a regular series of changes in the microscopic appearance of natural bone surfaces (Figures 5-5–5-7). These changes are visible in bones or teeth heated to as little as 185°C. At 350–400°C, all of the organic material in bone is driven off, producing frequent cracking, which tends to produce rectangular segments separated by deep cracks perpendicular to the bone's surface. At 750–800°C, bone undergoes a profound change in microscopic appearance, accompanied by a reorganization of the hydroxyapatite into a form with a larger crystal size, as shown by powder X-ray diffraction studies. Progressive heating is also accompanied by a marked decrease in strength and an increase in brittleness.

PIEZO-ELECTRICITY

One of the more unusual properties of bone is that it generates electricity when deformed. This phenomenon is commonly attributed to piezoelectricity, a property of many crystalline substances, such as quartz, and of collagen itself, whereby they produce electricity under pressure. Apparently the pressure deforms the structure of piezoelectric substances, separating the positive and negative ions and thereby producing a current. The electrical potential generated by pressure is proportional to the force applied to the bone.

The significance of piezoelectricity in bone is unclear. Early studies by Bassett and co-workers suggested that piezoelectricity provides a mechanism for the remodeling of bone in response to stress. Areas of bone samples subjected to compression generate negative charges, while areas of bone samples subjected to tension generate positive

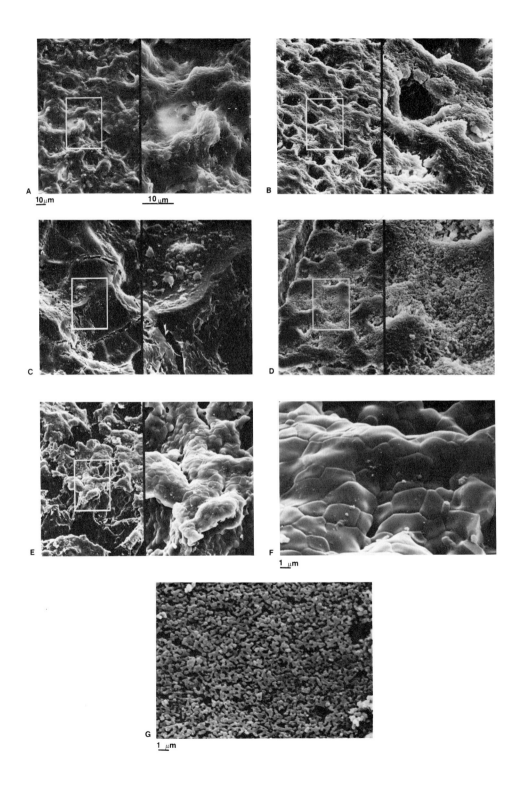

A

10 μm   10 μm

B

C

D

E

F

1 μm

G

1 μm

charges. The negative charges stimulate bone deposition in experimental animals, apparently by triggering osteoblast activity. The precise mechanisms are unknown. The effect is to thicken, and strengthen, bone that is being compressed. The positive charges generated by tension do not have the opposite effect of stimulating bone resorption. Since contracting any muscle produces tension at the insertion site, bone resorption at such points would be maladaptive. Remodeling, however, as measured by the frequency of young osteons, is correlated with positive charges.

If the natural electrical activity of bone is related to bone deposition or remodeling activity, it may have a clinical application, for artificially produced electrical activity could be used to stimulate repair of fractures. Experiments in which electrodes are attached to fractured bones show some acceleration of healing and new bone growth indeed occurs at the negative electrode. Problems with experimental design invalidated the results of the initial studies, although later work confirmed that growth is accelerated, if not as dramatically as originally suggested. It is not yet clear whether the effect is clinically significant.

An alternative hypothesis is that the electricity produced by bending bone is due to streaming potential, or the production of electrical charges by the movement of fluid. The focus of this hypothesis is on hydrated bone, which is saturated with physiological fluid as in life, rather than on dry bone. Although dry bone also generates electricity under experimental conditions, probably because of the piezoelectric properties of collagen, this effect may be so slight as to have no relevance to the functioning of bone in vivo. In hydrated bones, bending generates electricity by forcing the fluid through the various canals and holes in the bone. If the channel walls preferentially attract ions of one sign, positive or negative, then ions of the opposite sign are concentrated in the fluid. Streaming potential may be the best explanation for the generation of electricity under physiological conditions, but the function of piezoelectricity in living tissues is still unclear.

Figure 5-5

Effects of heating on the microscopic morphology of normal bone surfaces. In this split-image micrograph the same area is shown at two different magnifications. All bones except (g) are subchondral. (a) Unheated bone. (b) Heating to 185–< 285°C produces a more granular surface covered in tiny surface asperities. (c) Heating to 285–< 440°C creates a glassy, vitrified surface. (d) Temperatures of 440–< 800°C create a frothy-looking surface. (e) Temperatures of 800–< 940°C make the particles melt and coalesce into undulating polygonal structures. (f) The same bone sample at a higher magnification. (g) In cortical bone heated to 940°C similar particles melt into nodular structures.

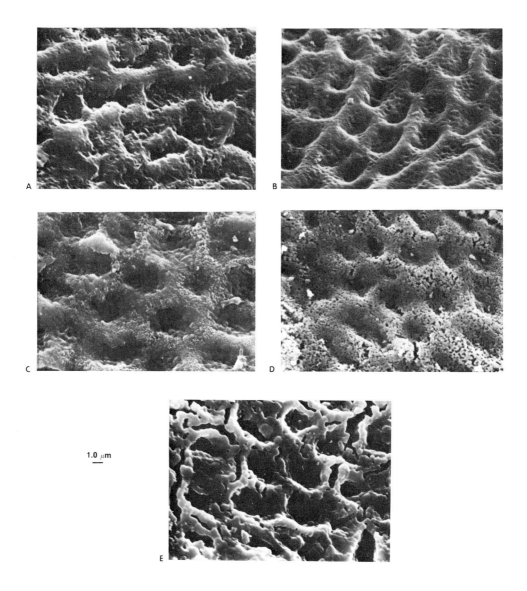

1.0 μm

Figure 5-6

Effects of heating on the microscopic morphology of normal enamel surfaces. *(a)* Unheated enamel typically has a honeycomb pattern. *(b)* At 185–< 285°C the surface texture is more irregular and dimpled. *(c)* At 285–< 440°C rounded particles appear, covering the surface. *(d)* At 440–< 800°C there are many vitrified particles separated by pores and fissures. *(e)* At 800–< 940°C these particles coalesce into smooth globules.

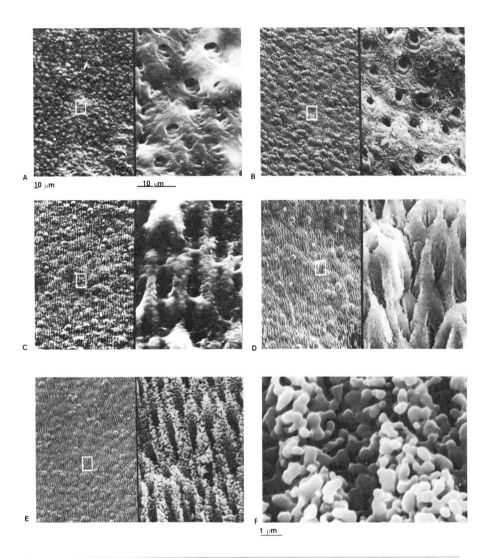

Figure 5-7

Effects of heating on the microscopic morphology of normal dentin surfaces. In this split-image micrograph the same area is shown at two magnifications. *(a)* An unheated dentinal surface in the pulp cavity has an array of tubules and calcospherites typical of young animals. *(b)* At 185–< 285°C the peritubular matrix has shrunken away from the intertubular matrix and the surface looks particulate. *(c)* At 285–< 440°C the asperities have smoothed out and the openings of the tubules have elongated. *(d)* At 440–< 800°C the openings of the tubules are further elongated and the surface is glassy and vitrified. *(e)* At 800–< 940°C the vitrified particles have melted into nodular spikes in a staggered array. *(f)* At a higher magnification these nodular structures resemble the structures in Figures 5-4*f*–*g* and 5-5*e*.

6
JOINTS AND LUBRICATION

Joints are essential structures that permit movement of the different parts of the body or of the body itself. Simply put, a joint is any place, point, or junction at which two bones meet and are joined together or articulate with each other.

BASIC TYPES OF JOINT

Structurally, there are three main types of joint in the body: fibrous, cartilaginous, and synovial. Fibrous joints, also called synarthroses, are the least mobile type of joint. Two bones are united by a fibrous connective tissue, containing many tough, collagen fibers. This fibrous connective tissue binds the bones closely together in an essentially fixed position. There are three major examples of fibrous joints in the body: sutures, such as those between the vault bones of the cranium; syndesmoses, in which the fibrous tissue forms an interosseous membrane, such as the membrane stretching between the tibia and fibula in humans; and gomphoses, a special type of peg-in-socket joint seen in humans only between the teeth and the alveoli or bony sockets that hold them.

The second type, a cartilaginous joint, which is also known as an amphiarthrosis, is generally more mobile than a fibrous joint. There are two types of cartilaginous joint in humans: synchondrosis and fibrocartilaginous. The most common type is the synchondrosis, which involves a layer of hyaline cartilage between two bones or parts of bones. Such joints persist in the growing human as the epiphyseal growth plates between the diaphyseal and epiphyseal centers of ossification. Although growth plates are not designed to permit movement, limited sliding of one part of the bone relative to the other occurs, in part because hyaline cartilage is somewhat elastic.

The other type of cartilaginous joint found in humans, fibrocartilaginous, occurs at symphyses, such as between the left and right pubis. In the pubic symphysis, each bony surface is covered with hyaline cartilage; between the two hyaline cartilage layers is a layer of fibrocartilage, which is stiffer and less flexible. Before childbirth, the mother secretes a special hormone, relaxin, which relaxes these fibers and permits a limited degree of opening of the symphysis. Other examples of fibrocartilaginous joints are the joints between the vertebral bodies, which are bound to each other by intervertebral disks made of fibrocartilage, and the joint between the superior and inferior parts of the sternum. Typically, cartilaginous joints occur on the midline of the body.

Synovial joints, also known as diarthroses, are the third major type of joint. They are the most freely mobile joints in the body, permitting most of the actions undertaken by an individual to occur. In any joint at which two substances move freely past each other, movement is hindered by the friction between the substances. Special lubrication is needed both to lessen this friction, making motion freer, and to prevent the elements of the joint from deteriorating due to friction and wear. All synovial joints are enclosed in a capsule made of connective tissue and are reinforced by tendons and ligaments. The nonarticulating parts of the joint capsule are lined with synovial membrane, a special tissue that produces synovia, the fluid that lubricates the joint. Synovial membrane and fluid are also involved in lubricating other moving structures of the body, such as tendons, which run in grooves in bones, and bursae, the sack-like structures filled with synovia that ensure free motion of a tendon, muscle, or skin over a bone.

LUBRICATION

The lubrication of synovial joints poses a special and demanding problem. Motion must be allowed among different parts of the skeleton in order to apply forces to the environment or to other parts of the body and to attenuate and absorb environmental forces applied to the body. Both of these functions are important for sustaining life and minimizing injury. But the human body makes more rigorous demands upon its joints than does any machine. Human joints must withstand great forces, up to about 600 lbs at the hip, and must last 70–80 years, during which time thousands of movements are made daily. They are often comprised of two incongruent structures, the opposing surfaces of which are microscopically rough, not smooth. Furthermore, human joints must remain adequately lubricated and mobile at velocities ranging from low to high, with a potential for rapid acceleration.

The way in which lubrication of synovial joints solves this problem is illustrated by the knee joint (Figure 6-1). The two main structural elements are the femur and tibia, which at the knee are each comprised of a complex network of cancellous bone covered by a thin skin of cortical

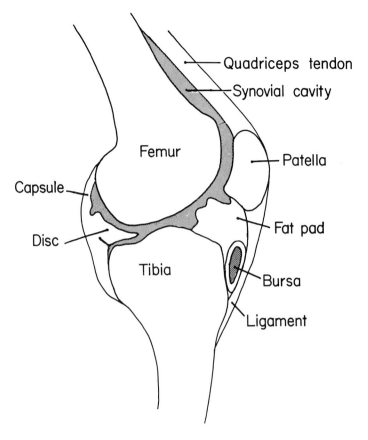

Figure 6-1

The knee joint, showing the three bony elements and various soft tissues.

bone. A third bone, the patella, is an integral part of the joint but bears no weight. One of the main functions of cancellous bone is to absorb forces put on the joint and to enable rapid remodeling of microfractures so that the bone can better withstand future forces. Typically, the articular surfaces of the opposing bones are not highly congruent. Thus, the distal femur, patella, and proximal tibia do not fit together tightly. The articular surfaces of these bones are overlaid with hyaline cartilage, which plays an important role in lubrication.

The hyaline cartilage that covers the articular surfaces of each bone is grossly smooth, shiny, and somewhat deformable, yet brittle. It is comprised of two layers. Immediately adjacent to the surface of the cortical bone are long columns of chondrocytes arranged perpendicular to the bony surface. Close to the bone's surface, these chondrocytes are fat, swollen, and hypertrophied, but at the top of the columns they are still healthy, actively producing more cartilage. Overlying the chondrocyte layer is the superficial tangential zone, which is a fibrous collagen sheet that also sends arcades of collagen fibers vertically down between the columns of chondrocytes through the gel-like matrix to the subchondral bone. Although theoretically the surface of the hyaline cartilage, the superficial tangential zone, ought to be extremely smooth in order to lessen friction during movement, hyaline cartilage is microscopically rough. The surface asperities on hyaline cartilage are 2–20 microns. Under the scanning electron microscope these asperities show up as pits separated by raised areas. Apparently these pits overlie the top chondrocyte in a column (Figure 6-2). The intervening raised areas overlie the matrix of the cartilage. The lower parts of the cartilage are nourished from subchondral bone vessels leading from nutrient arteries in the bone, while the upper parts are nourished from the synovia itself.

The nonarticulating parts of the joint capsule are lined with synovial membrane, a highly vascularized tissue through which blood is dialyzed to yield synovial fluid. Synovia is basically composed of serum — the clear, watery part of blood — with two additional substances. These substances are produced by the two types of cell, A and B, that are present in synovial membrane. A cells produce hyaluronic acid, a large molecule that gives synovia its viscosity and slipperiness, and B cells produce a double glycoprotein, a much smaller molecule. Synovial fluid is thick, slippery, and rich in nutrients needed by the cartilage. It has another important property in that, like ketchup, it is thixotropic, or much less viscous once movement has been initiated. There is very little synovial fluid in joints, despite the fact that it is the only lubricant present; only 0.5 ml is found in the knee. However, synovial fluid is absolutely essential for lubrication and normal joint function. Joints lacking synovia for some pathological reason rapidly and painfully deteriorate.

The other major components of the knee joint are the fat pads and the menisci or discs. Fat pads are normal features of synovial joints and increase the congruency of the two opposing surfaces. They also help spread synovial fluid throughout the joint space. Fat pads are so important to the normal functioning of joints that in cases of starvation they are among the last sources of fat to be utilized by the body. Menisci are found in several synovial joints in the body, including the knee, the sternoclavicular, and the temporomandibular joints. Like fat pads, the menisci increase joint congruency and separate the joint into two com-

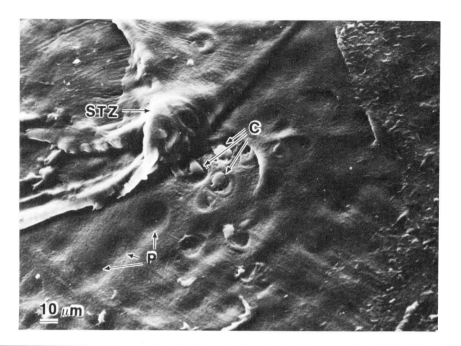

Figure 6-2

Surface structure of cartilage, showing the shallow pits *(P)* characteristic of hyaline cartilage. In this micrograph the superficial tangential zone *(STZ)* of the cartilage is peeled back at upper left to reveal the top chondrocytes *(C)* in the underlying columns.

partments in which independent motions can be carried out. Menisci are made of fibrocartilage, not hyaline cartilage, and are not covered with synovial membrane.

Finally, the joint capsule itself is a thick, fibrous bag that totally encloses the joint. Thickenings of the capsule are called capsular ligaments. Usually there are also extracapsular ligaments and tendons that provide the limits of normal joint motion as well as the basic stability and integrity of the joint. Trauma can tear or stretch the extracapsular ligaments, which are not easily restored to their original state, leading to chronic joint instability. Muscles provide and control the movement at joints; their tendons maintain joint integrity; and their actions place the highest stresses on joints.

Theoretically, lubrication of the joints could be achieved by one of three basic modes of lubrication as understood by engineers: boundary, hydrodynamic, or hydrostatic lubrication. Boundary lubrication depends upon the surface molecules that interact to produce low frictional forces as the two surfaces move past each other. Teflon is a familiar material in which a molecule is used to produce boundary lubrication. In boundary lubrication, the total area of the articulating surfaces is not directly related to the amount of friction produced. Only the high points of those surfaces actually touch each other, and these represent a small proportion of the total area. The force produced by friction in boundary lubrication is usually a function of the weight applied. That is, the actual contact area between two deformable surfaces, as opposed to their total surface area, increases as more weight is applied and the surfaces deform.

The two other types of lubrication, hydrodynamic and hydrostatic, involve a fluid film that lies between the two opposing surfaces, separating them and reducing the friction to that within the fluid itself. For fluid film lubrication, a compromise must be reached between highly viscous fluids, which more easily form films and are more easily drawn into the correct position, and less viscous fluids, which have much less internal friction during movement.

One of the types of fluid film lubrication, hydrodynamic lubrication, depends upon the relative motion of the two surfaces to pull a fluid film between them. Like a ball bearing in a socket, the spinning of the surfaces drags lubricant into the joint. To be successful as a lubricant, this film must be thicker than the irregularities on the surfaces being lubricated, so that the film can separate them from each other. Important factors in hydrodynamic lubrication are the speed at which the two surfaces move past each other, the viscosity of the fluid, the thickness of the fluid, the area of contact between the surfaces, and the congruency of those surfaces.

The other type of fluid film lubrication, hydrostatic lubrication, also depends upon a fluid film to separate the two opposing surfaces from each other and thus to lessen friction. But whereas in hydrodynamic lubrication this film is drawn between the surfaces by their motion, in hydrostatic lubrication the fluid film is forced between the surfaces by some type of pump or pumping mechanism.

The type or types of lubrication that apply to human joints are not fully known. Since synovial fluid is both present in joints and essential for their lubrication, much research has focused on the two types of fluid film lubrication. However, the properties of anatomical joints do not match those that would be expected in a hydrodynamically lubricated joint.

Since the object of lubrication is to produce freer motion by lessening friction, features that reduce friction are important. In hydrodyna-

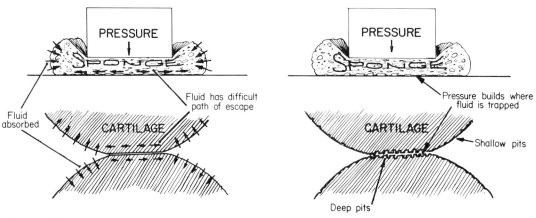

Figure 6-3

Models of joint lubrication. *(Left)* In McCutcheon's weeping model, pressure squeezes fluid laterally within the cartilage, like water within a sponge. Fluid is weeped out from the load-bearing region, creating a fluid film between the cartilage or sponge and the surface upon which it rests. Fluid soaks back into the cartilage or sponge at the edges. *(Right)* In Walker's model, pits on the surface of cartilage enlarge their volume under pressure, trapping the lubricating fluid between the sponge or cartilage and the surface upon which it rests.

mic lubrication, the most obvious way to reduce friction is to increase the thickness of the fluid film that works to separate the two surfaces. Several features maximize the fluid film thickness. First of all, a thick film is most easily formed by a highly viscous fluid, since viscosity makes it easier to drag the fluid between the opposing surfaces. Second, fluid film thickness is greater in joints with highly congruent surfaces, because their relative movement past each other drags more fluid between them. To increase film thickness still further, these surfaces need to be very smooth, because this increases congruency. In addition, hydrodynamic lubrication works best on joints that generally bear low loads, since high loads tend to force the fluid back out from between the articulating surfaces. Finally, the fluid film thickness is increased by increasing the velocity at which the two opposing surfaces move past each other, since more rapid movements drag in more fluid.

Unfortunately, real joints have few of these properties. They are neither congruent nor smooth; they move at both high and low velocities and high and low loads; and the lubricating fluid is thixotropic rather than being consistently viscous. In other words, human joints do not show the properties necessary for successful hydrodynamic lubrication, and this model probably does not apply.

The fluid film thickness in synovial joints also gives evidence that hydrodynamic lubrication does not occur. Since film thickness is difficult to measure in an intact joint, it must be estimated from other known factors, such as the velocity at which joints move, the curvature of their surfaces, the viscosity of synovia, and the applied load. If average values for these factors are used in the calculations, fluid film thickness is about 0.0123 microns. Since the irregularities on the surface of cartilage are 2–20 microns in height, a film thickness of much less than 1 micron cannot possibly be adequate for hydrodynamic lubrication. Therefore, the features needed for hydrodynamic lubrication are not present in real joints.

Hydrostatic lubrication is more likely to occur in human joints, although the pumping mechanism responsible for such lubrication is still unclear. There are two possibilities (Figure 6-3). McCutcheon proposed that cartilage is lubricated by a combination of weeping and resoaking, actions that can be observed in simple experiments with an ordinary sponge. For example, when pressure is applied to a soaked sponge in the shower, the sponge weeps fluid. Even if the pressure is applied at the center of the sponge, the fluid can escape readily only at the edges, because the structure of the sponge makes it difficult for water to travel laterally within the sponge. Thus, the applied pressure creates a thin layer of fluid between the sponge and the shower tile. Cartilage might respond similarly, with synovial fluid weeping out of the cartilage in regions where it bears a load and soaking back into the cartilage in its unloaded regions.

Experiments with cartilage soaked in synovia on glass demonstrate that the lubricating properties of synovial fluid are in fact superior to those of water and that weeping and resoaking do occur. But there are problems with this model. One is that resoaking takes too long to account for lubrication under natural conditions; hydrostatic lubrication may occur, but not in quite this way. Another problem is that Walker has recently demonstrated that synovial fluid does travel laterally within cartilage in the load-bearing region. The final difficulty is that, despite the fluid film, the high points of the cartilage may still come into contact.

A more likely pumping mechanism for the hydrostatic lubrication of synovial joints, proposed by Walker, involves the pits on the cartilage surface that overlie the columns of chondrocytes. Apparently the columns of chondrocytes are more compressible than is the cartilage matrix between them. As pressure is applied, these pits may deepen, trapping synovial fluid between their surface and the opposing cartilage. Once the pit deepens to a hemisphere, fluid is passively pumped out from the pits to lubricate the high points between pits.

Hydrostatic lubrication involving the pits on the cartilage surface may be combined with boundary lubrication. Although viscous fluids work well as lubricants, hyaluronic acid, which makes synovia viscous, is not responsible for lubrication. Radin and his co-workers reached this conclusion by treating synovia with an enzyme, hyaluronidase, that destroys hyaluronic acid and then using it to lubricate cartilage-on-cartilage movements in vitro. Lubrication was unimpaired. Despite the destruction of the hyaluronic acid and the low viscosity of the treated fluid, the coefficient of friction remained constant before and after treatment of the synovia. Hyaluronic acid thus is not directly involved in lubricating joints, although it lubricates the synovial membrane that covers the nonarticulating parts of the joint. But when they injected a joint with hyaluronidase and then with trypsin, an enzyme that destroys the double glycoprotein in synovia, lubrication ceased. The double glycoprotein alone accomplishes lubrication of the hyaline cartilage surfaces. Since synovia containing only the double glycoprotein feels thin and nonslippery, like water, the double glycoprotein is unlikely to act as a fluid film lubricant and must be a boundary lubricant. These experiments show that lubrication in anatomical joints, though not yet fully understood, probably involves a combination of boundary and hydrostatic lubrication.

CRACKING JOINTS   One interesting feature of some synovial joints is that they can be pulled apart until they create a cracking noise. Joints that are not synovial may also produce cracking noises, but the phenomenon in their case is different. In nonsynovial joints, the noise is usually produced by a tendon or ligament slipping over a bony projection. This kind of cracking can be repeated at frequent intervals, but cracking of synovial joints can be repeated only after about 15 minutes. The more congruent synovial joints, such as those between metacarpals and phalanges, crack more readily than the less congruent joints.

As a synovial joint is pulled on, the two opposing surfaces show little separation, despite the negative pressure being formed in the synovial fluid. Negative pressure draws carbon dioxide out of synovia, until it eventually forms a large bubble of gas, in a step called cavitation.

Abruptly, the opposing surfaces of the joint separate until limited by the joint capsule. Once the surfaces are separated, the ambient pressure within the joint exceeds that within the bubble. This pressure difference causes the bubble to collapse, creating a cracking noise. The implosion of the large bubble of gas creates a set of smaller bubbles, which gradually go back into solution. Until these small bubbles disappear and the gas is once again completely dissolved, the joint cannot be cracked again. Habitual cracking may damage the hyaline cartilage of the joint, leading to joint degeneration, arthritis, and dysfunction.

JOINTS AS LEVERS   Joints serve as parts of a lever system. A lever is any rigid bar or strut that moves about an axis. In the body, muscles produce actions by contracting and thus pulling on bones, the stiff struts, which in response move around joints, the axes. Any lever system has three components: the power, load, and fulcrum or point at which movement occurs. In the human body, the power is provided by the muscle at its point of attachment, the load is usually a part of the body weight, and the fulcrum is the joint.

Depending on the relative placement of its three components, a lever is classified as first-order, second-order, or third-order (Figure 6-4). First-order levers work like seesaws or crowbars. By definition, the fulcrum lies between the power and the load. Such a lever in the body is the muscles of the neck that act to prevent the head from dropping forward. The fulcrum is the atlas or first vertebra. Second-order levers have the load interposed between the fulcrum and the power. For example, the Achilles tendon joining the calf muscles to the calcaneum is such a lever as it lifts the body weight of an individual onto the toes. Third-order levers are those in which the power lies between the fulcrum and the load. The biceps muscle on the front of the upper arm is such a lever as it acts to raise a weight in the hand. The fulcrum is the elbow.

The amount of force or power needed to produce a given movement in a lever is a simple function of the resistance to the movement, called the load, the distance between the power and the fulcrum, called the power arm, and the distance between the load and the fulcrum, called the load arm: power = (load × load arm)/power arm. The longer the distance between the fulcrum and the power, the less power is needed to achieve a given result. Even a small change in the length of the power arm can have a significant effect. Consider the effect of increasing the power arm when a small child tries to seesaw with a much larger child.

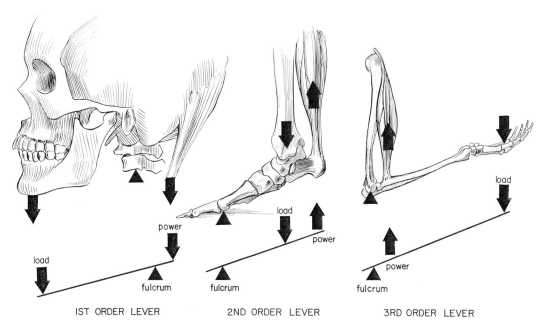

IST ORDER LEVER   2ND ORDER LEVER   3RD ORDER LEVER

Figure 6-4

Orders of levers. *(a)* First-order levers are like the neck muscles that hold the head level. Their fulcrum is between the load and the power. *(b)* Second-order levers are exemplified by lifting the body on tiptoe. The power (gastrocnemius muscle) is separated from the fulcrum (proximal interphalangeal joint) by the load (body weight). *(c)* Third-order levers work like the biceps as it lifts a weight in the hand. The power (biceps) lies between the fulcrum (elbow) and the load (in the hand).

Seesawing works well only if the two loads balance or nearly balance each other. If the small child sits at one end of the seesaw and the large child sits closer to the fulcrum, the two are balanced. Then their relative positions can be controlled by a relatively slight muscular effort on the part of whichever child is touching the ground. That child, by gently extending his knees and pushing off with his feet, can raise his end of the seesaw into the air. Similarly, an animal dependent on digging will need to extend its arm powerfully. Therefore, the olecranon, a process on the proximal ulna to which the main elbow extensor is attached, is elongated to lengthen the power arm of that muscle.

The speed with which a lever produces movement also depends on the length of the power and load arms. Increasing the total lever length, which is the sum of the power arm and the load arm, increases the speed with which the end of the lever moves. Since levers are rigid, the end of a lever moves over a greater distance than a point on the lever closer to the fulcrum (Figure 6-5). In other words, the end of the lever moves faster than a point near the fulcrum because the end moves farther in the same amount of time. However, power is a trade-off for speed; speed is enhanced by a short power arm, and power is enhanced by a long one.

SESAMOIDS

Sesamoids are bones, such as the patella, that grow within tendons. Sesamoids play an important role in lubricating areas where a tendon bends around a joint. The patella protects the joint capsule of the knee by spreading the force of the large muscle of the anterior thigh, the quadriceps femoris, over a broader area than that of the tendon. This effect decreases the pressure on the capsule. The patella is an integral and strong part of the capsule itself, rather than being extracapsular. Further, the patella acts as a pulley, to move the line of action of the quadriceps muscle farther away from the fulcrum. In this case, the center of the condylar curve is the fulcrum about which the condyle rotates. This, the patella lengthens the power arm and improves the efficiency of the quadriceps in producing motion at the knee joint.

Sesamoids may function to increase the area of muscle attachment in constricted areas. An example is the thumb, where the sesamoids at the proximal metacarpophalangeal joint give partial insertion to the adductor pollicis, the muscle that adducts the thumb. Also, sesamoids may help to guide tendons along the appropriate pathways. For example, there are two sesamoids on the plantar surface or sole of the foot, which lie at the distal end of the first metatarsal and keep the tendon of a long flexor muscle of the big toe, the flexor hallucis longus, in the appropriate orientation. Continual wearing of high-heeled shoes may deflect this tendon from its proper course in a lateral direction, ultimately displacing the toe's phalanges painfully from the head of the metacarpal.

AXES OF MOVEMENT

Synovial joints permit movement of the body parts or of the body itself. A maximum of three mutually perpendicular axes of movement are possible. Joints are therefore classified as uniaxial, biaxial, and multiaxial, according to the number of axes about which independent movement is permitted.

Uniaxial joints work like hinges, with only a single axis or degree of movement. The movement involved may be flexion or extension, such

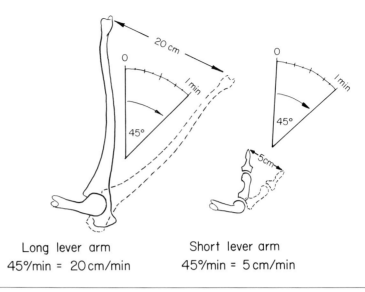

Long lever arm
45%/min = 20 cm/min

Short lever arm
45%/min = 5 cm/min

Figure 6-5

Speed of movement related to lever length. When the input power and the degree of movement at a joint are equal, *(left)* a long lever arm moves through a larger arc than *(right)* a short lever arm. Therefore, lengthening a lever arm increases its speed of movement.

as occurs at the humeroulnar joint, or a pivotal movement, such as occurs between the first two cervical vertebrae or at the proximal radioulnar joint. Uniaxial joints may also involve sliding in one plane, as at the intercarpal joints. Uniaxial joints are said to possess one degree of freedom. Since in reality, joint surfaces are curved rather than perfectly flat, motion in uniaxial joints often involves some rotation as well as some change in the angle formed between the two bones. Nonetheless, since these movements in a secondary axis are both inadvertent and impossible to produce independently, such joints are not considered biaxial.

Biaxial joints have two degrees of freedom; that is, independent movements can occur in either of two perpendicular axes. An example of a biaxial joint is the knee, at which both flexion or extension and a limited degree of medial or lateral rotation occur. Multiaxial joints have three degrees of freedom in that independent movements can occur in each of three perpendicular axes, as well as through a range of axes intermediate in position. Examples include the ball-and-socket joints of the body, such as the hip and shoulder.

The degree of freedom of a joint is in part a function of the shape of that joint. Joint shapes fall into one of seven general categories. Planar joints have only slightly curved surfaces and are likely to show gliding or sliding movements in a single axis. Hinge joints have more congruent surfaces than average. These joints permit only a single axis of movement, whose orientation is tightly controlled by shape. Condylar joints have spindle- or spool-shaped surfaces, like the distal femur and proximal tibia. Two or three axes of movement are often possible at condylar joints. Spheroidal joints are classic ball-and-socket joints, like the hip, and show all three degrees of movement.

Ellipsoidal joints have articulating surfaces that are longer in one direction than the other, giving an outline like an ellipse. These joints are commonly biaxial, like the radiocarpal joint. Pivotal joints, also called trochoid, are uniaxial, but the axis of rotation is parallel to the long axis of the rotating member. An example is the proximal radioulnar joint, in which the head of the radius spins in a ligamentous ring attached to the ulna. Finally, saddle-shaped or sellar joints permit biaxial or triaxial movement. An example is the carpometacarpal joint at the base of the thumb. Opposition of the thumb involves flexion and adduction at the first carpometacarpal joint and rotation of the thumb about its long axis, so that in anatomical position the nail of the thumb faces laterally, but in flexion it rotates 90° and faces anteriorly.

PART TWO
THE FUNCTION
OF BONES

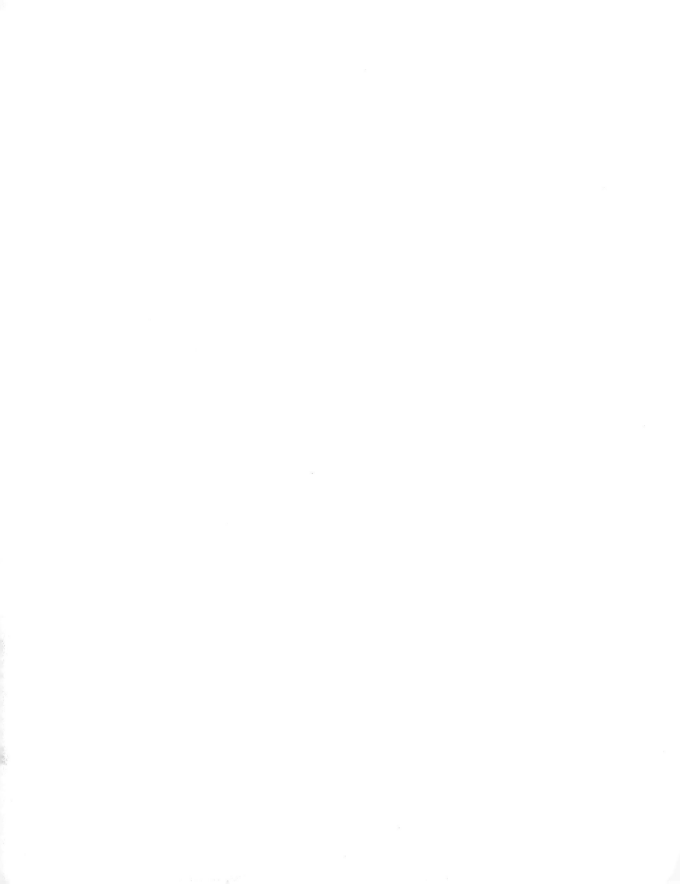

7
THE AXIAL SKELETON

The axial skeleton comprises the vertebrae, the sacrum, the ribs, and the sternum. Structurally, these elements play a major role both in supporting the head and upper limbs and in supporting and protecting the organs of the thorax. The vertebral column itself encloses and protects the spinal cord and the spinal nerves that enter and leave the cord to innervate the body. In addition, the axial skeleton provides attachments for the muscles involved in respiration and in movement of the torso.

THE VERTEBRAL COLUMN AND SACRUM

The vertebral column makes up about two-fifths of the total height of the body. The column has five distinct regions, going from superior to inferior: the cervix or neck, thorax, lumbar or loins, sacrum or pelvis, and coccyx or caudal extremity. The vertebrae include seven cervical (C1–7), twelve thoracic (T1–12), and five lumbar (L1–5) vertebrae (Figure 7-1). Prior to adulthood, there are also five sacral (S1–5) and three to five coccygeal (Co1–5) vertebrae. The twenty-four cervical, thoracic, and lumbar vertebrae are often called presacral or true vertebrae, to distinguish them from the eight to ten sacral and coccygeal vertebrae, which are fused in adults to form the sacrum and coccyx.

In lateral view, a normal adult vertebral column shows four characteristic curvatures. The cervical and lumbar curvatures are concave posteriorly, whereas the intervening thoracic and sacral curvatures are concave anteriorly. The concave curvatures are considered primary, as they are present even during fetal life. The primary curvatures are formed largely by the differing shapes of the vertebral bodies, which are the columnar, weight-bearing portions of the vertebrae. In contrast, the cervical curvature develops at about three months after birth, when a baby begins to hold up its head, and the lumbar curvature develops at about six months, with the onset of sitting up. At about one year of age, when a child begins to walk, the lumbar curvature is often accentuated. The secondary curvatures are largely the result of the

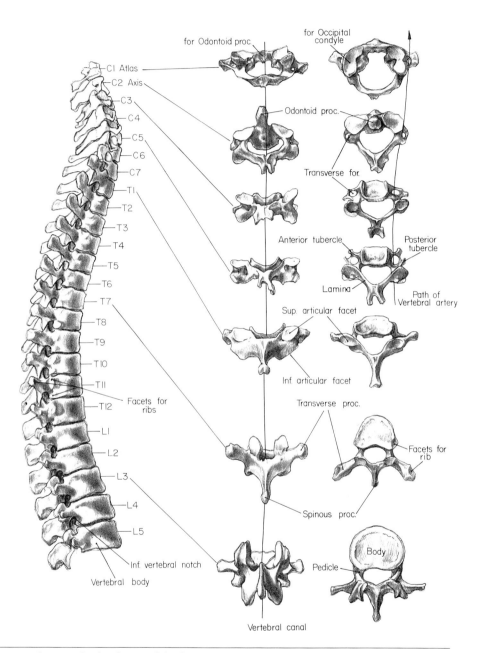

Figure 7-1

The vertebral column: *(left)* the entire column from C1 to L5 and *(right)* selected vertebrae, showing the typical body, spinous process , and articular facet in posterior and superior view.

shape of the fibrocartilaginous discs that are interposed between each adjacent pair of vertebral bodies.

Although the vertebrae of each region of the column differ somewhat in shape, they are constructed along a common plan (Figure 7-2). Anteriorly, nearly all vertebrae have an approximately columnar portion, called the body or centrum. The body of a vertebra is made up of coarse cancellous bone and bears the body's weight; its function is primarily supportive. For this reason, both the height and the overall dimensions of the bodies increase from superior to inferior, until the level of the hip joint is reached, after which the body dimensions decrease. In addition, the vertebral body in adults is filled with marrow and serves as one of the sites for red blood cell production. Differences between the anterior and posterior height of individual bodies cause the thoracic and sacral curvatures of the column. The superior and inferior surfaces of the body are ossified from thin epiphyseal plates which fuse to the rest of the vertebral body at about 25 years.

The body of each vertebra is connected to the bodies of the adjacent vertebrae by intervertebral discs. Each disc consists of a semifluid mass of tissue, called the nucleus pulposus, surrounded by a ring of fibrocartilaginous tissue, the anulus fibrosus. The anulus fibrosus binds adjacent vertebral bodies together, and the nucleus pulposus it contains deforms and compresses in response to movements. Thus, the intervertebral discs help the vertebral column function as a spring to attenuate the forces of locomotion and other movements. Slight movements between each adjacent pair of vertebrae give flexibility to the column as a whole, although movement is freer in the cervical and lumbar regions than in the thoracic region.

Projecting posteriorly from each vertebral body is an arch, enclosing the vertebral foramen through which the spinal cord passes. The anterior portion of this arch is the pedicle, a name derived from the Greek word for "root," and the posterior portion of the arch on each side is the lamina. Each pedicle bears both an inferior and superior notch, so that when two adjacent vertebrae are articulated, the inferior notch of one vertebra joins the superior notch of the subadjacent vertebra to form the intervertebral foramen. The intervertebral foramen is the bony hole through which spinal nerves exit from the spinal cord. Hence, a small displacement of the vertebral column can pinch and damage the spinal nerves.

Where the right and left laminae of a vertebra meet posteriorly at the midline, a spinous process or neural spine projects downward and backward from the vertebral arch. In addition, a vertebra typically has

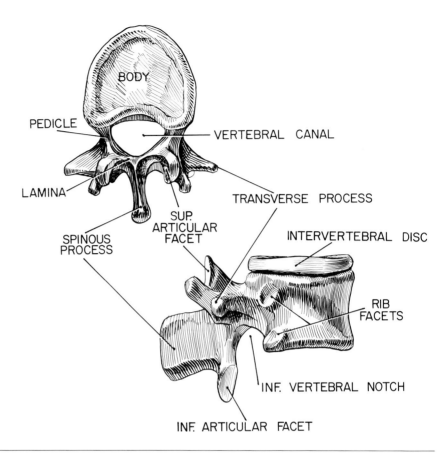

Figure 7-2

The thoracic vertebra, showing the parts of a typical vertebra. *(Top)* In superior view, posterior is toward the bottom and anterior is toward the top. The pedicles and laminae together form the arch. *(Bottom)* In lateral view, posterior is to the left and anterior is to the right. A fibrocartilaginous intervertebral disc is interposed between the bodies of each pair of adjacent vertebrae.

two bony transverse processes, projecting laterally from the arch. The transverse and spinous processes give attachment to a complex series of ligaments and muscles responsible for both maintaining the integrity of the vertebral column and initiating and controlling movements of the column. Spinous processes can be readily felt in living humans, especially the process of C7, which is unusually prominent.

The vertebral arch also gives rise to paired superior and inferior articular process; each process articulates, in a synovial joint, with a corresponding process on the subjacent or superjacent vertebra. Thus the superior articular process of one vertebra articulates with the inferior process of the vertebra above it. The angle and shape of the articular facets of these processes differ in different regions of the vertebral column. The superior articular facets face superiorly at the top of the cervical region, gradually reorienting to face posteriorly in the thoracic region, and then reorienting again to face medially in the lumbar region. Similarly, the inferior articular facets face inferiorly in the cervical region, anteriorly in the thoracic region, and laterally in the lumbar region. The angle and curvature of these articular facets and processes dictate both the axes of movement possible between adjacent vertebrae and the freedom of those movements.

Several abnormal conditions of the vertebral column are sufficiently common to warrant mention here. The condition called hunchback, or kyphosis, is an exaggerated thoracic curvature. Scoliosis is a lateral curvature or assymmetry of the vertebral column and ribs, which appears most often in teen-age girls and can cause considerable pain and deformity if not corrected. Spina bifida is caused by the failure of the vertebral arch or arches surrounding the spinal cord to fuse properly, which leaves the spinal cord and its surrounding membranes unprotected. Finally, a so-called slipped disc is usually a herniation or rupture of the nucleus pulposus out of the anulus fibrosus. Because the displaced nucleus may press upon the spinal nerves as they exit from the spinal cord, this condition is painful and potentially dangerous.

The seven cervical vertebrae show several modifications of the basic vertebral plan. Cervical vertebrae are the only vertebrae with foramina piercing their transverse processes in a superior-inferior plane. Through these foramina run the two vertebral arteries, which branch from major arteries close to the heart: the subclavian artery on the left and the brachiocephalic trunk on the right. The vertebral arteries then run upward through the canal formed by the transverse foramina to the superior surface of C1, where each artery swings laterally and posteriorly around the superior articular process and passes up into the skull through the foramen magnum. These arteries supply the posterior portion of the brain.

The first two cervical vertebrae are readily recognizable because of their distinctive shapes. C1 is called the atlas because it articulates superiorly with the occipital condyles of the skull. The atlas has no body; it is a bony ring with a lateral mass on either side from which the transverse process projects. At midline on the anterior surface of the anterior arch is the anterior tubercle or swelling. On the posterior surface of the anterior arch is an articular facet for the odontoid process of C2. On the posterior surface of the posterior arch is the posterior tubercle, which is a rudimentary spinous process. The lateral masses lie between the superior articular facets, which are kidney-shaped in outline and concave, and the inferior facets, which are flatter and oval in outline. The motion of nodding the head occurs at the joint between the occipital condyles and the superior articular facets of the atlas.

The second cervical vertebra is called the axis. Unlike the atlas, the axis possesses a body, the distinguishing feature of which is the odontoid process, or dens. This process projects superiorly from the body and bears on its anterior aspect a convex, oval facet for articulation with the odontoid facet on the atlas. The superior articular facets of the axis, also called atlantal facets, slope downward from medial to lateral. The atlas can pivot on the axis around the odontoid, producing the motion of shaking the head. This movement gives rise to the name "axis" for C2. The axis has a short, thick spinous process that is often bifid or separated into two parts.

The third through seventh cervical vertebrae are more similar to the typical vertebra. Their bodies are usually somewhat rectangular in outline, and their spinous processes are often bifid. On their transverse processes are small anterior and posterior tubercles on either side of the transverse foramen. The seventh cervical vertebra most closely resembles a thoracic vertebra. Its spinous process is prominent, downward sloping, and not usually bifid; its transverse foramina are small; and its inferior articular facets face posteriorly. There is only a posterior tubercle on the transverse process, although a common abnormality is for the anterior tubercle to be enlarged into a cervical rib.

The twelve thoracic vertebrae are less specialized morphologically than are the cervical vertebrae. A major distinguishing feature of a thoracic vertebra is the presence of one or two facets for the heads of ribs. These facets are found on the posterolateral aspects of the body. A typical thoracic vertebra bears two demifacets, which make complete facets when the adjacent vertebrae are in articulation. T1 bears a complete facet for the first rib and a demifacet for the second; T10–12 may sometimes bear only the upper facet, which extends onto the transverse process.

The body of a thoracic vertebra changes from an oval outline at T1, with its long axis running mediolaterally, to a heart-shaped outline with the point placed anteriorly in T6–10. In T9–12, the point of the heart is blunted and rounded. From superior to inferior, the vertebral bodies of thoracic vertebrae deepen and the vertebral foramen decreases in size. The spinous processes elongate and show an increasingly downward slope in T1–T10. In T11–12, the spinous processes shorten, thicken, and become more horizontal in course. The superior articular facets, which face posteriorly at the top of the thoracic region, reorient to face somewhat medially by T12; similarly, the inferior facets go from facing anteriorly to facing more laterally. The transverse processes are long and laterally directed in the upper thoracic vertebra but are shorter and thicker in the lower thoracics. The anterior aspect of the transverse processes of T1–10 bear facets for the tubercle of the rib.

The five lumbar vertebrae are the largest and deepest of the free vertebrae. Their bodies range from kidney-shaped at L1 to a broad oval at L5, and they do not bear rib facets. Their transverse processes are short, thick, and strong. The superior articular facets of lumbar vertebrae are strongly concave and the inferior facets are strongly convex, with the result that most intervertebral movement in this region is limited to a superior-inferior axis. L1–2 have bodies that are deeper posteriorly than anteriorly, whereas the situation in L3–5 is the converse. This body depth disproportion gives rise to the posteriorly concave lumbar curvature. The opening of the vertebral foramina diminishes among the lumbar vertebrae, since the spinal cord proper stops at L1–2 and a set of thin nerve roots, called the cauda equina or horse's tail, continues to travel downward through the foramina.

The five sacral vertebrae are strongly altered from the typical vertebral pattern (Figure 7-3). The body of S1 is a large oval in outline with its long axis oriented mediolaterally; the bodies of S2–5 decrease in size. The lip of the body of S1 protrudes anteriorly, which is called the sacral promontory. The superior articular facets of S1 persist in adults to articulate with the inferior articular facets of L5. In all sacral vertebrae, the pedicle and transverse process on each side are fused into a single broad structure called the ala or wing. One ala arises from each lateral aspect of the body. The vertebral arch is small, defining the sacral canal through which the cauda equina runs.

The sacral vertebrae begin to fuse into a single unit at 16–18 years, and fusion is usually complete by the mid-twenties. Even in an adult sacrum the divisions between the originally separate sacral vertebrae are often apparent as transverse ridges on the pelvic or anterior surface. Just lateral to each of these ridges are the anterior sacral foramina, through which emerge parts of the first four sacral nerves. The pelvic surface is strongly concave anteriorly, especially in females.

The dorsal surface of the sacrum is convex posteriorly and shows a series of tubercles, equivalent to the spinous processes, which join

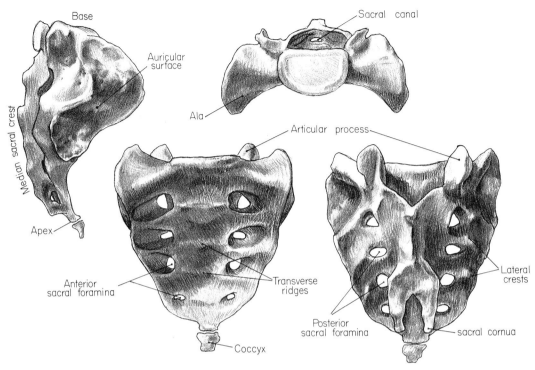

Figure 7-3

The sacrum: *(clockwise from upper left)* lateral, superior, posterior, and anterior view. The base of the sacrum is joined to the body of L5 by an intervertebral disc, not shown here, and the articular processes of the sacrum articulate with the inferior articular facets of L5.

together to form the median crest. Lateral to this crest is a flat area, representing the fused laminae. Farther lateral to the flat area are three or four articular tubercles that make up the intermediate crest; these tubercles are homologues of the articular processes in the juvenile. Lateral to these tubercles are both the four dorsal sacral foramina, through which exit additional parts of the sacral nerves, and the lateral crest, which is made up of transverse tubercles. The dorsal sacral foramina correspond to the superior sacral notches found lateral to the superior articular facets; the transverse tubercles represent the fused transverse processes of S2–5. At the apex of the sacrum, on the dorsal surface, is the sacral hiatus, an opening into the sacral canal, which is bounded laterally by the sacral cornua, or bony horns. The sacral cornua articulate with the coccygeal vertebrae inferiorly.

The lateral or auricular surfaces of the sacrum articulate with the ilia or upper portions of the innominates. These somewhat triangular surfaces are roughened for the attachment of the sacroiliac ligaments that bind the sacrum to the ilia.

The coccygeal vertebrae, which vary in number from three to five, are much smaller than the other vertebrae. They have vestigial bodies and only traces of the vertebral arches. The coccygeal vertebrae fuse to form the coccyx at 20–30 years of age. Like the sacrum, the coccyx is concave anteriorly and convex posteriorly. Co1 articulates with the sacrum, from which it is separated by a thin intervertebral disc. This coccygeal vertebra retains transverse processes, which are absent or much diminished in size in the other coccygeal vertebrae.

THE RIBS

Normal humans have twelve pairs of ribs to protect the thoracic organs and give attachment to the muscles of respiration and thoracic movement (Figure 7-4). Only thoracic vertebrae normally carry ribs, although cervical and lumbar ribs occasionally do. Each rib has a head, the enlarged and rounded end that articulates with a vertebral body; a constricted region or neck that joins the head to a curved shaft; and an anterior end where the costal cartilage attaches to the rib. The other end of the costal cartilage articulates with the sternum.

The head typically bears two facets, separated by a crest. Each facet articulates with a demifacet on a separate vertebral body. These facets form synovial joints. The neck of the rib is elongated and compressed anteroposteriorly. Its lower border is rounded, but the superior border is sharp. The tubercle intervenes between the neck and the curved shaft of the rib. On the tubercle is an articular facet for the synovial joint with the facet on the transverse process of a vertebra. In upper ribs, the tubercular facet is convex and faces posteriorly, but in lower ribs it is more planar and faces inferiorly and posteriorly. The shaft of the rib is flattened anteroposteriorly and follows a spiral course downward and forward from the articulation with the vertebra. This spiraling course is more pronounced in lower than in upper ribs. The inferior border of the rib shows a groove for the intercostal artery, nerve, and vein. This groove is an important feature in orienting isolated ribs because there are few other obvious differences between the superior and inferior borders of a rib. The anterior end of the rib is oval in section and roughened for attachment of the costal cartilage, which may ossify in elderly people.

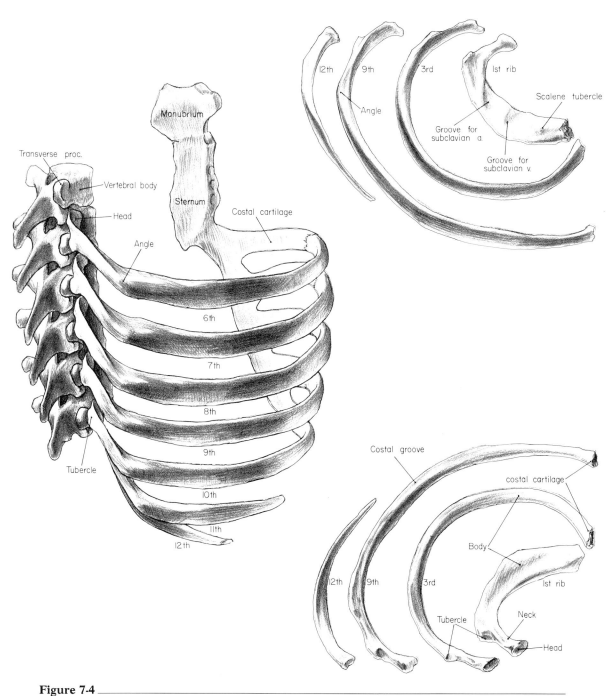

Figure 7-4

The ribs: *(clockwise from left):* their attachment to the thoracic vertebrae and sternum, superior view of selected ribs, and inferior view of selected ribs.

Particular ribs have distinguishing features. The first rib is the short-est, broadest, and least spiral in course. It is sharply curved in superior view, and its flattened surfaces face superiorly and inferiorly, not ante-riorly and posteriorly. It bears only a single articular facet on its head, corresponding to the single facet on the body of T1. The superior sur-face of the first rib is marked by two shallow grooves for the subclavian vessels, separated by the scalene tubercle, to which a neck muscle, the scalenus anterior, is attached in life. The inferior surface of the first rib is smooth.

The tenth, eleventh, and twelfth ribs are all short and bear only single facets on their heads. Neither the eleventh nor the twelfth rib articulates with costal cartilage. These are rather the "floating ribs" that terminate in the muscles of the abdominal wall. The twelfth rib in particular shows neither a marked angle in its shaft nor a groove for the intervertebral vessels and nerve. These ribs also lack tubercles, since their heads articulate with vertebral facets that emerge onto the trans-verse processes rather than being confined to the vertebral bodies.

Ribs ossify from cartilaginous models. During the eighth week of fetal life, primary centers of ossification for the ribs appear at the angle of the shaft, slightly distal to the tubercle. Secondary centers, one for the head and two for the tubercle, appear at about 16 years of age, and these fuse to the shafts by age 25. In adults, ribs are comprised primar-ily of spongy bone, filled with marrow, covered by a skin of compact cortical bone.

THE STERNUM

The sternum is an elongated, flat bone that lies on the midline of the anterior thorax (Figure 7-5). It is divided into three sec-tions from superior to inferior: the manubrium, the body, and the xiphoid process. The manubrium is roughly quadrilateral in out-line and flattened anteroposteriorly. Its superior border shows a pro-nounced curvature, called the jugular notch. Lateral to this notch on either side is the clavicular notch, an articular facet that forms a syn-ovial joint with the head of the clavicle. This joint is the only bony attachment of the entire shoulder girdle to the trunk. Immediately inferior to the clavicular notch on either side of the manubrium is the articulation for the costal cartilage of the first rib. This articulation is one of the few synchondroses in the human body. The inferior border of the manubrium articulates with the body of the sternum at a slight angle, called the sternal angle, which is readily observed on slender people. At the lateral edges of the inferior border of the manubrium

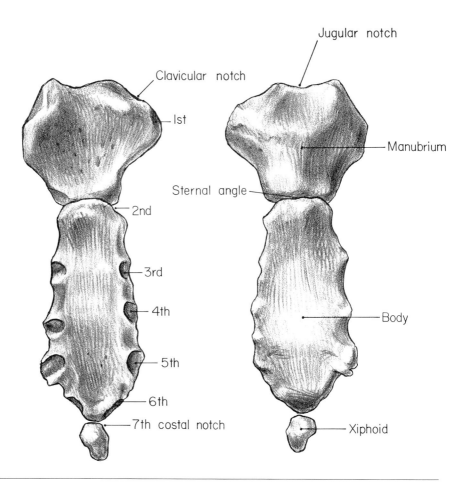

Figure 7-5

The sternum, showing the seven articulations for the costal cartilages of different ribs: *(left)* posterior and *(right)* anterior view.

and continuing onto the body of the sternum are the roughened depressions for attachment of the second costal cartilages. Ossification centers for the manubrium appear in a cartilage model during the sixth fetal month. The manubriosternal joint may fuse partially in older adults.

The body of the sternum is also flattened in an anteroposterior plane. In juveniles, the body of the sternum ossifies from four centers which complete fusion at about 21 years; transverse ridges across the anterior face of adult sterna are remnants of the junctions between these segments. Down the lateral borders of the sternal body lie the articulations with the second through seventh costal cartilages. The depression for the seventh costal cartilage extends onto the xiphoid process inferiorly.

The xiphoid process is a small flat bone ending in a point that is occasionally bifid or perforated. On each lateral and superior aspect, the xiphoid bears a partial facet for the seventh costal cartilage, the other part of the facet being on the body of the sternum. The ossification center for the xiphoid appears at about 3 years of age. Fusion to the body is completed at about 40 years.

Like the ribs, the entire sternum is filled with spongy bone and marrow. In the adult, the sternum produces red blood cells.

8
BREATHING

A major bodily function involving the axial skeleton is breathing or respiration. Through movements of the thoracic cage, fresh air is brought into the lungs, where it oxygenates the blood and is exchanged for waste carbon dioxide. In addition to protecting the lungs from injury, the thoracic skeleton plays a primary role in their functioning by providing attachments for the muscles involved in respiration. Respiration involves a manipulation of the intrathoracic pressure to create pressure differentials between it and the atmospheric pressure. Like water that always seeks its own level, air moves in and out of the lungs in an attempt to equilibrate pressures.

The lungs are paired, spongy organs that occupy most of the thoracic cavity from the level of the first rib to between the seventh and eighth ribs anteriorly and from the first to the tenth rib posteriorly in mid-respiratory cycle. In line with their function, lungs are highly elastic and capable of great changes in capacity. Inspiration always requires muscular effort to increase the volume of the rib cage, thereby lowering the intrathoracic pressure to below atmospheric pressure and drawing air into the lungs. In contrast, quiet expiration is a passive action that is caused by the elastic recoil of the lungs and thoracic tissues; contraction of these tissues decreases the thoracic cavity, thus increasing intrathoracic pressure and causing air to move outward. Vigorous expiration, such as coughing or sneezing, requires muscular effort to decrease thoracic capacity suddenly, increase intrathoracic pressure, and forceably expel air.

Each lung is surrounded by a thin, slippery membrane called the pleural sac. Part of the pleural sac encloses the lung. This portion, called the visceral or pulmonary pleura, adheres closely to the surface of the lung itself. Another portion of the pleural sac, called the parietal pleura, lines the thoracic cavity. The parietal pleura meets the pulmonary pleura at midline, where the lungs branch off from the bronchi, the tubes leading from the trachea, the larynx, and the nose and mouth. The parietal and pulmonary pleura slide freely past each other during inspiration and expiration because they are lubricated by a thin fluid film. Normally the two pleura resist separation because of the viscosity of the fluid film, and there is only a potential space between them, the pleural cavity. Puncture injuries to the thoracic wall may introduce air or fluid into the pleural cavity, which then expands because the pressure in the pleural cavity is much lower than the atmospheric pressure. Expansion of the pleural cavity by fluid or gas, called pneumothorax, causes the lung on that side to collapse.

The total lung capacity of an adult human is about 7 liters (1.8 gallons). The maximum volume expelled in a single breath, called the vital capacity, is about 5.6 liters (1.5 gallons), which leaves a residual volume of about 1.4 liters (0.3 gallons) of air that does not leave the lungs. In normal, quiet respiration the difference between lung capacity during inspiration and expiration, called the tidal volume, is much less than the maximum possible, being about 0.5 liters (0.52 quarts). Quiet respiration involves about 12 breaths per minute in adults and 39 breaths per minute in newborns. Inspiration is accomplished in about 1 second, expiration in 3 seconds.

THE RIB CAGE

Respiration occurs because of pressure differentials between the atmosphere and the thorax. The pressure changes that cause inspiration or expiration are a direct result of movements of the components defining the thoracic cavity. The ribs, sternum, and vertebral column are the scaffolding for the walls and roof of the thoracic cavity.

Thoracic volume is increased in two major ways, by movement of the ribs on the vertebral column and by contraction of muscles in the thorax and abdomen. The rib cage differs in shape and volume in full inspiration and in exhalation (Figure 8-1). With each inhalation, the ribs move, expanding the thoracic volume. As the internal thoracic volume expands, the pressure inside drops below that outside the body and the air rushes in to equilibrate the two.

Two motions create this pressure differential (Figure 8-2). First, the anteroposterior dimension of the thorax is increased as the second to sixth ribs rotate about an axis passing horizontally through each head and tubercle. At the costovertebral joint, each rib rotates about its head, which is strongly convex, so as to lift its end. The combined action of all of the ribs lifts the manubrium upward and forward. This action is called the pump-handle movement because the sternal end of the rib is pumped upward and downward by the rotations at its head.

The transverse diameter of the thorax is increased by a different motion, called the bucket-handle movement. This movement is pro-

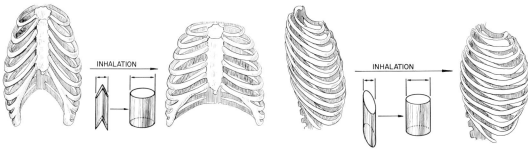

Figure 8-1

Change in thoracic volume as the ribs move from exhalation to inhalation in *(left)* anterior and *(right)* lateral view.

duced by a gliding motion that occurs primarily at the planar joints between the transverse processes of the vertebrae and the articular tubercles of the seventh to tenth ribs. The result of this motion is that the lower ribs, which angle sharply downward in the resting position, move to a more nearly horizontal position and thus widen the total transverse diameter of the thorax. The bucket-handle movement tends to pull the body of the sternum posteriorly. Since pump-handle and bucket-handle movements produce opposing pulls on the sternum, inspiration accentuates the sternal angle by flexing the manubriosternal joint. To accommodate the movements of normal breathing, some twisting of the costal cartilages is also needed.

In deep or forceable breathing, the vertebral column itself may undergo movements. The thoracic curvature may be somewhat straightened, and the back extended. The entire rib cage may be lifted upward by muscles in the neck and upper thorax, such as the sternocleidomastoid and the scalenus anterior, to increase thoracic capacity still further.

THORACIC AND ABDOMINAL MUSCLES

The differences in thoracic volume that result in breathing are created by remarkably small movements of the rib cage. For example, in quiet inspiration the circumference of the chest increases by only 1.2 cm (0.5 in), although the total volume increases by 0.5 liters (0.52 pints). Thus, additional factors are needed to account for the large increase in thoracic volume during inspiration. These factors are the thoracic and abdominal muscles.

The muscle that produces the most dramatic effect on thoracic

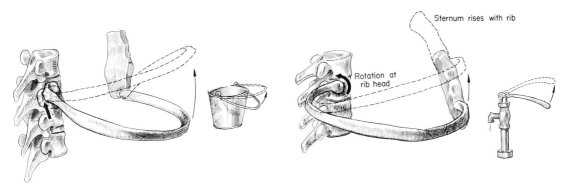

Figure 8-2

Movements of the rib that produce expansion of the thoracic volume, drawing air into the lungs. *(Left)* The bucket-handle movement, in which the rib rotates about the anterior-posterior axis, increases the transverse diameter of the thorax. *(Right)* The pump-handle movement, in which the rib rotates about the medial-lateral axis, increases the anteroposterior diameter of the thorax.

volume is the diaphragm (Figure 8-3). The diaphragm is a dome-shaped sheet of muscle that separates the thoracic and abdominal cavities; in effect, it defines the floor of the thoracic cavity into which the lungs expand. In a standing individual, the dome of the diaphragm is at about the level of the fifth costal cartilage at its attachment to the sternum. In contraction, the dome of the diaphragm moves downward, usually by a few centimeters, but in vigorous breathing it moves by more than 10 cm (4 in). The downward movement of the diaphragm increases the su-peroinferior dimension of the thoracic cavity, which in turn decreases the intrathoracic pressure. Although the diaphragm is often the only muscle that contracts during quiet inspiration, individuals with para-lyzed diaphragms can breathe using the other thoracic muscles.

The diaphragm is divided into three parts: sternal, costal, and lumbar. The sternal part arises from the posterior surface of the xiphoid process. The costal part arises from the posterior surfaces of the six costal cartilages and from the lower four ribs. The lumbar part originates from the two upper lumbar vertebrae, both from their bodies and from the fibrous arches extending from their bodies to their transverse processes. All three parts insert into the central tendon, which has no bony attachments.

Two other sets of thoracic muscles contribute to respiration: the external and internal intercostals. The eleven external intercostals arise from the inferior margin of the first through the eleventh ribs.

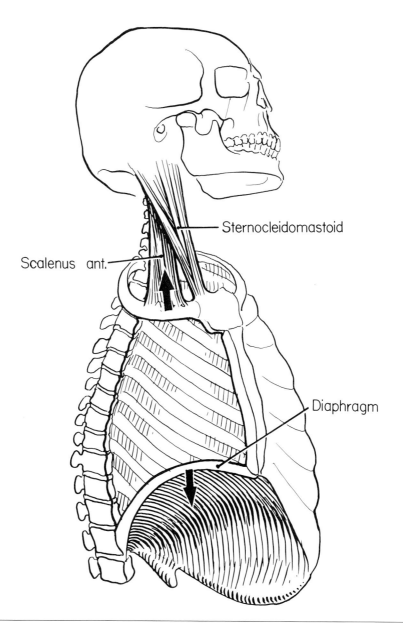

Figure 8-3

Actions of the diaphragm and sternocleidomastoid in respiration. In vigorous inspiration, the sternocleidomastoid pulls upward on the first rib. In all inspiration, vigorous or quiet, the diaphragm moves downward, increasing the superoinferior dimension of the thoracic cavity.

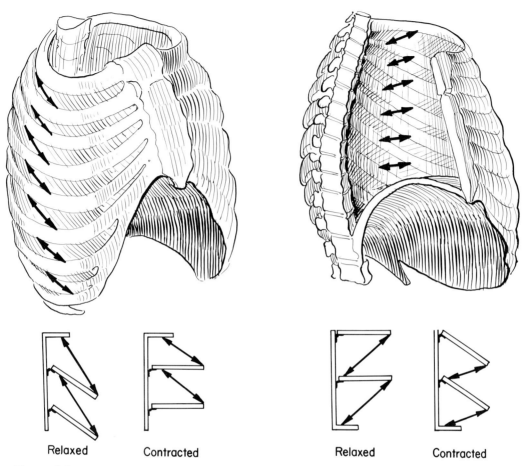

Figure 8-4

Actions of the internal and external intercostals in respiration. *(Left)* The external intercostal muscles help lift the rib cage during inspiration. *(Right)* The internal intercostals depress the rib cage and strengthen the intercostal spaces to prevent bulging outward of the wall of the thoracic cavity during expiration.

Their fibers run downward and medially, to insert into the upper margin of the subjacent rib (Figure 8-4). These muscles form the outermost wall of the thorax from the rib tubercles posteriorly to the junction with the costal cartilages anteriorly. From the junction with the costal cartilage to midline, the outer wall of the thorax is comprised of external intercostal membranes. Contraction of the external intercostals elevates the entire rib cage and forces it into a cylindrical shape, thus increasing the thoracic capacity. Both pump-handle and bucket-handle movements are produced by the external intercostals.

The internal intercostals have an antagonistic action to the externals, as they depress the rib cage and strengthen the intercostal spaces to prevent outward bulging of the wall during forceable expiration. They arise, like the external intercostals, from the lower margins of the first through eleventh ribs and the costal cartilages, and they lie internal to the external intercostals. However, the fibers of the internal intercostals run downward and laterally to insert into the superior margin of the subjacent rib. Thus, the fibers of the external and internal intercostals run nearly perpendicular to each other. The internal intercostals extend from the sternum anteriorly to near the tubercles of the ribs, where muscle fibers are replaced by the internal intercostal membrane.

The most important muscles involved in forceable expiration are those in the abdomen or visceral cavity, such as the external obliquus, the rectus abdominus, and the internal oblique muscles. As a group, these form an anterior muscular wall to the abdominal cavity which runs from the twelfth rib downward to attach to the pelvis. Contraction of these muscles increases abdominal pressure until it exceeds intrathoracic pressure and forces the diaphragm upward. Elevation of the diaphragm decreases the thoracic cavity and forces out the air. This group of abdominal muscles also serves to depress the rib cage by pulling on the twelfth rib.

9
THE UPPER LIMB

In humans, the upper limb is primarily an organ of manipulation. Anatomically, the upper limb is divided into three basic regions: the arm, the forearm, and the hand. The arm includes the shoulder girdle and the portion of the limb proximal to the elbow; the forearm is the region distal to the elbow and proximal to the wrist; and the hand is the region from the wrist to the fingertips. There are 32 major bones in the upper limb and two sesamoids (Figure 9-1). The articulations of these bones are complex, permitting a wide range of motion.

Most of the major bones of the upper limb ossify from cartilaginous precursors starting at about the eighth week of fetal life. The primary center of ossification is usually in the shaft, with two or more secondary centers in the proximal and distal epiphyses. Fusion of the epiphyses to the shaft occurs at about 14–20 years. The exception to this cartilaginous model is the clavicle, which ossifies intramembranously during the sixth week of fetal life.

The carpus, or wrist, ossifies in cartilage beginning in the first year of life. Most of the carpals are ossified by the fourth year; the last carpal to ossify, the pisiform, is complete by 10 years of age. The metacarpals and phalanges also undergo cartilaginous ossification. Like the major long bones, their ossification begins at about 8 fetal weeks with a primary center in the shaft of each bone. Fusion of the epiphyses with the shaft occurs at about 17 years.

THE ARM

The arm has three bony elements: the clavicle and the scapula, which comprise the shoulder girdle, and the humerus, which is the major bone of the arm. The clavicle, or collar bone, provides the only bony articulation of the upper limb with the thorax. The paired clavicles each articulate with the manubrium near the midline at a synovial joint. The clavicle can pivot around this joint, an action important in throwing. Each clavicle proceeds laterally from the manubrium to articulate with the acromion of the scapula. The clavicle lies on the anterior surface of the thorax, crossing over the first rib in its course, whereas the scapula lies on the posterior thoracic surface. Thus, the

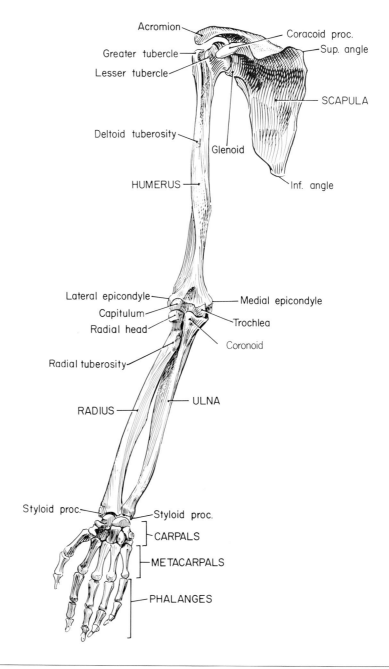

Figure 9-1

Bones of the upper limb in anterior view. The clavicle is omitted to show the articulation of the humerus and scapula. The position of the clavicle is shown in Figure 1-1.

shoulder girdle embraces the entire thorax. The major function of the clavicle is to hold the shoulder joint and the upper limb away from the thorax, permitting free movement of the limb. This function is immediately apparent in individuals with fractured clavicles, since their affected shoulder and upper limb collapse across the chest. The clavicle is absent in many mammals that use their forelimbs for terrestrial locomotion, but it persists in species that use their forelimbs for grasping.

The clavicle is basically an S-shaped cylinder, flattened on the superior and inferior surfaces (Figure 9-2). Going from medial to lateral, the clavicle is first convex forward and then concave forward. The medial end or sternal extremity is enlarged and rounded for articulation with the manubrium. Medially, the articular surface for the sternoclavicular joint extends onto the inferior surface. In contrast, the lateral end, or acromial extremity, is flattened superoinferiorly; as a result, the anterior and posterior borders are more clearly demarcated. The articulation for the acromion is flattened and slightly beveled, so that a displaced clavicle overrides the acromion rather than vice versa.

The superior surface of the clavicle is relatively smooth compared to the inferior surface. Its major feature is the deltoid tuberosity, which marks the most medial attachment of the deltoid, a major shoulder muscle. Because the small sternoclavicular joint is the only bony attachment of the upper limb to the thorax, the two clavicular joints, along with the sternum and the scapula, are reinforced by three different ligaments that leave their markings on the inferior clavicular surface. Just lateral to the sternoclavicular joint lies a roughened impression for insertion of the costoclavicular ligament. This ligament originates on the first costal cartilage and helps maintain the integrity of the sternoclavicular joint by binding the clavicle to this extension of the first rib. Laterally and somewhat posteriorly, the inferior surface bears the conoid tubercle, to which the conoid ligament attaches. This ligament runs from the coracoid process of the scapula, inferior to the clavicle, up to the inferior clavicular surface, thereby reinforcing the joint between the acromion of the scapula and the clavicle. Leading laterally from the conoid tubercle is the trapezoid ridge, also called the oblique ridge, to which attaches the trapezoid ligament. Like the conoid ligament, the trapezoid ligament runs from the coracoid process of the scapula superiorly to the inferior clavicular surface and helps prevent displacement of the acromioclavicular joint. The lateral third of the inferior clavicular surface shows a depression or groove for the subclavius muscle that links the clavicle to the rib cage.

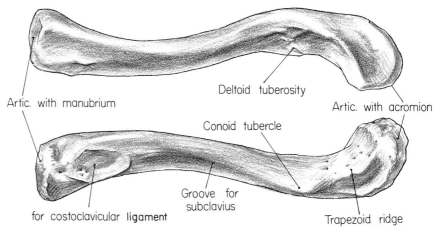

Figure 9-2

The clavicle: *(top)* superior and *(bottom)* inferior view.

The scapula is a large, flat bone that combines with the clavicle to make up the shoulder girdle (Figure 9-3). Basically triangular in shape, the scapula moves freely across the posterior surface of the rib cage, to which it is attached by many muscles. The body of the scapula has a costal, or anterior, surface and a dorsal, or posterior, surface. The costal surface is concave forward to accommodate the curvature of the rib cage. The three angles of the body are called the superior, inferior, and lateral angles. The adjacent borders are known as the superior, medial or vertebral, and inferior or axillary borders respectively.

Three major projections are found on the scapula. At the lateral angle, the scapula bears the glenoid fossa, a shallow, cup-shaped depression for articulation with the head of the humerus. This ball-and-socket joint is responsible for the great freedom of movement possible at the shoulder. Running roughly horizontally in a mediolateral direction is the spine of the scapula, terminating at its lateral end in the acromion process. The spine is a strong bony bar projecting posteriorly from the body of the scapula, which provides attachment for a variety of muscles. The acromion is a subrectangular expansion of the end of the spine presenting a gently rounded superior surface and a gently concave inferior surface. Laterally, the acromion articulates with the clavicle. The third projection, the coracoid process, arises just medial and superior to the glenoid fossa. The coracoid is a short, curved bony bar that arches laterally and medially from its origin. The coracoid serves as the attachment for a variety of ligaments and muscles that reinforce the shoulder joint and produce motion.

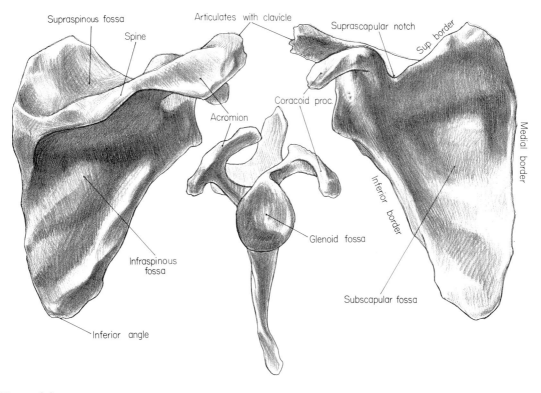

Figure 9-3

The scapula: *(left to right)* dorsal or posterior, lateral, and costal or anterior view.

The posterior surface of the scapula is divided into two major regions by the spine. Superior to the spine, and incorporating its superior surface, is a large concave depression called the supraspinous fossa. Within the supraspinous fossa and just medial to the glenoid, the superior border of the scapula is marked by the suprascapular notch, through which passes a nerve and its accompanying blood vessels. Inferior to the spine is a large convex area which, together with the inferior surface of the spine, is called the infraspinous fossa. The costal surface of the scapula is not similarly divided, its entire concave surface forming the subscapular fossa.

The humerus is the bone of the arm. Like other long bones, it is basically cylindrical in shape with rounded articular surfaces at either end (Figure 9-4). At the proximal end, the head of the humerus has a hemispherical surface that articulates with the glenoid of the scapula. The head faces medially in anatomical position. Anterior and lateral to

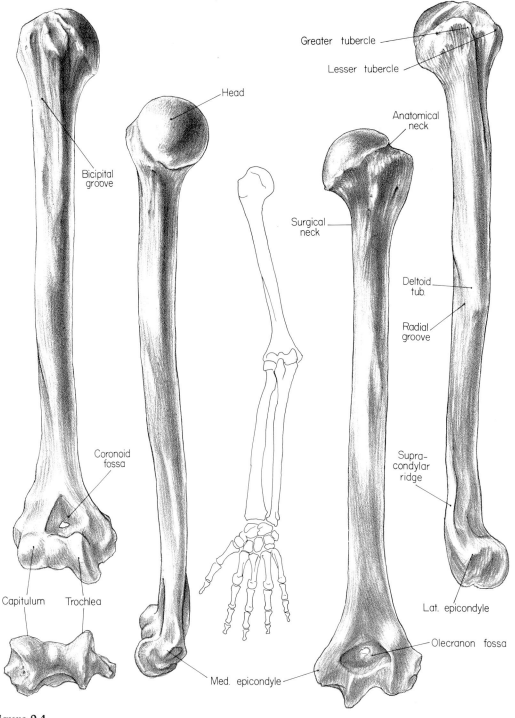

Figure 9-4

The humerus: *(left to right)* anterior view, medial view, placement relative to other bones, posterior view, and lateral view.

the head, two projections are located: the greater and lesser tubercles. The greater tubercle is the most lateral of these and projects beyond the acromion. The lesser tubercle lies medially and anteriorly to the greater tubercle and projects less; its crest runs distally down the shaft. Separating the greater tubercle from the lesser tubercle is the bicipital groove, a strongly demarcated furrow that continues distally down the humeral shaft. Its edges are defined by two crests, one running from the greater tubercle and one from the lesser. The anatomical neck of the humerus is a constriction demarcating the borders of the articular surface, in contrast with the surgical neck, which runs transversely through the shaft about 2 cm (0.8 in) below the head.

The shaft of the humerus has three surfaces that face anterolaterally, anteromedially, and posteriorly. The upper part of the shaft is roughly cylindrical, but the distal third is compressed anteroposteriorly. About halfway down the shaft, the anterolateral surface is marked by a large roughened area, the deltoid tuberosity, onto which the deltoid muscle inserts. The deltoid tuberosity follows a spiral course, traveling downward from posterior to anterior. The posterior surface of the humerus may show a feature called the radial or spiral groove that runs downward and laterally across this surface. Distal to the deltoid tuberosity and the spiral groove, the medial and lateral borders thin and flare to form the medial and lateral supracondylar ridges. Immediately proximal to the distal condyle, these ridges lead into blunt projections, the medial and lateral epicondyles, the medial being more pronounced.

The distal condyle has a complex surface for articulation with the radius on the lateral side and the ulna medially. Laterally, the condyle presents a spherical surface, called the capitulum, that articulates with the head of the radius. The articular surface of the capitulum does not extend onto the posterior surface of the condyle. The shape of the capitulum permits flexion or extension of the radius on the humerus as well as rotation of the radius about its long axis. The medial section of the condyle is pulley-shaped, consisting of two rounded ridges or lips separated by a groove; this section, called the trochlea, articulates with the ulna. The medial lip of the trochlea is more prominent than the lateral; thus, the long axis of the ulna is set at an angle, called the carrying angle, to the axis of the humerus. The articular surface of the trochlea extends onto the posterior surface, where it is set off from the shaft by a marked, oval depression called the olecranon fossa. In full extension of the elbow, the olecranon fossa accommodates the olecranon process at the proximal end of the ulna. A corresponding fossa, the coronoid fossa, is on the anterior surface just proximal to the trochlea and capitulum.

THE FOREARM

Two long bones, the radius and the ulna, comprise the skeleton of the forearm. Proximally, each articulates with the humerus and with each other. A single, complex joint capsule encloses the humeroradial, humeroulnar, and radioulnar joints. Distally, the radius articulates with the ulna and with two carpal bones, the scaphoid and lunate. Since the scaphoid indirectly supports the first metacarpal, the radius is commonly said to "carry the thumb." Distally, the ulna articulates only with the radius; it is separated from the triquetrum, the nearest carpal, by an articular disc.

The radius is the larger and most laterally placed of the two forearm bones (Figure 9-5). Proximally, the radius has a head that is circular in outline and concave upward. The concave surface articulates with the capitulum of the humerus, while the circumference articulates with the ulna at its radial notch. The neck of the radius is a constriction just distal to the head. Distal to the neck and on the anteromedial side of the radius lies the bicipital or radial tuberosity. Proceeding laterally and inferiorly from the bicipital tuberosity is the anterior oblique line, a ridge that meets the lateral border of the radius at about midshaft. On the posterior surface is the posterior oblique line, a similar ridge that runs laterally and inferiorly at about midshaft.

The interosseous crest of the radius is a ridge defining the medial border of the shaft from the bicipital tuberosity to the distal end. It is sharpest in its middle third. Distally it divides into two ridges that define the anterior and posterior margins of the ulnar notch, where the distal radius and ulna articulate.

The distal end of the radius is a broad pentagon in inferior view. The gently concave, distal articular surface is divided into two sections. Laterally, there is a triangular area for articulation with the scaphoid. This scaphoid articulation is divided from the medial, rectangular area for the lunate by a ridge. The anterior surface of the distal end is mildly concave and does not articulate with any other bone. Medially, the distal radius bears the concave ulnar notch. On the posterior surface of the radius are four grooves for the tendons of the extensor muscle of the fingers. Projecting downward from the posterior surface is the styloid process of the radius.

The radius undergoes cartilaginous ossification. The primary center is in its shaft. There are two secondary centers for the proximal and distal epiphyses, which fuse to the shaft at 18 and 20 years respectively.

The ulna is slenderer and slightly shorter than the radius. The proximal end of the ulna is considerably thicker than the distal end (Figure

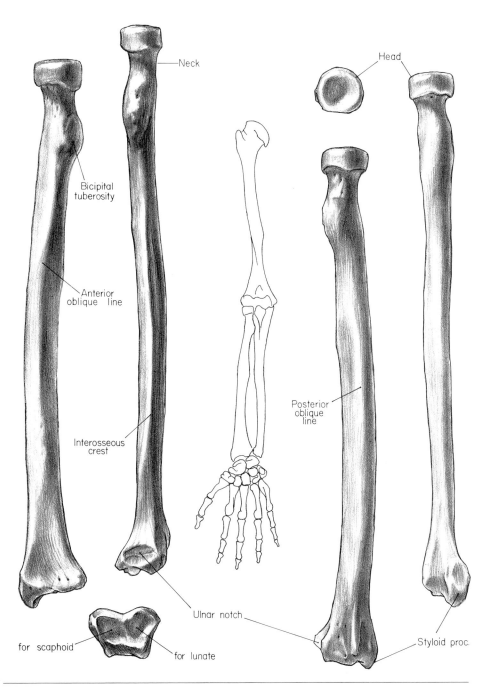

Figure 9-5

The radius: *(left to right)* anterior view, medial view and inferior view of distal end, placement relative to other bones, posterior and superior view of head, and lateral view.

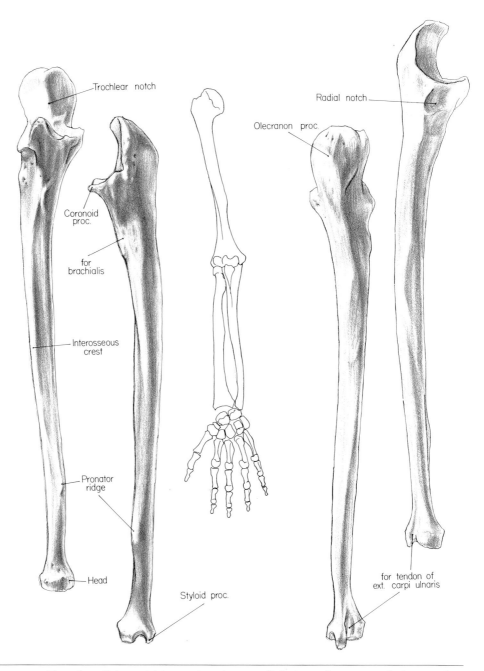

Figure 9-6

The ulna: *(left to right)* anterior view, medial view, placement relative to other bones, posterior view, and lateral view.

9-6). The most proximal portion of the ulna is the olecranon, a roughened process that provides attachment for the triceps muscle. Distal to the olecranon, on the anterior surface of the ulna, is the coronoid process, which provides the inferior edge of the trochlear or semilunar notch. This strongly concave notch is roughly hourglass-shaped in outline and articulates with the trochlea of the humerus. Continuous with the surface of this notch on the lateral side is the radial notch, into which the head of the radius fits.

The shaft of the ulna is triangular in section and diminishes in size from superior to inferior. Along the lateral border of the shaft is the sharp interosseous crest, which directly opposes the interosseous crest of the radius. In life, a tough, fibrous sheet, the interosseous membrane, connects these two crests. Distally on the medial border is the pronator ridge for the pronator quadratus muscle. The distal end or head of the ulna, which is rounded, articulates laterally with the distal radius, and distally it contacts the articular disc of the wrist. Projecting distally from the posterior surface is the styloid process of the ulna.

THE HAND

Eight carpal bones, arranged in two rows of four each, form the skeleton of the wrist. The hand is made up of a row of five metacarpals, which underlie the palm, and fourteen phalanges, the bones of the fingers. Three phalanges are located on each digit with the exception of the pollex, or thumb, which has only two phalanges (Figure 9-7). The hand has two aspects, the palmar or anterior and the volar or posterior.

All eight carpals are small and generally rounded (Figure 9-8). In general, carpals have six surfaces — anterior, posterior, lateral, medial, proximal, and distal — all of which, except the anterior and posterior surfaces, are usually articular. The first or proximal row of four carpals, from lateral to medial, consists of the scaphoid, lunate, and triquetrum; the fourth carpal, the pisiform, lies anterior to the triquetrum. The carpals are named for their shapes. The scaphoid resembles a boat and in other mammals is often called the navicular; the lunate in its anteroposterior aspect resembles a crescent moon; the triquetrum has three articular surfaces; and the pisiform is pea-shaped. The scaphoid, lunate, and triquetrum form an anteriorly concave bony surface, with the small pisiform placed anteriorly on top of the triquetrum. The pisiform is exceptional in having only a single articular surface posteriorly. Because it grows in a tendon, the pisiform is technically a sesamoid. Distally, the three larger carpals comprise a

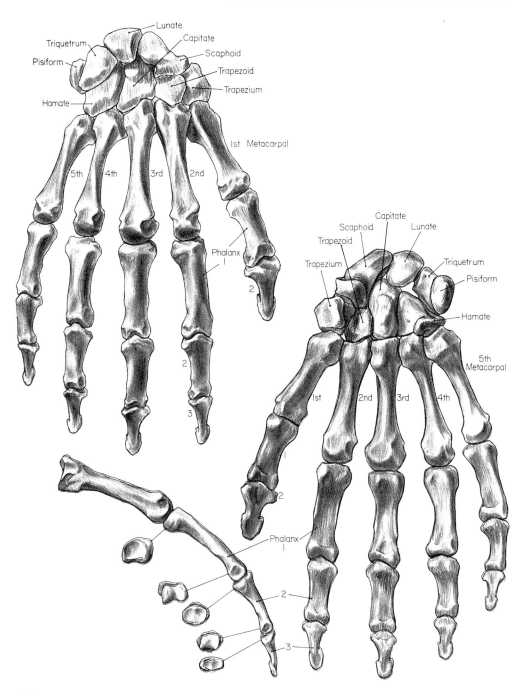

Figure 9-7

Bones of the hand: *(clockwise from top left)* posterior or volar view, palmar or anterior view, and lateral view of the second finger with proximal and distal articular surfaces of the three phalanges.

strongly convex articular surface that meets the radius and the articular disc of the ulna.

The second row of four carpals, from lateral to medial, are the trapezium, trapezoid, capitate, and hamate. The placement of the trapezium and the trapezoid is indicated by the nonsense rhyme:

The trapezium
Supports the thumb;
The trapezoid
Lies insoid.

Both the trapezium and the trapezoid are four-sided, giving rise to their names. The capitate is named for its rounded projection, called the head, which articulates proximally with the lunate. The hamate is named for the large hook-shaped projection on its anterior surface. The scaphoid articulates with both the trapezium and the trapezoid, thus supporting the thumb.

Anteriorly, there are four projections from the carpals. In the first row, the tubercle of the scaphoid and the pisiform project on the lateral and medial sides respectively. In the second row, a pair of projections is formed by the crest of the trapezium laterally and the hook of the hamate medially. Between these four projections stretches a dense, fibrous band called the flexor retinaculum, which holds the carpals in an anteriorly concave position. Through the carpal tunnel created by the flexor retinaculum — that is, between the retinaculum and the carpals — run the tendons of the muscles that flex the fingers.

Posteriorly, the carpals present a convex surface. The articular surfaces of the proximal row of carpals extend onto the proximal surface, permitting extension of the wrist at the radiocarpal joint. Flexion of the wrist occurs primarily at the midcarpal joint.

The second or distal row of carpals supports five metacarpals (m/c I–V), one for each digit starting with the thumb (Figure 9-9). Each metacarpal has a base proximally, where it articulates with the carpals, a shaft, and a rounded head at the distal end. The base of each metacarpal has a proximal-facing articular surface and often has medial or lateral articular surfaces where it contacts other metacarpals. The anterior shaft surface of a metacarpal is mildly concave. Medially and laterally, there are ridges for the attachment of various muscles that flex, extend, abduct, and adduct the fingers. The anterior surface of the head shows a shallow groove for the tendons. Medially and laterally on the head are tubercles for the attachment of ligaments.

M/c I, for the thumb, is noticeably shorter, broader, and stronger

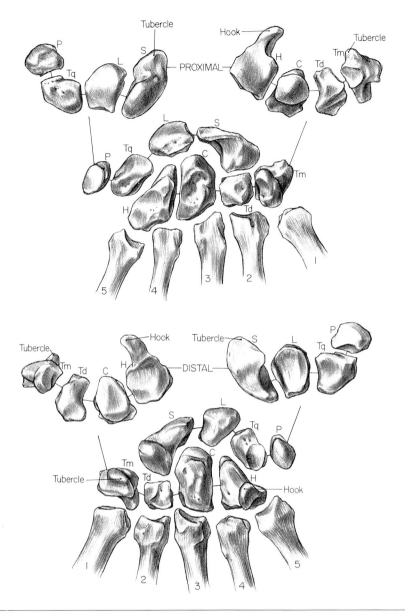

Figure 9-8

The carpals. *(Top left)* The proximal row in proximal view shows articulations for the radius: pisiform *(P)*, triquetrum *(Tq)*, lunate *(L)*, scaphoid *(S)*. *(Top right)* The distal row in proximal view shows articulations for the proximal row of carpals: hamate *(H)*, capitate *(C)*, trapezoid *(Td)*, trapezium *(Tm)*. *(Top center)* The wrist in posterior view shows metacarpal bases in position. *(Bottom left)* The distal row of carpals in distal view shows articular surfaces for the metacarpal bases. *(Bottom right)* The proximal row of carpals in distal view shows articulations for the distal row. *(Bottom center)* The wrist in anterior view shows metacarpal bases in position.

than the other metacarpals. Its base carries a saddle-shaped articular facet for the trapezium. This facet is oriented so that its concave surface faces laterally and inferiorly and its convex surface faces anteroposteriorly. On the anterolateral surface of m/c I is a ridge for the insertion of the opponens pollicis. Its origin is medial, on the trapezium and the flexor retinaculum. Thus, contraction of the opponens pollicis rotates m/c I medially 180° about its long axis, in an action called opposition. The head of m/c I bears two facets on its anterior surface, one medially and one laterally, for the two sesamoids of the hand.

M/c II is usually the longest metacarpal. Like all metacarpals, the shape and number of its basal facets enable identification. Proximally, m/c II presents two broad planar facets that intersect each other at a clearly marked angle and articulate with the trapezoid laterally and the capitate medially. In addition, it has a medially facing facet for articulation with m/c III. Finally, m/c II has a small laterally facing facet where it articulates with the trapezium.

M/c III is readily identified by its styloid process. This projection, which arises on the radial or lateral side of the posterior aspect of the base, is useful in distinguishing between left and right third metacarpals. Proximally, m/c III shows an articular facet for the capitate that is longer anteroposteriorly than it is broad. Laterally, the base shows a two-humped facet for m/c II; medially, it bears two distinct but closely spaced facets for articulation with m/c IV.

M/c IV has a smaller base than either the second or the third. The proximal facet is quadrangular and articulates with the hamate. To the lateral side are oval articular facets for m/c II and the capitate. Medially, m/c IV sometimes has an elongated facet for m/c V.

M/c V is the smallest of the metacarpals. Proximally, it articulates with the hamate. Laterally, it has a facet for m/c IV. There is a prominent tubercle on the medial side of the base for attachment of the extensor carpi ulnaris muscle, which is an extensor of the wrist.

Distal to the metacarpals are the phalanges of the fingers. The first digit has only a proximal and a terminal or distal phalanx; the other digits each have proximal, middle, and distal or terminal phalanges. Like the metacarpals, each phalanx has a base proximally, for articulation with its metacarpal or phalanx, connected by a shaft to a head distally. Phalanges are generally mildly concave anteriorly and convex posteriorly. The length of the phalanges of any digit decreases from the proximal to the distal row.

The proximal phalanges have concave articular facets for the meta-

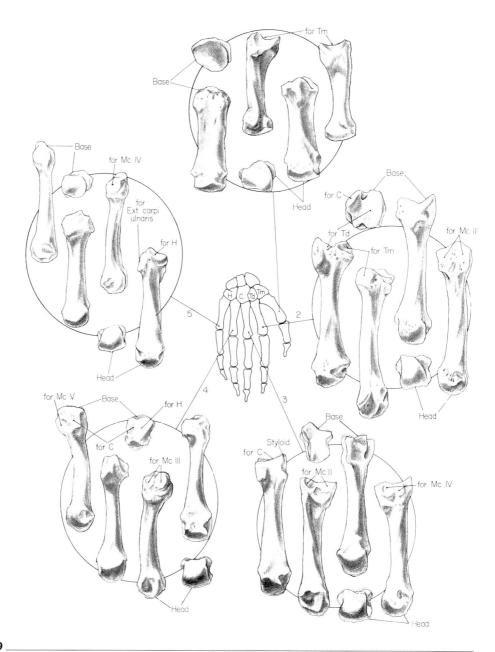

Figure 9-9

The metacarpals: *(clockwise from upper left)* m/c I in proximal, lateral, medial, anterior, distal, and posterior view; m/c II-III in proximal, anterior, lateral, distal, medial, and posterior view; m/c IV in proximal, anterior, distal, lateral, posterior, and medial view; and m/c V in proximal, medial, anterior, distal, posterior, and lateral view.

carpal heads and sharp medial and lateral borders. Their heads bear a
shallow groove that divides the articular facets into medial and lateral
condyles. The articular facets extend onto the anterior surface farther
than onto the posterior surface. Middle phalanges are similar in shape
to proximal phalanges but are shorter, broader in the shaft, and larger
at the base. The articular facets on the bases of middle phalanges are
divided into lateral and medial halves by a low ridge. Again, the anterior articular surface of the head is larger than the posterior. Distal
phalanges are distinguished both by their small size and by their distal
tuberosity. The distal tuberosity is a roughened surface that is broad-
ened and flattened anteroposteriorly into a semicircular shape. It
underlies the fleshy ball of the finger and anchors the fingernail. Distal
phalanges are flatter anteroposteriorly than other phalanges.

10
MANIPULATION

The upper limb functions as an organ of manipulation. The movements of the upper limb that are important in manipulation are caused by the actions of muscles upon bones that articulate at joints. Each joint has a potential for movement defined by the shapes of the bones participating in the joint, by the structure of the joint capsule, and by the placement of muscles about the joints. All of the possible movements are reciprocal.

JOINTS OF THE UPPER LIMB

There are eight joints or sets of joints in the upper limb: the shoulder, elbow, distal radioulnar, radiocarpal, midcarpal, carpometacarpal, metacarpophalangeal, and interphalangeal. Different types and ranges of movement are possible at each joint.

The most proximal joint, the shoulder, is a relatively incongruent ball-and-socket joint that permits a wide range of movements (Figure 10-1). There are four primary, reciprocal pairs of movements at the shoulder: abduction and adduction of the arm, flexion and extension at the shoulder, medial and lateral rotation of the arm, and elevation and depression of the shoulder. The fifth pair of movements, circumduction, is secondary because it is a combination of the other movements; it can occur in either direction. For these movements, the body is envisioned as starting not in the standard anatomical position but from a position in which the arms hang freely at the side with the palms facing medially. Abduction at the shoulder moves the arm upward and laterally from the body; adduction is the return from an abducted position to its starting point. However, abduction and adduction can occur in two different planes: the plane of the thorax, a coronal plane in which the arm moves either directly laterally (abduction) or medially (adduction); or the plane of the scapula, in which the arm moves either forward and laterally (abduction) or backward and medially (adduction.)

Flexion and extension at the shoulder occur on a different plane from abduction and adduction. Flexion occurs when the arm is moved

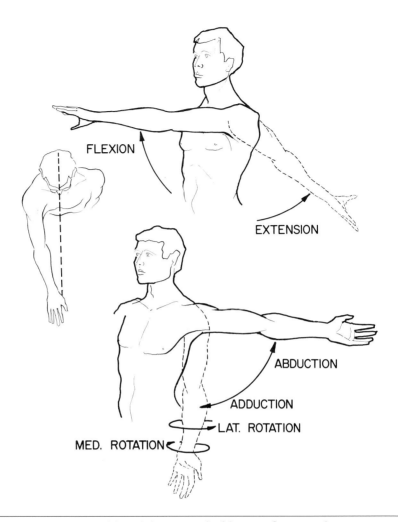

Figure 10-1

Movements at the shoulder: abduction and adduction, flexion and extension, medial and lateral rotation.

medially in front of the body until the arm makes an angle of about 45° to the coronal plane in superior view. Extension occurs when the arm is moved laterally and posteriorly along the same plane. Flexion and extension thus occur on a plane that is perpendicular to the scapular plane of abduction and adduction. In other terms, flexion is an action that decreases or makes more acute the angle between the clavicle or scapula and humerus, and extension is an action that increases that angle or makes it more nearly straight. The changing angle is best visualized in anterior view.

Rotation of the upper limb at the shoulder may occur in a medial or lateral direction. In either case, the limb is spun about its long axis. In standard anatomical position, the upper limb is already laterally rotated, although it is possible to rotate the arm laterally still farther. This can be verified by standing in anatomical position, flexing an elbow so that the palm faces upward, and then laterally rotating the arm at the shoulder. In this sequence, the movement of the hand makes readily apparent the lateral rotation at the shoulder. Medial rotation with a fixed, extended elbow brings the palm of the hand to face medially and somewhat posteriorly.

Circumduction with a fixed elbow causes the hand to describe the base of a wide cone, the apex of which is the shoulder. The shoulder can also be elevated, as in shrugging, or depressed, relative to anatomical position.

During the various movements of the arm at the shoulder, the bony elements of the shoulder girdle move as well. The most important movements involve the scapula. During flexion, the scapula moves so that the glenoid faces more anteriorly; in extension the glenoid moves to a more posterior-facing position. In the early stages of abduction, the scapula may not move, for elevation of the arm is produced by the movement of the head of the humerus in the glenoid. However, abduction above shoulder height cannot occur without rotation of the scapula, in which the inferior angle swings laterally to make the glenoid face more superiorly. If such rotation does not occur, further elevation of the humerus is prevented because the greater tuberosity and the overlying soft tissues cannot underride the acromion. During circumduction, the scapula rotates both upward and downward and moves anteriorly and posteriorly. Elevation and depression of the shoulder are accomplished primarily by muscle actions that move the entire scapula upward or downward. Equally important to the movement of the shoulder is the clavicle, which pivots about the sternoclavicular joint and permits the entire shoulder girdle to move anteriorly or posteriorly.

The elbow is a complex set of three joints: the humeroradial, radioulnar, and humeroulnar. These joints allow three different kinds of reciprocal action. The most restricted joint in terms of movement is the tightly congruent humeroulnar, at which the primary movements are flexion or bending the elbow and extension or straightening the elbow.

The humeroradial and radioulnar joints permit the second pair of reciprocal movements to occur: supination and pronation. In anatomical position the hand is supinated, or palm forward, with the shafts of the ulna and radius lying parallel to each other. In pronation, the radius is rotated medially about its long axis, so that its head spins against both the capitulum and the radial notch of the ulna. In the fully pronated position, the palm faces posteriorly. In this position, the proximal radius is lateral to the ulna, the midshaft of the radius is anterior to the ulna, and the distal radius is medial to the ulna (Figure 10-2). Supination is the action of returning the forearm to anatomical position.

These two actions of the elbow — flexion or extension and pronation or supination — can occur independently of each other and of the lateral or medial rotation at the shoulder. Abduction and adduction constitute the third reciprocal action of the forearm at the elbow. This movement is slight, occurring through minor movements of the ulna on the trochlea.

The distal radioulnar joint is involved in pronation and supination. In pronation, the distal radius moves anteriorly and medially around the distal ulna, producing the crossing over of the shafts and the reorientation of the hand.

The radiocarpal and midcarpal joints act as part of the same complex called the wrist. Adduction occurs primarily at the radiocarpal joint, whereas abduction occurs mostly at the midcarpal joint. These two movements at the wrist are also referred to, respectively, as radial and ulnar deviation from anatomical position. A greater degree of ulnar than of radial deviation is possible, for the reason that the distal radius articulates directly with the carpals while the distal ulna is separated from the carpals by a compressible, articular disc.

The radiocarpal joint also permits extension, but little flexion. Extension of the wrist involves moving the hand posteriorly from anatomical position, so that the palm faces downward and forward instead of forward only. People who slip often brace themselves by extending their wrists, the result being a fracture of the scaphoid, which is exposed as the primary weight-bearing bone in extension. Flexion of the wrist, in which the hand is brought forward so that the palm faces upward, occurs primarily at the midcarpal joint. The wrist can be flexed to a greater degree than it can be extended, indicating that the midcarpal joint can open more widely without damage than can the radiocarpal joint.

The carpometacarpal joints permit little movement, with the exception of the joint at the base of the thumb. This special, saddle-shaped joint has a capsule that permits a wide range of movements, including flexion and extension, abduction and adduction, and rotation about the long axis of the thumb.

At the metacarpophalangeal joints a much wider range of movement

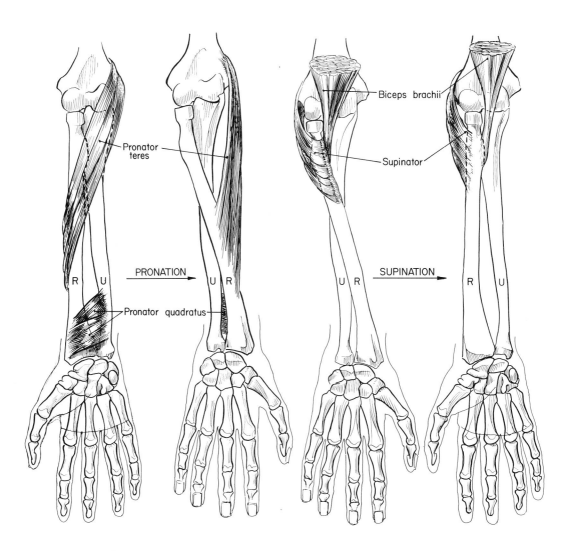

Figure 10-2

Pronation and supination: *(left to right)* the right forearm in supinated (standard anatomical) position, showing the pronators; after pronation, showing the pronators and the altered positions of the hand, the radius *(R)*, and the ulna *(U)*; after pronation, showing the supinators; and after supination, showing the return to standard anatomical position and the supinators.

is possible. The proximal phalanges are readily flexed and extended upon the metacarpals at this joint. In addition, abduction and adduction of the fingers are accomplished by motion at the metacarpophalangeal joints. In the hand, abduction and adduction are considered to occur as movements away from or toward a longitudinal plane through the third or middle finger because some of the important hand muscles are arranged symmetrically around this finger. In addition, the third finger can itself be abducted either laterally or medially from its standard position. The degree of abduction and adduction that is possible at the metacarpophalangeal joints is much greater in extension than in flexion.

Finally, the interphalangeal joints each permit flexion and extension to occur. These are primarily hinge joints.

MUSCLES OF THE SHOULDER

The major muscles acting upon the shoulder joint fall into three groups: those acting to move the scapula upon the thorax, those acting to move the humerus upon the scapula in rotation and abduction or adduction, and those acting to flex or extend the shoulder. In life these different muscle groups work smoothly together, and many motions of the upper limb involve the action of muscles in all three groups.

Rotation of the scapula so that the glenoid faces upward is required in any action that raises the arm above the shoulder. An important muscle involved in scapular rotation is the trapezius, a large triangular muscle found on the back of the neck and thorax. The trapezius originates from the skeleton along its midline, extending from a bony ridge called the nuchal line on the occipital of the skull to the spines of C7–T12. The trapezius inserts on the spine of the scapula, along the acromion, and onto the lateral third of the clavicle. Different parts of the trapezius can contract separately, so that it can elevate the scapula in a shrug, rotate the scapula to make the glenoid face upward, or depress the scapula (Figure 10-3).

Working with the trapezius muscle in rotating the scapula is the serratus anterior. The serratus anterior originates from the external surfaces of the upper eight ribs just anterior to their extreme lateral curvature. In inserts on the medial edge and inferior angle of the costal surface of the scapula. Thus, contraction of the serratus anterior swings the inferior angle of the scapula in a lateral direction along the rib cage and simultaneously works to keep the scapula close to the rib cage. These actions permit abduction of the arm above the horizontal.

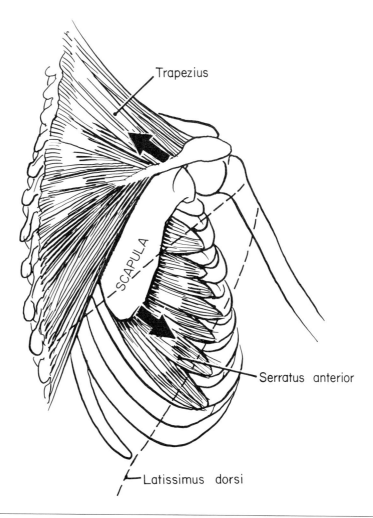

Figure 10-3

Major muscles for rotating the scapula: trapezius, serratus anterior, and latissimus dorsi *(dashed lines)*, which overlies the serratus anterior.

The primary muscle that works to abduct the humerus is the deltoid (Figure 10-4). This is the large, fleshy muscle that gives the shoulder and proximal humerus their rounded shape. The origin of the deltoid closely parallels the insertion of the trapezius. The deltoid arises from the spine of the scapula, the acromion, and the lateral third of the clavicle, in each case lying just lateral or just inferior to the trapezius insertion. It inserts on the deltoid tuberosity of the humerus, which lies about halfway down the shaft. The deltoid muscle is multipennate, or

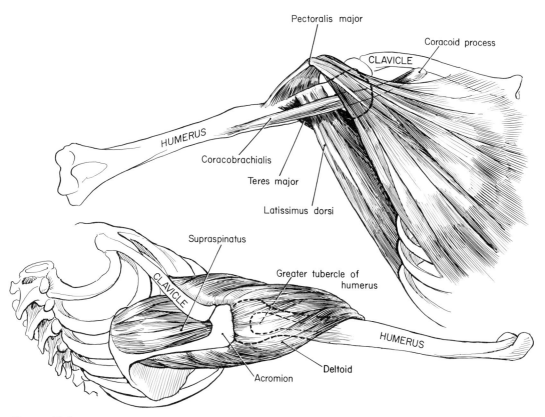

Figure 10-4

Major muscles for flexion or extension and abduction or adduction at the shoulder: deltoid, pectoralis major, latissimus dorsi, coracobrachialis, and supraspinatus.

comprised of several different parts: clavicular, scapular, and acromial. As a result, portions of the muscle can contract separately or in concert. Thus, when the entire deltoid or just the acromial portion contracts, the effect is to abduct the humerus powerfully. When the clavicular portion alone contracts, the deltoid helps to rotate the humerus medially. When the scapular portion alone contracts, the deltoid helps to rotate the humerus laterally.

Two muscles play the major role in flexion and extension of the arm at the shoulder. Flexion is brought about in large part by the actions of a muscle on the anterior surface of the rib cage, the pectoralis major. This muscle originates from the medial half of the clavicle, the surface of the sternum, and the six costal cartilages. The tendon of the pectora-

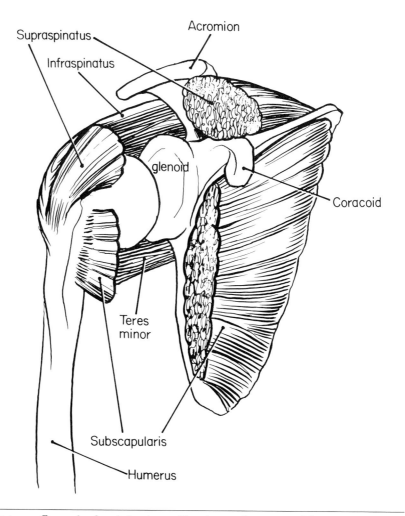

Figure 10-5

Rotator cuff muscles for abduction, adduction, and rotation of the arm in anterior view: subscapularis, supraspinatus, infraspinatus, and teres minor.

lis major inserts on the lateral lip of the bicipital groove, which is also called the crest of the greater tubercle. Therefore, the pectoralis major acts as either a powerful medial rotator of the humerus or, when rotation is resisted by antagonistic muscles, a flexor of the humerus.

Extension is produced by the actions of a muscle of the back, the latissimus dorsi. The latissimus originates from the spines of T6–L5, the sacrum, and the iliac crest of the innominate. It proceeds laterally from its origin, incorporates additional muscle fibers originating from the inferior angle of the scapula, passes medial to the humerus, and inserts on the floor of the bicipital groove on the anterior, proximal humerus. In contraction, the latissimus dorsi has three possible actions: rotating the arm medially, adducting the humerus, and extending the shoulder.

Four other major muscles are involved in abduction, adduction, medial rotation, and lateral rotation of the arm: the subscapularis, supraspinatus, infraspinatus, and teres minor. These four muscles are collectively called the rotator cuff muscles, because they form a cuff of tendon and muscle that protects the shoulder joint on the anterior, superior, and posterior sides (Figure 10-5). The ring of muscle and tendon is incomplete inferiorly, which is why dislocations of the shoulder almost always involve the head of the humerus slipping downward out of the glenoid.

The rotator cuff muscles originate in an incomplete ring or horseshoe around the glenoid. From anterior to superior to posterior, the muscles arise from the subscapularis fossa, the supraspinatus fossa, the infraspinatus fossa, and the dorsal surface of the inferior border of the scapula. Their insertions upon the humerus also form a horseshoe. Thus, the subscapularis inserts on the lesser tubercle, the supraspinatus on the greater tubercle, and the infraspinatus on the posterior side of the greater tubercle. The teres minor inserts on the posterior humerus on the crest of the lesser tubercle, just inferior to the subscapularis insertion and paralleling its course.

The tendon of each of these muscles blends with and reinforces the joint capsule of the shoulder. All of the rotator cuff muscles therefore help to stabilize and strengthen this joint. The action of each muscle is dictated by its site of insertion. The subscapularis inserts anteriorly, rotates the humerus medially and functions in adduction; the supraspinatus, which inserts superiorly, initiates abduction of the humerus; and the infraspinatus and teres minor, which insert posteriorly, rotate the humerus laterally. All of these muscles participate in complex actions, such as circumduction.

MUSCLES OF THE ELBOW

Because the elbow has a more restricted range of movements than the shoulder, fewer muscles are involved. A single, antagonistic pair of muscles, the biceps and triceps brachii, are primarily responsible for flexion and extension at the elbow. Three other major muscles are involved in pronation and supination: the pronator teres, pronator quadratus, and supinator, along with the biceps brachii.

The major flexor of the elbow is the biceps brachii (Figure 10-6). This

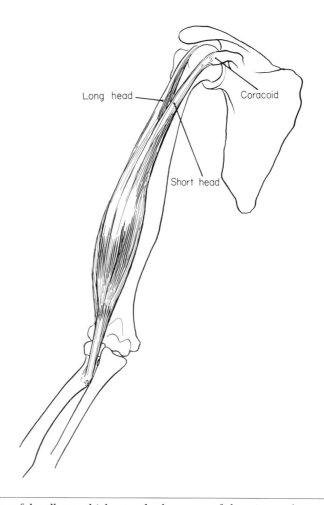

Figure 10-6 _____

Major flexor of the elbow, which may also be a powerful supinator: biceps brachii.

muscle has two separate origins, called the long and short heads. The long head arises just superior to the glenoid, and the short head arises from the tip of the coracoid process. The tendon of the long head lies in the bicipital groove on the proximal humerus. The two heads unite into a single fleshy region called the belly, which inserts, via a tendon, onto the bicipital tuberosity of the radius. Thus, the biceps crosses two joints, the shoulder and the elbow. Although the biceps assists in actions at the shoulder, such as abduction, its primary action takes place at the elbow. In anatomical position, contraction of the biceps flexes the elbow. In pronation, the radius rotates medially, winding the biceps

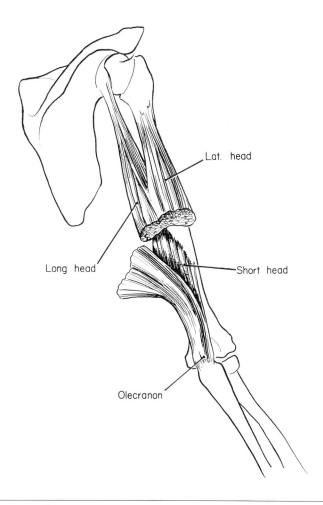

Lat. head

Long head

Short head

Olecranon

Figure 10-7

Major extensor of the elbow: triceps brachii.

tendon about the proximal radius by means of its bicipital tuberosity. Contraction of the biceps alone, with the forearm in a pronated position, produces supination rather than flexion. However, if other muscles are used to hold the forearm in pronation, contraction of the biceps produces flexion.

The major extensor of the elbow is the triceps brachii, a muscle that occupies the posterior and medial part of the arm and has three heads: the long, lateral, and medial or short (Figure 10-7). The long head of the triceps arises from a tubercle just inferior to the glenoid. The lateral head originates from the posterior surface of the humerus, lateral and superior to the radial groove. The medial head arises on most of the posterior surface of the distal humerus, starting from just inferior and medial to the radial groove and terminating above the joint capsule of the elbow. These three heads unite to insert on the olecranon process of the ulna. Contraction of the triceps produces a powerful extension of the elbow.

Two muscles are primarily responsible for pronation: the pronator teres and the pronator quadratus (Figure 10-2). Of these, only the pronator teres crosses the elbow joint. The pronator teres arises from the medial supracondylar ridge and the medial epicondyle of the humerus. This muscle runs diagonally downward and laterally, to insert on the lateral edge of the midshaft of the radius. In contraction, the pronator teres pulls the radius shaft anteriorly and medially, producing the crossing of the radius over the ulna. Distally, the pronator quadratus has a similar action. This muscle arises from the anterior surface and medial border of the distal ulna and inserts on the anterior surface and lateral border of the radius. Again, contraction of the pronator quadratus pulls the distal radius across the ulna to produce pronation.

Supination is the work of two muscles: the biceps brachii and the supinator muscle. The supinator arises from the lateral epicondyle of the humerus and parts of the lateral surface of the proximal ulna. It inserts on the anterior oblique line of the proximal radius. Contraction of the supinator and biceps when the forearm is pronated spins the radius laterally about its long axis to restore normal anatomical position.

EXTRINSIC MUSCLES OF THE HAND

Some of the important muscles producing movements of the wrist and hand originate above the elbow. These muscles, considered extrinsic hand muscles, produce flexion and extension of the wrist, abduction and adduction of the wrist, and flexion and extension of the fingers. The five muscles with the most proximal origins are the two flexors and three extensors of the wrist (Figure 10-8). The combined action of these five muscles produces circumduction of the hand at the wrist. The three muscles responsible for flexion and extension of the second through fifth fingers originate slightly distal to those that move the wrist. Additional muscles for the thumb, second or index, and fifth or little fingers arise within the forearm.

The two flexor muscles of the wrist are the flexor carpi ulnaris and the flexor carpi radialis. As their names indicate, these lie on the ulnar

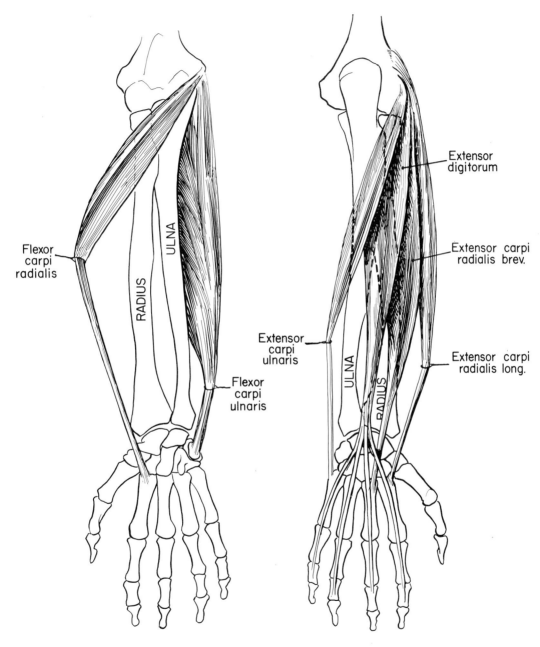

Figure 10-8

Extensors and flexors of the wrist: extensor carpi ulnaris, extensor carpi radialis brevis, extensor carpi radialis longus, flexor carpi ulnaris, and flexor carpi radialis. The extensor of the fingers, extensor digitorum, is also shown.

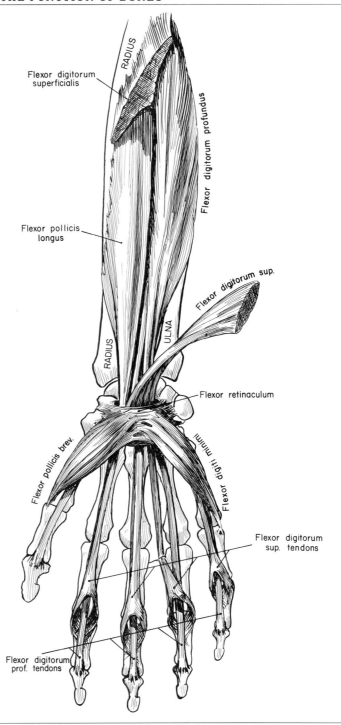

Figure 10-9

Flexors of the fingers: flexor digitorum superficialis, flexor digitorum profundus, flexor pollicis longus, flexor pollicis brevis, and flexor digiti minimi.

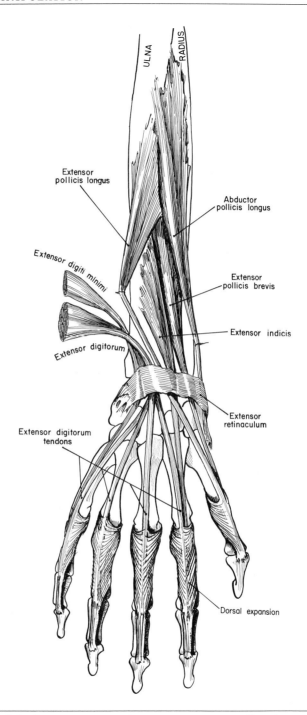

Figure 10-10

Extensors of the fingers: extensor digitorum, extensor pollicis longus, extensor pollicis brevis, extensor indicis, and extensor digiti minimi. The long abductor of the thumb, abductor pollicis longus, is also shown.

or medial and radial or lateral sides of the anterior surface of the forearm. They arise respectively from the medial and lateral epicondyles of the humerus. The flexor carpi ulnaris inserts on the pisiform, the hook of the hamate, and the base of m/c V. The flexor carpi radialis inserts on the bases of m/c II and III. When both of these muscles contract, the wrist flexes.

The three extensor muscles of the wrist are the extensor carpi ulnaris and the extensor carpi radialis brevis and longus (Figure 10-8). The extensor carpi ulnaris arises from the lateral epicondyle and inserts on the base of the fifth metacarpal, almost paralleling the course of the flexor carpi ulnaris. The extensor carpi radialis brevis and longus also arise from the lateral side of the humerus, from the supracondylar ridge and epicondyle respectively. They insert on the back of the second and third metacarpal bases. Contraction of all three extensor muscles extends the wrist.

Abduction at the wrist is produced by contracting the radial flexor and extensor muscles simultaneously. Adduction is produced by contracting the ulnar extensor and flexor simultaneously.

In addition to flexors and extensors of the wrist, the distal humerus also gives rise to the major flexors and extensors of the fingers (Figure 10-9). While the thumb has its own flexor and extensor, the second through fifth fingers share two flexors, one superficial and the other deep, and one extensor. The relative position of the two flexors within the forearm explains their designation as either superficial or deep. The medial epicondyle of the humerus bears the common flexor tendon, from which come the two flexors of the wrist and the superficial flexor of the fingers, called the flexor digitorum superficialis. The deep flexor of the fingers, called the flexor digitorum profundus, arises from the proximal two-thirds of the anterior surface of the ulna. From the lateral epicondyle of the humerus comes the common extensor tendon, from which originate the ulnar and the short radial extensors of the wrist, the extensor of the second through fifth fingers, called the extensor digitorum, and the special extensor of the fifth or little finger, called the extensor digiti minimum (Figure 10-10).

Both the superficial and deep flexors of the fingers lie on the anterior surface of the forearm and hand, the deep flexor lying underneath the superficial flexor. Each muscle has a fleshy belly that then divides into four tendons, one for each finger. At the wrist, these tendons pass under the flexor retinaculum, a fibrous sheath anchored to the carpals. In flexion of the wrist and fingers, this arrangement prevents tendons from bowstringing, or going directly from the distal humerus to the phalanges without following the curvature of the forearm and hand bones. The flexor retinaculum also protects these important tendons. The tendons then pass along the appropriate metacarpal. Anterior to the proximal phalanx, each superficial flexor tendon divides into two parts which then pass laterally and medially around the deep flexor tendon to reunite beneath it. The superficial flexor tendon inserts on the anterior surface of the middle phalanx, whereas the deep flexor tendon continues distally to insert on the base of the terminal phalanx. Thus, the superficial flexor flexes the joint between the proximal and middle phalanges, whereas the deep flexor flexes the joint between the middle and distal phalanges. Both tend to act together to flex the metacarpophalangeal joints as well.

The extensor digitorum, for the fingers, lies on the posterior surface of the forearm and hand. Like the flexors, this muscle divides into four distinct but connected muscle bellies which give rise to four tendons at the wrist. The tendons pass under the extensor retinaculum and then diverge to insert on the different fingers. In each finger, the extensor tendon dives under a dorsal expansion, or hood, of connective tissue that lies posterior to the metacarpophalangeal joint. Each tendon is divided into lateral and medial parts under this hood, where it also receives fibers from tendons of intrinsic hand muscles. Ultimately, the terminal portion of each extensor tendon inserts on the base of the distal phalanx of a single digit. The extensor digitorum muscle simultaneously extends the metacarpophalangeal and all interphalangeal joints.

The thumb, index, and fifth fingers have a number of special muscles of their own. The thumb is the most heavily muscled, having a long flexor, the flexor pollicis longus; a long abductor, the abductor pollicis longus; and a short and long extensor, the extensors pollicis brevis and longus. The flexor and the extensors arise from the anterior and posterior surfaces of the radius and ulna. The long flexor and long extensor insert on the distal phalanx of the thumb, while the short extensor inserts on the proximal phalanx. The abductor arises from the interosseous membrane to insert on the trapezium and the lateral side of the first metacarpal. The index and little fingers also have their own extensors.

INTRINSIC MUSCLES OF THE HAND

The hand is capable of an unusually wide range of finely controlled movements, as a consequence of the many intricately arranged muscles of the hand and their elaborate neural control. Four muscles account for many movements of the thumb: the abductor pollicis brevis, the flexor pollicis, the opponens

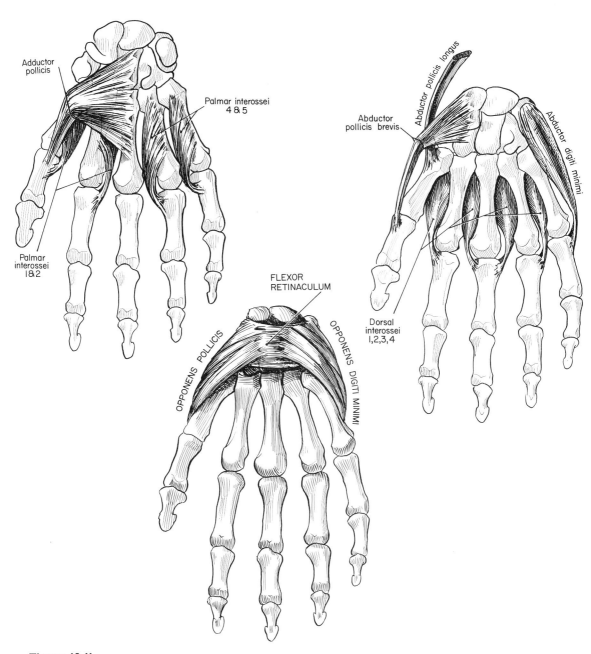

Figure 10-11

Some intrinsic muscles of the hand: *(top left)* palmar interossei, which adduct the fingers, and adductor pollicis in anterior view; *(top right)* dorsal interossei, which abduct the second–fourth fingers, abductor pollicis longus and brevis, and abductor digiti minimi, which abducts the fifth finger, in dorsal view; and *(bottom)* opponens pollicis, which flexes and rotates the thumb about its long axis, and opponens digiti minimi, which has a similar action on m/c V, in anterior view.

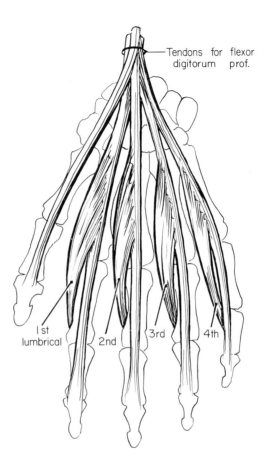

Tendons for flexor
digitorum prof.

1st
lumbrical   2nd   3rd   4th

Figure 10-12

Other intrinsic muscles of the hand: the lumbricals, which arise from the lateral
side of the deep flexor tendons and insert on the extensor tendons of the same
finger, in anterior view. When contracted, the lumbricals short-circuit the contraction of the flexors to the extensors, so that the metacarpophalangeal joints flex
but the interphalangeal joints extend.

pollicis, and the adductor pollicis. Three sets of muscles, the lumbricals
and palmar and dorsal interossei, are the intrinsic hand muscles for the
second through fifth fingers.

Three of the four intrinsic hand muscles to the thumb — the short
abductor or abductor pollicis brevis, the short flexor or flexor pollicis
brevis, and the opponens pollicis — arise from the flexor retinaculum
or various protuberances on the nearby carpals (Figure 10-11). The
short flexor and the short abductor insert on the lateral sesamoid and
the adjacent base of the proximal phalanx of the thumb. The opponens,

which runs deeper, inserts on the lateral side of the shaft of m/c I and can therefore produce medial rotation of the thumb about its long axis during opposition. Some individuals, particularly those engaged in manual labor, have very pronounced flanges on their first metacarpals for the opponens muscle. The fourth muscle of the thumb is the adductor pollicis, which arises from two heads. One of these heads originates from the base of m/c II and the capitate and trapezoid; the other head arises from the front of m/c III. They insert with a common tendon onto the medial sesamoid and the medial side of the base of the proximal phalanx of the thumb.

Like the thumb, the second through fifth fingers are capable of movements in addition to flexion and extension. The four lumbricals arise from the flexor tendons of these fingers in a complicated pattern and insert upon the dorsal expansion of the extensor tendons on the posterior side of the hand (Figure 10-12). The lumbricals flex the metacarpophalangeal joints and, because they insert on the dorsal extensor expansion and contribute fibers to the extensor tendons, simultaneously extend the two interphalangeal joints.

The four palmar interossei arise from the medial sides of the shafts of m/c I and II and from the lateral sides of m/c III and IV. They also insert onto the dorsal extensor expansions. They serve to adduct the metacarpal, and thus the finger, from which each one arises.

The four dorsal interossei have the opposite function of abducting the fingers when they are extended. Each dorsal interosseous muscle arises by two heads, from the sides of the shafts of two adjacent metacarpals, and inserts onto the side of the dorsal extensor expansion that will enable it to abduct the finger. The third finger has a dorsal interosseous muscle on each side and can therefore be abducted in either direction. Both palmar and dorsal interossei assist the lumbricals in flexing the metacarpophalangeal joints while extending the interphalangeal joints.

11
THE LOWER LIMB

In many ways, the lower limb is similar in structure to the upper. Both limbs are attached to the trunk by a girdle: the shoulder girdle in the case of the upper limb, the pelvic girdle in the case of the lower limb. Both limbs are divided into three similarly arranged units: the arm, forearm, and hand for the upper limb; the thigh, leg, and foot for the lower limb. The skeleton of the proximal part of each limb is comprised of a single large bone: the humerus in the upper limb, the femur in the lower limb. The middle part of each limb is comprised of a pair of bones: the radius and ulna in the forearm, the tibia and fibula in the leg. And the distal unit of each limb, the hand and the foot, includes many small bones. Beyond this simple level, however, there are major differences between the two limbs, because the upper limb is adapted as an organ of manipulation, while the lower limb is adapted as an organ of locomotion and support (Figure 11-1).

The lower limb contains 31 major bones, including the sacrum, and one large sesamoid, the patella. The long bones in the thigh and leg ossify first, generally from cartilaginous precursors, starting during the eighth week of fetal life. The primary centers of ossification are in the shafts, with two or more secondary centers in the proximal and distal epiphyses. The final fusion of the various epiphyses to the shaft in long bones occurs at 18–20 years of life. The innominates, the large bones of the pelvic girdle, ossify later, starting in the second to fifth months of fetal life. Fusion of the elements of the innominate into a whole is completed by 20 years of age.

The tarsal bones ossify slowly, their centers of ossification appearing from the sixth fetal month through the third year of life. The calcaneus is the only tarsal with a secondary center of ossification, which appears at about 8 years and fuses to the primary center by about 16 years. The metatarsals and phalanges all ossify cartilaginously from three centers of ossification. The primary centers appear in their shafts in the ninth fetal week. Fusion of the secondary centers, for the heads and bases, with the shafts is complete at about 18 years of age.

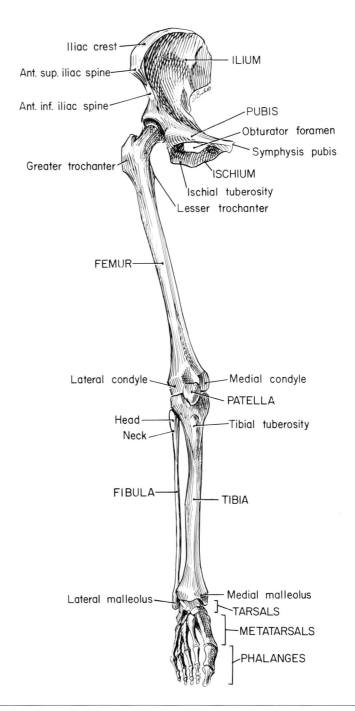

Figure 11-1 ————————————————————————————

Bones of the lower limb in anterior view.

THE PELVIC GIRDLE

The pelvis or pelvic girdle consists of three different bones: the sacrum at midline and one innominate on each side. The sacrum is an integral part of the pelvic girdle and plays an important role in the functioning of the lower limb. Through the sacrum, the lower limb is firmly fixed onto the axial skeleton in a manner far less mobile and far more stable than the manner in which the shoulder girdle is affixed to the thorax.

Each innominate ossifies from three major centers, which give rise to its three major regions: the ilium, ischium, and pubis (Figure 11-2). Another major feature of the innominate is the acetabulum, which is the socket for the head of the femur. The acetabulum is formed by the fusion of the ilium, ischium and pubis, each of which carries part of the socket. Prior to skeletal maturity, the region of the acetabulum where fusion will occur has a special cartilage plate, called the triradiate growth plate. Evidence of the triradiate growth plate may persist as roughened lines for some time after fusion has occurred. The triradiate growth plate is structurally the same as an epiphyseal growth plate, although it is located between three parts of the innominate, none of which can be considered to be an epiphysis. The last major feature of the innominate is the obturator foramen, a large hole through the inferior part of the innominate.

The ilium is the broad blade of the superior innominate that gives the pelvis its bowl-like shape. The ilium includes the superior third of the acetabulum. It provides support for the pelvic and abdominal organs as well as giving attachment to many of the important muscles of the abdomen and lower limb. The curvature and mediolateral flattening of the ilium in humans are striking, making even fragments of ilium readily recognizable.

The ilium has two surfaces, the gluteal or external surface and the medial or interior surface. The gluteal surface is strongly convex, and the medial surface is strongly concave. The gluteal surface is crossed from superior to inferior by two raised ridges, the anterior and posterior gluteal lines. A third ridge, the inferior gluteal line, runs roughly horizontally just superior to the acetabulum. The anterior two-thirds of the medial surface of the ilium is occupied by the iliac fossa, a smooth concavity. The posterior third of the medial surface is raised and roughened. The auricular or ear-shaped surface is the strongly marked area where the innominate articulates with the sacrum. Superior to this surface lies a rougher area for the attachment of the strong sacroiliac ligaments that bind the sacrum and ilium together. Also on the posterior third of the medial surface is the large iliac tuberosity. Inferi-

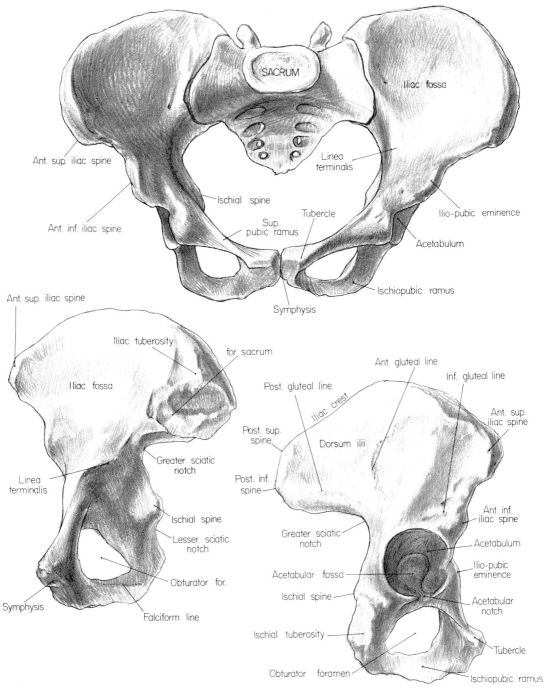

Figure 11-2

The bony pelvis: *(clockwise from top)* superior view, with anterior toward the bottom; the right innominate in internal view; and the right innominate in external view.

orly, the medial surface is crossed by the linea terminalis, or arcuate line, which runs from the auricular surface to the superior pubic ramus, where it is also known as the pectineal line.

The iliac crest forms the superior border of the ilium and has its own epiphysis. Anteriorly, the iliac crest terminates in the anterior superior iliac spine. Below this spine and just superior to the acetabulum is the anterior inferior iliac spine. Posteriorly, the iliac crest terminates in the posterior superior iliac spine, which is paired with the posterior inferior iliac spine. The pronounced indentation in the posterior border of the ilium that lies medial to the posterior inferior iliac spine is the greater sciatic notch. The walls of this notch make a broader angle in females than in males and thus provide a major clue in sexing skeletons.

The acetabulum is a large, cup-shaped socket. The rim of the acetabulum is incomplete inferiorly at the acetabular notch. In anatomical position, the entire pelvis is oriented so that the anterior superior iliac spines and the pubic symphysis, where the right and left pubic articulate, form a vertical plane. Thus, the acetabulum faces laterally and inferiorly. Within the acetabulum is a horseshoe-shaped region of subchondral bone with which the head of the femur actually articulates. The middle and inferior area, called the acetabular fossa, is not articular. In life, this fossa is occupied by a fat pad, covered in synovial membrane, and gives rise to the ligament called the ligamentum teres that attaches to the femoral head. This ligament carries the blood supply to the femoral head and ensures that the head stays firmly in the acetabulum; it also partly limits the mobility of the femur.

The ischium is the posterior segment of the innominate. It consists of the posteroinferior third of the acetabulum and its surrounding bone, called the body; the ischial tuberosity, which is the posteriormost portion of the ischium; and a ramus, or arm of bone, that projects anteriorly to join the inferior pubic ramus. The posterior border of the body forms one wall of the greater sciatic notch. The sharp ischial spine separates the greater from the lesser sciatic notch. The inferior border of the body forms part of the superior border of the obturator foramen. Immediately inferior to the lesser notch is the ischial tuberosity, a large, roughened protuberance that supports the body's weight in sitting and is especially apparent to individuals sitting on hard surfaces. Like many of the tuberosities of the innominate, the ischial tuberosity also gives rise to various muscles of the thigh. Like the iliac crest, the ischial tuberosity ossifies as an epiphysis. The ischial ramus is much more flattened mediolaterally than either the tuberosity or the body of the ischium. It meets the inferior pubic ramus below the acetabular notch. Together, the two rami form the ischiopubic ramus, which is the inferior border of the obturator foramen. Both have thinner, sharper superior borders and thicker, more rounded inferior borders.

The pubis is the anteroinferior segment of the innominate. It bears a superior and an inferior ramus that meet each other in the symphyseal region. The superior ramus terminates in the acetabulum, where it fuses to the portions of the acetabulum carried by the ilium and ischium. The inferior ramus passes inferolaterally from the symphysis to meet the ischial ramus in the ischiopubic ramus. In addition to being the region where the superior and inferior rami of the pubis meet each other, the pubic symphysis is also where each pubis articulates with its opposite member. The pubic symphysis marks the anterior border of the entire pelvis.

The angle formed by the inferior pubic rami of a pelvis indicates the sex of the individual: females have a wide subpubic angle of about 90°, and males have a much narrower one, about 60° (Figure 11-3). The symphysis itself is flat in both the superoinferior and anteroposterior planes, and the symphyseal surface of each pubis is roughened. The extent of roughening and ridging on the pubic symphysis corresponds to the age of the individual. The superior ramus of the pubis angles upward and backward from the symphysis. It is more rounded in section than the inferior ramus and becomes wider near the acetabulum. The superior pubic ramus forms the anterior border of the obturator foramen. The pubic tubercle is a small bump on the superior border of the superior ramus close to the symphysis. In females, the superior pubic ramus tends to be relatively longer than in males.

Despite its large size, the obturator foramen does not transmit any large structures. In life, the foramen is mostly closed by a membrane. Only a small nerve, artery, and vein pass out of the pelvis through the foramen. The shape of the obturator foramen is more oval in males and more triangular in females.

An innominate or pelvis provides the strongest indicator of sex in the entire skeleton. The pronounced pelvic differences are determined by function. The major reason that male and female skeletal anatomy differs so strongly in the pelvic region is that only females must carry and bear large-brained infants. In the course of human evolutionary history, the selective pressures for increasing brain size have altered the pelvic structure in ways that actually impair human efficiency in bipedal locomotion. To bear big-brained babies, a human female needs

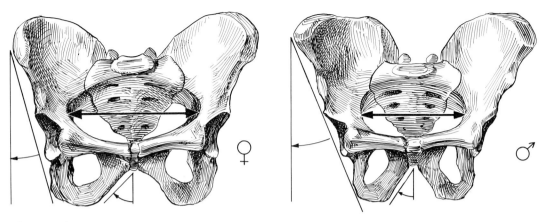

Figure 11-3

Sexual dimorphism in the pelvis. *(Left)* The female pelvis in anterior view shows a greater transverse diameter of the pelvic inlet, shallower and less flared shape, and greater subpubic angle. *(Right)* The male pelvis in anterior view shows a narrower transverse diameter of the pelvic inlet, greater iliac flare and superoinferior depth of the pelvis, and lesser subpubic angle.

a broad pelvis with a large pelvic inlet and outlet. In contrast, to be an efficient biped, a human needs a narrow pelvis that places the hip joints closer both to each other and to the body's midline. Such an arrangement minimizes the side-to-side displacement of the body during walking and helps to maximize mechanical efficiency. Thus, the demands of bipedal locomotion and childbirth conflict, yet each is important in human evolution.

The compromise that has been achieved is biologically and mechanically complex. One consequence of these conflicting demands is that human infants are less physically mature at birth than other mammals. Thus, a greater proportion of the growth in brain size comes after birth in humans than in most mammals. While this places a tremendous burden on the mother during lactation, when she must provide sufficient energy for the infant to grow such a large brain, it greatly alleviates her obstetrical difficulties, since the infant's brain is relatively small at birth. A second consequence is that, on average, human female pelvic structure is less efficient for bipedalism than human male structure. As a result, females of unusual locomotor efficiency, such as Olympic runners or speed skaters, are noticeably masculine in general body build, being wide-shouldered and narrow-hipped. Although the seriousness of the consequences of being ill-adapted for childbearing are more obvious than those of being ill-adapted for locomotion, the maintenance of such striking sexual dimorphism attests to the strength of selection for locomotor efficiency.

THE THIGH

The only bone of the thigh is the femur. The femur is the largest and longest bone in the human skeleton. It provides the structural support for the entire body weight in standing and walking. At the proximal end of the femur is the large spherical head (Figure 11-4). The clearly demarcated pit in the head is the fovea capitis, which is the area of insertion of the ligamentum teres that arises in the acetabulum. The articular surface of the femoral head is highly congruent with that of the acetabulum.

The neck joins the head to the shaft. The bone of the neck is a somewhat flattened cylinder set at an angle of about 125° to the long axis of the shaft. Its superior and posterior surfaces are typically fibrous in appearance and show many nutrient foramina. The neck is constricted near the head and broadens as it approaches the shaft.

The proximal shaft bears several major features. Rising above the level of the neck is the greater trochanter. On the anterior shaft, the greater trochanter is set off from the neck by the trochanteric line, a bony ridge running medially and downward from the greater trochanter. The lesser trochanter is visible from the anterior view as a bump on the medial shaft below the level of the neck. However, the lesser trochanter clearly arises from the posterior shaft. On the posterior surface of the proximal femur, the intertrochanteric crest runs between the greater and lesser trochanters. This crest separates the neck from the shaft and is a much more pronounced feature than the trochanteric line on the anterior surface. Medial to the superior end of the intertrochanteric crest, and at the base of the greater trochanter, lies a deep, smooth depression called the trochanteric fossa.

Leading downward from the greater and lesser trochanters are two small ridges to which muscles attach. These join each other at midline in the thick, compound bony ridge called the linea aspera. Structures that contribute to the linea aspera are the spiral line, the pectineal line, and the gluteal ridge. The linea aspera appears on the posterior surface of the femur down to about the distal third of the shaft, where it divides into the medial and lateral supracondyloid ridges. Distally, the posterior surface of the shaft shows many nutrient foramina in the region called the popliteal surface. The anterior surface of the shaft is generally smooth and mildly convex, although it, too, is marked by nutrient

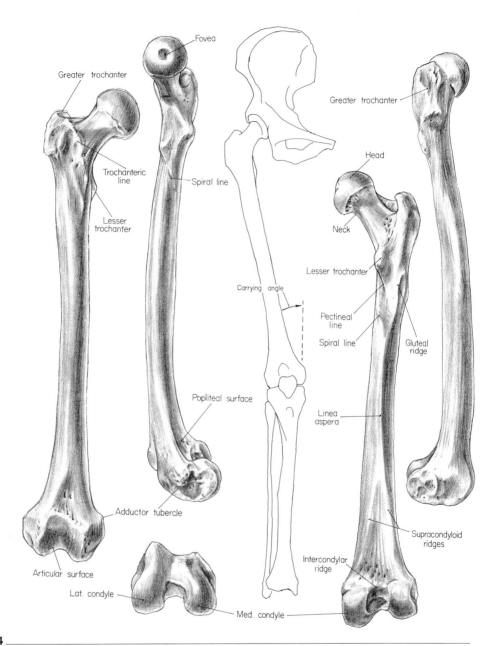

Figure 11-4

The femur: *(left to right)* anterior view with distal view of femoral condyle, medial view, placement relative to other bones, posterior view with superior view of head, and lateral view. The carrying angle of the femur is greater in females than in males.

foramina at the distal end, just superior to the articular surface. The shaft broadens distally into medial and lateral epicondyles, roughened surfaces just proximal to the condyles themselves. The adductor tubercle is a particularly pronounced tubercle on the medial epicondyle to which the adductor magnus muscle attaches. The cross-sectional area of the femur is closely correlated with both the weight and stature of the individual during life. The geometry of femoral cross-sections may also reflect the stresses imposed by a particular lifestyle.

The distal end of the femur bears two condyles, medial and lateral, for articulation with the tibia. The articular surface for the tibia continues upward onto the anterior surface, where it becomes the patellar surface, a grooved region onto which the patella rides in full flexion of the knee. The lateral edge of the patellar groove or surface protrudes farther anteriorly than the medial edge, and this increased height helps prevent the patella from being dislocated laterally during extension of the knee. On the posterior surface, the articular surfaces of the two condyles curve tightly upward. Between them lies the deep intercondyloid fossa, bounded superiorly by the intercondylic ridge.

The role of the femur in bipedalism is revealed by many of its features. In anatomical position, as in efficient bipedal locomotion, the knees are closer together than the hips. In order for the femur to pass from the knee at midline to the laterally placed hip joint, it must be set at an angle to the vertical, with the proximal end sloping outward. The carrying angle of the femur varies from about 14° in males, whose hips are relatively narrow, to about 17° in females, who have wider hips. The angle is produced by the greater protrusion of the medial condyle relative to the lateral. The presence of this angle is diagnostic of bipedalism in fossil species. The thick cortical walls of the shaft also reflect the femur's important role in support and locomotion.

The patella, the largest sesamoid in the body, is triangular in anteroposterior outline, (Figure 11-5). It rides in the tendon of the quadriceps femoris, the large muscle of the anterior thigh. The patella is covered on its anterior surface by the quadriceps tendon. The quadriceps femoris arises on the anterior femur and innominate and inserts via the patellar ligament on the tibial crest of the proximal tibia. Because the hip joint, near the origin of the quadriceps, is more laterally placed than the insertion of the quadriceps, contracting this muscle yields a diagonal pull which tends to displace the patella laterally from its groove. For this reason, the lateral lip of the patellar groove is more built up than the medial lip. Although the anterior surface of the

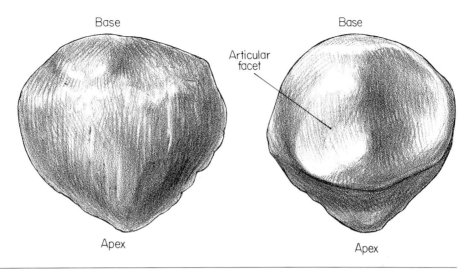

Base   Base

Articular
facet

Apex   Apex

Figure 11-5

The patella, showing the articular surface for the femur: *(left)* anterior and *(right)* posterior view.

patella is fibrous and bears many nutrient foramina, the posterior surface is given over to smooth, subchondral bone. The articular facet for the lateral condyle and surface of the lateral side of the groove is larger than the medial and can be used to distinguish left from right patellae.

THE LEG

The tibia and fibula are the paired bones of the leg. They are disparate in size, the tibia having a much greater diameter and a somewhat greater length, as befits the major weight-bearing bone of the pair. The tibia lies medial to the fibula. The tibia articulates with the femur proximally, the fibula laterally, and the talus inferiorly. The fibula articulates only with the tibia and talus.

The tibia has an enlarged proximal end bearing a pair of flattened condyles, which receive the femoral condyles (Figure 11-6). The articular surface of the medial condyle is both oval in outline, with its long axis oriented anteroposteriorly, and mildly concave. The lateral condyle has a smaller, more nearly circular articular surface, and it is also slightly concave. Separating the two condyles is a raised area, the intercondylar eminence, marked with two distinct intercondylar tubercles. Anterior and posterior to the intercondylar eminence are the anterior and posterior intercondylar fossae, both of which are perforated by

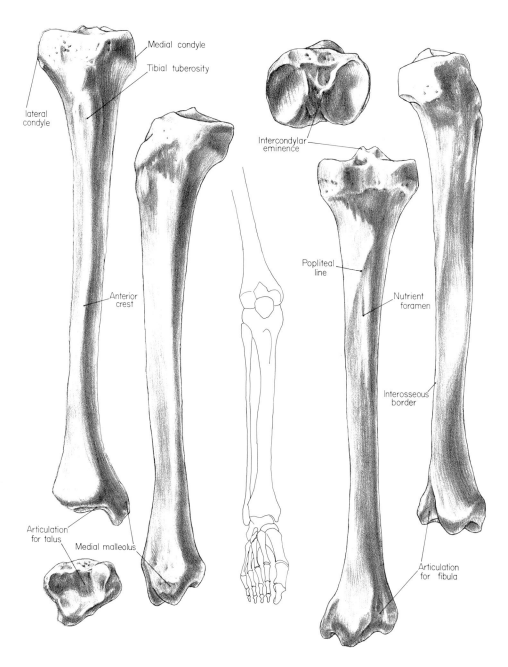

Figure 11-6

The tibia: *(left to right)* anterior view with distal view of distal articulation, medial view, placement relative to other bones, posterior view with superior view of head, and lateral view.

nutrient foramina. On the lateral, posterior side of the tibial head is a small articular facet for the proximal fibula.

The tibial shaft is triangular in section, having medial, lateral, and posterior surfaces. The sharp anterior crest forms the border between the lateral and medial surfaces. At its proximal end is an enlarged, roughened protuberance called the tibial tuberosity, into which the patellar ligament of the quadriceps femoris inserts. The medial surface of the shaft is smooth and slightly convex; the lateral surface is concave and marked by the interosseous crest. A corresponding interosseous crest appears on the medial surface of the fibula, and as in the forearm, a tough interosseous membrane stretches between these crests on the two bones. The posterior surface of the tibial shaft is overhung proximally by the tibial head. Running diagonally downward from lateral to medial is a bony ridge called the popliteal line. Usually just below this line and nearer to the lateral side of the posterior surface is a large nutrient foramen that opens upward so that the vessel entering it points downward or away from the knee joint.

The distal end of the tibia is smaller than the proximal end but larger than the shaft. The distal end bears the medial malleolus, a large rounded projection perforated by many nutrient foramina that forms the bony bump on the medial ankle in life. On its lateral surface, the medial malleolus has an articular surface for the side of the talus. This articular surface is continuous with the main inferior articular surface, although the medial malleolus projects farther inferiorly than the rest of the surface. From the inferior view, the inferior articular surface is quadrilateral in outline. The lateral side of the distal extremity is concave, to receive the fibula, and is marked by nutrient foramina. The articular surface for the fibula is often not readily apparent.

The fibula is markedly slenderer than the tibia (Figure 11-7). The proximal end bears a rounded, enlarged head with an articular facet for articulation with the proximal tibia. Projecting upward from the posterior part of the lateral or nonarticular surface of the head is the apex or styloid process. The slender shaft has four surfaces — medial, anterior, lateral, and posterior — and three crests that serve as borders separating those surfaces. These different borders and surfaces are relatively difficult to distinguish. The medial surface is concave and faces the tibia. It is strongly demarcated proximally but becomes less distinct distally. The interosseous or medial crest, which faces its counterpart on the tibia, is the sharpest border and separates the medial from the anterior surfaces. The anterior surface is very narrow and flat proximally, where the anterior and interosseous crests closely

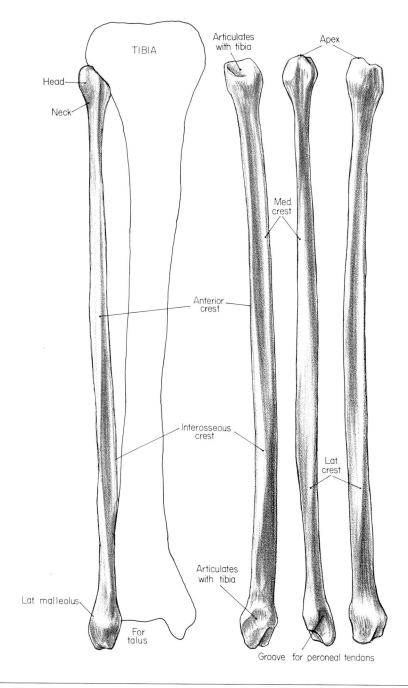

Figure 11-7

The fibula: *(left to right)* anterior view in relation to tibia, medial view, lateral view, and posterior view.

approximate each other. In the distal third of the fibula, the anterior surface becomes broader and then tapers sharply just above the distal extremity. Separating the anterior from the posterior surfaces is the anterior crest, which divides into two branches about two inches above the distal extremity, enclosing a flat, elongated triangular space between its branches. The lateral surface is concave proximally and convex distally. It is separated from the posterior surface by the lateral crest, which is less sharp than the other borders. The lateral crest spirals around the shaft, being lateral at the proximal end and posterior at the distal end. Thus, the posterior and lateral surfaces also follow a spiral course. The distal end of the fibula is larger and heavier than the proximal end. When a complete fibula is balanced at midshaft, its distal end invariably points downward. The distal extremity bears the lateral malleolus, the rounded, bony bump on the outer side of the ankle. On the medial surface of the distal fibula is the articular surface for the talus and, posterior to it, the deep malleolar fossa. This fossa enables ready identification of the side from which a fibula comes, since it always occurs on the posterior, medial portion of the malleolus.

THE FOOT

The foot is comprised of seven tarsal bones that vary greatly in size, five metatarsals (m/t I–V), and fourteen phalanges (Figure 11-8). The big toe or hallux, like the thumb, has one less phalanx than the other digits. Unlike the hand, however, the foot is greatly modified to give stable support to the body's weight. Mobility and independence of the digits are therefore compromised.

One of the largest tarsal bones, and the most proximal, is the talus, called the astragalus in most other mammals (Figure 11-9). The main portion of the talus, which is wedge-shaped in superior view, is called the body. Protruding anteriorly from the medial side of the body are the neck and head of the talus.

The talus participates in a special joint with the tibia and fibula, called the ankle or the talocrural joint (crus is Latin for leg or limb). Although the tibia and fibula are separate bones, they are so firmly bound together at their distal ends, by anterior and posterior tibiofibular ligaments, that they function as a single unit with respect to the talus. From an anterior view, the distal articular surfaces of the tibia and fibula form the roof and two sides of a rectangle. The superior surface of the body of the talus is given over to an articular surface, the trochlea, that meets the distal articulation of the tibia, which is the roof of the rectangle. The trochlea is strongly convex anteroposteriorly but

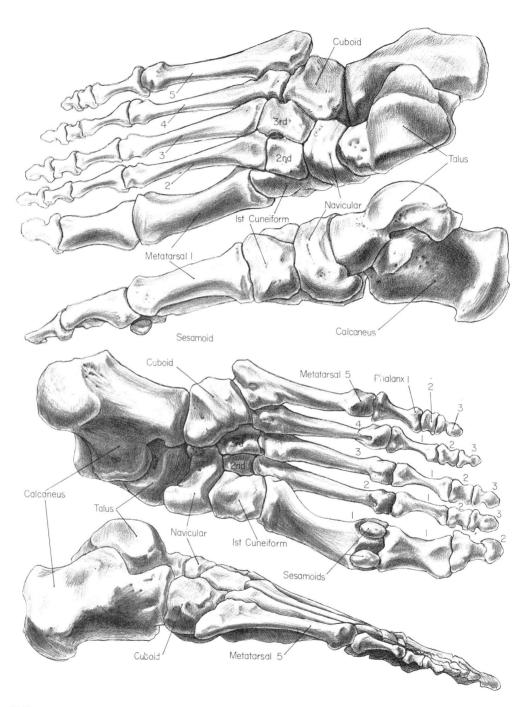

Figure 11-8

The bony foot: *(top to bottom)* superior, medial, inferior, and lateral view.

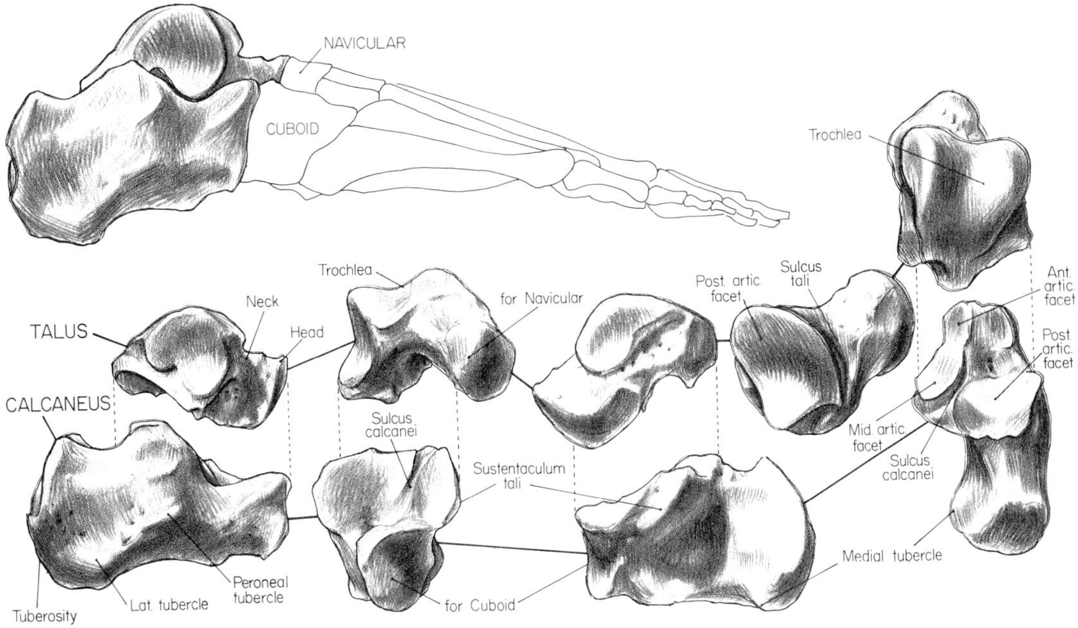

Figure 11-9

The talus and calcaneus: *(top)* placement in bony foot; *(middle, from left)* the talus in lateral, anterior, medial, inferior, and superior view; *(bottom, from left)* the calcaneus in lateral, anterior, medial, and superior view. Dotted lines show relation of the talus to the calcaneus.

gently concave mediolaterally. Articular surfaces on the lateral and medial sides of the talus articulate with the lateral malleolus of the fibula and medial malleolus of the tibia, which together make the two sides of the rectangle. Thus, the talocrural articulation resembles a mortice and tenon joint.

The lateral articulation of the talus is more extensive than the medial. In dorsiflexion, where the toes are pulled upward, the tibia and fibula ride forward and articulate with the anterior trochlea (Figure 11-10). In plantarflexion, where the heel is pulled upward and the toes move downward, the tibia and fibula ride backward and articulate with the posterior trochlea. Because the trochlea is broader anteriorly than posteriorly — a feature that gives this facet its wedge shape — the tibiofibular ligaments are stretched tighter in dorsiflexion than plantarflexion (Figure 11-11). This arrangement makes the talocrural joint more congruent and stable in dorsiflexion than in plantarflexion. As a result, lateral movements at the talocrural joint are limited, especially in dorsiflexion. In quadrupeds that are adapted for high-speed running,

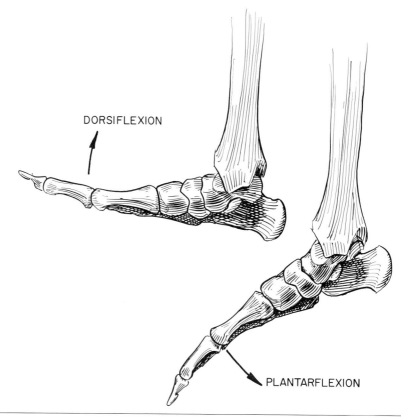

DORSIFLEXION

PLANTARFLEXION

Figure 11-10

Movements at the ankle: dorsiflexion and plantarflexion.

such as the horse, the trochlea is not merely gently concave mediolaterally but actually deeply grooved, producing a more tightly congruent joint with no capability for lateral movements.

The posterior body of the talus is marked by a deep, vertically oriented groove for the tendon of the flexor hallucis longus muscle, the long flexor of the big toe. The inferior or plantar surface of the body presents three articular facets for the calcaneus—posterior, middle, and anterior—which are separated by a deep groove. Although these facets are located on the talus, they articulate with the calcaneus and are thus called calcaneal. The joint between this facet and the calcaneus is called the subtalar joint. Anterior to this facet is a groove, the sulcus tali, the floor of which is marked by large nutrient foramina. The sulcus tali separates the posterior calcaneal facet from the middle calcaneal facet. The middle calcaneal facet lies anterior to the sulcus tali on the medial side of the inferior talus. Still farther anterior and lateral to the middle calcaneal facet is the anterior calcaneal facet,

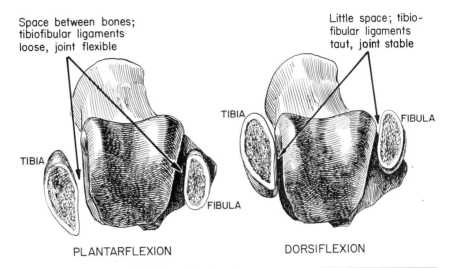

Space between bones; tibiofibular ligaments loose, joint flexible

Little space; tibio-fibular ligaments taut, joint stable

TIBIA

FIBULA

TIBIA

FIBULA

TIBIA

FIBULA

PLANTARFLEXION

DORSIFLEXION

Figure 11-11

Change in relations of the tibia, fibula, and talus in plantarflexion and dorsiflexion. In plantarflexion the tibia rides posteriorly on the talar trochlea. The ligaments binding the tibia to the fibula are loose, because the trochlea is narrower posteriorly, creating a less stable configuration of the talocrural joint. In dorsiflexion the tibia rides forward on the broader part of the talar trochlea, tightening the tibiofibular ligaments and stabilizing the ankle joint. Dorsiflexion is the position during heel strike, the onset of a walking stride.

which may be separated from the middle calcaneal facet by only a ridge. The anterior calcaneal facet is continuous with the articular facet of the talar head.

The head and neck of the talus are angled at about 15° to an anteroposterior plane bisecting the talus. The head is strongly convex, with an articular facet for the navicular, another tarsal bone, that extends from its anterior onto its inferior surface. The upper surface of the neck bears many nutrient foramina. In some individuals the upper, lateral region of the neck may bear two additional articular surfaces called squatting facets. These small facets indicate that the individual habitually maintains a squatting posture, and they are formed by the anterior edge of the distal tibia.

The calcaneus is the largest tarsal bone. It lies directly inferior to the talus and is therefore a major, weight-bearing bone. The long axis of the calcaneus is oriented almost directly anteroposteriorly. The calcaneus is much longer than it is broad, and it is flattened mediolaterally. Its elongated, posterior protuberance, the calcaneal tuberosity, forms the bony heel to which are attached many of the calf muscles. This tuberosity is rougher in its inferior third. On the dorsal surface of the calcaneus are the posterior, middle, and anterior facets for articulation with their corresponding facets on the talus. The posterior facet is strongly convex and fits congruently with the posterior calcaneal facet on the talus. Separating the posterior facet of the calcaneus from the other two facets is a deep groove, the sulcus calcanei. The middle and anterior facets are more nearly planar than the posterior facet. They are located on a large, medial projection from the body of the calcaneus called the sustentaculum tali. At the head or anterior end of the calcaneus is another almost vertically oriented articular facet for the cuboid, another tarsal bone. The medial surface of the calcaneus has no articular facets. Immediately below the sustentaculum tali, however, is a distinct groove for the ligament of the flexor hallucis longus muscle to the big toe. This is the same muscle that grooves the posterior talus. The lateral side bears the peroneal tubercle, which separates two shallow grooves. The superior groove is for the tendon of the peroneus brevis muscle, and the inferior groove is for the peroneus longus muscle. These two muscles evert the foot, or turn the sole laterally, and the peroneus longus also plantarflexes the foot. The plantar surface of the calcaneus bears no important features.

The remaining tarsal bones are the navicular, the cuboid, and the first or medial, second or intermediate, and third or lateral cuneiforms. Unlike the carpals, which are arranged in neat rows, the tarsals are arranged in a more complex fashion (Figure 11-12). Each of the remaining tarsals is roughly cuboidal and therefore has six surfaces: proximal, distal, superior, inferior, medial, and lateral.

The navicular lies directly distal to the talus and articulates with its head. The entire navicular is boat-shaped, being concave proximally and convex distally. The proximal surface has a single, oval facet for the head of the talus; the distal articular surface is divided into three facets, one for each cuneiform. The dorsal, plantar, and lateral surfaces are all rough and nonarticular. Even though the cuboid lies directly lateral to the navicular, the two bones do not articulate. The medial surface of the navicular bears a prominant, hooklike tuberosity than can be felt on living individuals and is of major use in siding naviculars, or distinguishing right from left.

The cuboid lies distal to the calcaneus and lateral to both the navicular and the third cuneiform. Its proximal, distal, and medial surfaces are all articular. Proximally, the cuboid articulates with m/c IV and V. This facet is therefore divided by a ridge into two regions. Medially, the

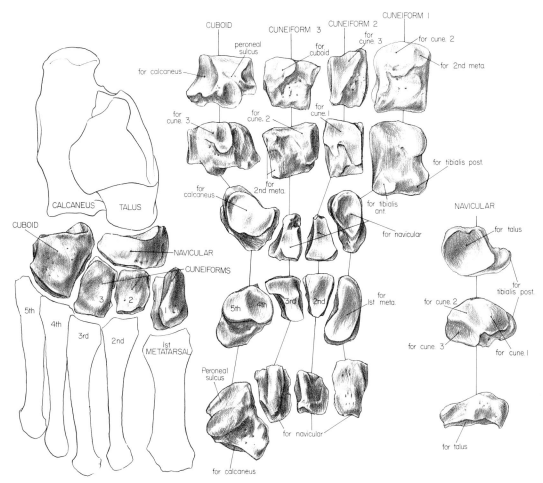

Figure 11-12

Tarsals of the foot: *(left)* position of the tarsals in superior view; *(center, from top)* surfaces of the cuboid, third or lateral cuneiform, second or middle cuneiform, and first or medial cuneiform in lateral, medial, proximal, distal, and inferior view; and *(right)* surfaces of the navicular in proximal, distal, and superior view.

cuboid articulates with the third cuneiform in a planar joint. Proximally, the cuboid meets the calcaneus. The dorsal surface is rough and nonarticular. The plantar surface is also rough, marked by a strong ridge, the tuberosity, that runs diagonally from proximal to distal and from medial to lateral. Proximal to the tuberosity is a groove for the peroneus longus muscle, which also marks the lateral calcaneus.

Sometimes the tendon of this muscle develops a sesamoid bone in this region, for which a small facet may be found in the lateral end of the groove on the plantar aspect of the cuboid.

The first, second, and third cuneiforms are arranged in a tidy mediolateral row distal to the navicular. Each bears an articular surface proximally for the navicular and one distally for the corresponding metatarsal. In addition, the first cuneiform bears only a lateral articular facet; the second cuneiform bears both medial and lateral articular facets; and the third cuneiform bears both medial and lateral facets.

The first cuneiform is the largest of the three and has a narrow, roughened dorsal surface. The facet for m/t I is kidney-shaped. On the medial surface, a smooth oval area is sometimes visible for attachment of the tibialis anterior muscle, a powerful dorsiflexor and inverter of the foot.

The second cuneiform is the smallest of the three and is the most nearly cuboidal in shape. Its dorsal surface is much broader than its plantar surface, a fact that is useful in orienting the bone correctly. The proximal portion of its lateral surface bears a facet for the third cuneiform, which can be used to side the bone once it is correctly oriented.

The third cuneiform is larger than the second and smaller than the first. Its dorsal surface is markedly broader than its plantar surface. Its proximal and distal surfaces articulate respectively with the navicular and m/t III. Medially, the third cuneiform bears three facets: two paired anterior ones for the lateral side of the base of m/t II and an unpaired posterior one for articulation with the second cuneiform. In contrast, the lateral surface bears one large facet for the cuboid and one small unpaired proximal facet for m/t IV. Thus, the difference in the arrangement of articular facets on the lateral and medial surfaces of the third cuneiform distinguishes left from right.

The five metatarsals form the next row of bones in the foot (Figure 11-13). Like the metacarpals, each has a proximal base, a shaft, and a rounded head for articulation with the proximal phalanges. Like metacarpals, metatarsals bear two prominent ridges, one on either side of the dorsal shaft just proximal to the head. Nonetheless, metatarsals differ from metacarpals in two ways. First, metatarsals are usually longer than metacarpals. Second, the overall shape of the bones is somewhat different. Metatarsals have large bases, mediolaterally compressed shafts, and small, mediolaterally compressed heads, whereas metacarpals have bases that are roughly equal in size to their heads and shafts that are flattened superoinferiorly. With the exception of m/t I, which is large and distinctive, the other four metatarsals differ

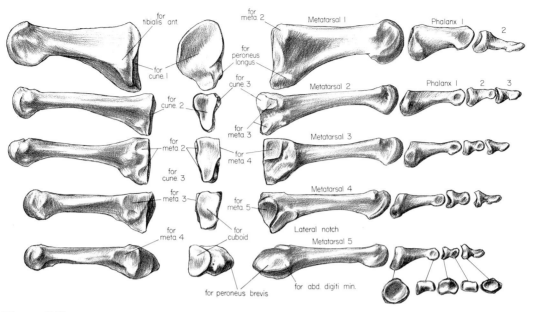

Figure 11-13

The metatarsals and phalanges: *(left to right)* metatarsals in medial, proximal, and lateral view; phalanges in lateral view.

from each other chiefly in the arrangement of articular facets on the medial and lateral sides of their bases.

M/t I is by far the largest and most robust of the metatarsals. Its base bears a large, concave facet for the medial cuneiform that is kidney-shaped in outline. The indentation on the kidney faces laterally and can be used to side an m/t I. The medial side of the base may show a small tubercle for attachment of the tibialis anterior muscle. The shaft is short, stout, and concave both laterally and inferiorly. The head has a strongly convex articular surface distally. The plantar surface of this articular surface bears two grooves that separate three ridges, one on either edge and one just lateral of the middle of the head. Into these grooves fit the two sesamoids of the flexor hallucis brevis, the short flexor of the hallux. These sesamoids also give insertion to other muscles. Attached to the lateral sesamoid is the adductor hallucis; attached to the medial is the abductor hallucis. These two muscles perform adduction and abduction of the big toe relative to a plane through the long axis of the second toe.

M/t II is much smaller than m/t I. It articulates with the third cuneiform via two small rounded facets, on the lateral side of its base, which are angled and continue distally for articulation with m/t III. This pair of angled facets is a distinguishing characteristic of m/t II. On the dorsal aspect of its medial side, m/t II bears a single facet for articulation with the first cuneiform. There is no articulation for m/t I. The base of m/t II articulates with the second cuneiform, and its head articulates with the second proximal phalanx. The base of m/t II, like the bases of m/t III – V, projects farther proximally on the lateral side than on the medial side, which can be used to side the bones. Also, the shaft of m/t II bears a strong dorsal ridge that lies to the lateral of midline.

M/t III is comparable in robustness to m/t II but is shorter. The medial side of its base bears two articular facets for m/t II, one of which is a nearly complete oval in outline and the other of which is smaller and hemispherical. The lateral side of m/t III bears a single, dorsally placed facet for m/t IV. Proximally, m/t III articulates with the third cuneiform, and distally it articulates with the third proximal phalanx. The dorsal ridge for m/t III lies just lateral of midline.

M/t IV is again shorter. Medially, it bears a single oval facet with a horizontal ridge across it for m/t III. This facet is placed somewhat dorsally and is well separated from the proximal facet for the cuboid. Laterally, there is a single, broad facet for m/t V that meets the cuboid facet proximally. The dorsal ridge on the shaft of m/t IV lies close to midline.

M/t V bears an obvious tuberosity, the styloid process, that projects proximally from the lateral and dorsal aspect of the base. It is also distinctive in having articular facets only on the medial and proximal surfaces of its base. Medially, there is a large facet for m/t IV that meets the facet for the cuboid at an angle of just more than 90°. The dorsal ridge on the shaft of m/t V lies toward the medial side.

The phalanges make up the bony structure of the toes. The hallux has only proximal and distal phalanges, but the other four digits each have proximal, middle, and distal phalanges. These phalanges closely resemble those of the hand, with a few significant differences. The foot phalanges are consistently shorter and slenderer than the hand phalanges, with the exception of the phalanges for the hallux which are longer and much stouter than any hand phalanges. The proximal phalanges of the foot have large bases and heads but slender, medio-laterally compressed shafts; the proximal phalanges of the hand are longer and have thicker shafts that are flat on the palmar surface and curved on the volar surface and often bear strong medial and lateral flanges for muscle attachments. In addition, the heads of proximal hand phalanges often show marked pits on the lateral and medial sides; in foot phalanges these pits are either absent or obscure. Middle and distal foot phalanges are very short and have shafts that are concave on both dorsal and plantar surfaces. In contrast, middle phalanges of the hand are longer and convex posteriorly. Terminal or distal phalanges of the foot are still shorter and have more pronounced tuberosities to support the end of the digit, in comparison with the distal phalanges of the hand. The distal phalanx of the hallux is particularly distinctive, being strongly built and unusually broad in its base relative to its head.

12
WALKING

The lower limb has essential functions in locomotion and postural support. The movements at the different joints are limited by both the arrangement of ligaments and the geometry of the joint surfaces. These movements are produced by the major muscles of the lower limb and are integrated in a complex pattern in walking.

JOINTS OF THE LOWER LIMB

There are nine joints or sets of joints in the lower limb: the sacroiliac joint, hip, knee, ankle or talocrural joint, intertarsal joints, tarsometatarsal joints, intermetatarsal joints, metatarsophalangeal joints, and interphalangeal joints. The sacroiliac joint is the most proximal in the lower limb. It is a synovial joint between the irregular but highly congruent auricular surfaces of the ilium and the sacrum. The articular capsule surrounding the sacroiliac joint is reinforced by strong ligaments. The strength of these ligaments and the congruity of the joint surfaces restrict motion at the sacroiliac joint. The most common movement at this joint is a slight rotation of the sacrum around a mediolateral axis during changes in posture and locomotion. The wedge-like shape of the sacrum and the congruency of the sacroiliac joint help to prevent the sacrum from being pushed downward by the weight of the body. Rotation of the sacrum so that its superior surface faces anteriorly is also resisted by two strong ligaments, the sacrotuberous and sacrospinous. The sacrotuberous ligament attaches to the posterior iliac spine and laterally to the dorsal surface of the sacrum and upper coccyx. Its major function is to prevent the dorsal and inferior sacrum from rotating upward. The sacrospinous ligament lies anterior to the sacrotuberous. It links the ischial spine with the lateral part of the lower sacrum and upper coccyx. It, too, helps hold the sacrum in a fixed position relative to the innominates.

In contrast, the hip is an unusually mobile joint. It is the classic ball-and-socket joint in the human skeleton. Although its movement is more restricted than that of its counterpart, the shoulder, this stability is needed. The body weight is displaced laterally from midline at the

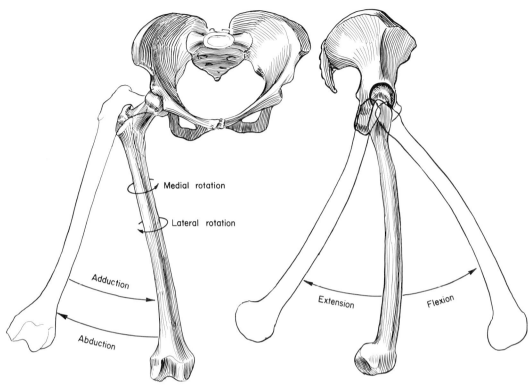

Figure 12-1

Movements at the hip: abduction and adduction, medial and lateral rotation, extension and flexion.

level of the sacrum and transmitted down through the lower limbs via the hip joints. Forces of from four to eight times body weight are experienced at the hip joint during normal walking.

Movements at the hip include flexion, extension, abduction, adduction, and medial and lateral rotation of the thigh (Figure 12-1). Circumduction is also possible, but it is more limited at the hip than at the shoulder, due in part to the arrangement of ligaments that bind the head of the femur into the acetabulum (Figure 12-2). In addition to the ligamentum teres, which runs from the acetabular fovea to the femoral head, three other ligaments reinforce the joint capsule: the iliofemoral, pubofemoral, and ischiofemoral ligaments. Each of these ligaments is named for its site of origin. The course of these ligaments on the right hip spirals in a clockwise direction from lateral view to insert onto the femur; the course of each ligament on the left hip spirals counterclockwise. Thus, the iliofemoral inserts on the intertrochanteric line on the

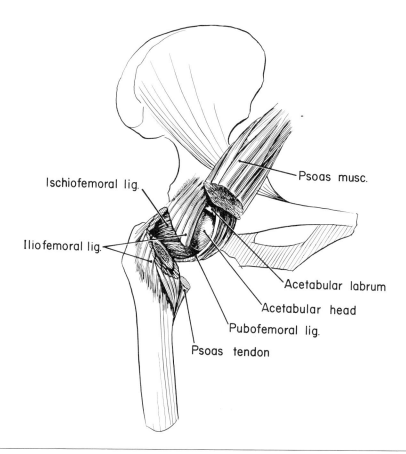

Figure 12-2

Ligaments of the joint capsule of the hip: ischiofemoral, iliofemoral, and pubofemoral. All three ligaments have a spiral course, so as to loosen in flexion and tighten in extension. The psoas muscle also reinforces this joint.

anterior femur; the pubofemoral inserts on the inferior portion of the trochanteric line near the lesser trochanter; and the ischiofemoral spirals around the posterior aspect of the femoral neck and inserts on the superior trochanteric line. As a result, the joint capsule of the hip loosens in flexion, thereby uncoiling the spiraling fibers, and tightens in extension of the thigh past vertical, thereby doing the opposite and coiling the fibers. None of these ligaments reinforces the inferior aspect of the hip joint, where the ring of the acetabulum is deficient. Commonly the femoral head is dislocated downward from the acetabulum, since at this point both the bony joint and the capsule are weakest.

The knee, like the elbow, is a complex joint that involves three differ-

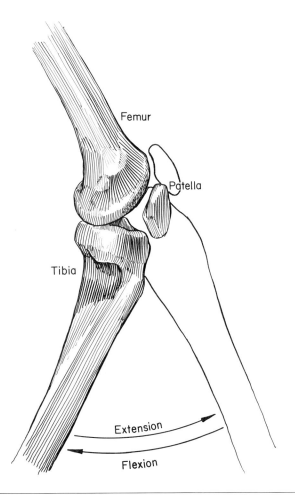

Figure 12-3

Position of the patella on the femur, which changes as the knee joint moves. In extension, the patella is high in the patellar groove; in flexion, it is more distally placed on the femur, near the condyles.

ent bones. The patella is an integral part of the joint, even though it articulates only with the femur. The patella rides in the patellar groove on the anterior femur. Its position in the groove varies with action: it lies in the superior part of the groove in extension and down on the femoral condyles in flexion (Figure 12-3). In effect, the patella lengthens the lever arm of the quadriceps in extension and protects the knee joint from damage from the anterior direction in flexion. The major movements of the knee occur between the distal femur and proximal tibia. The primary movement is flexion or extension. A lim-

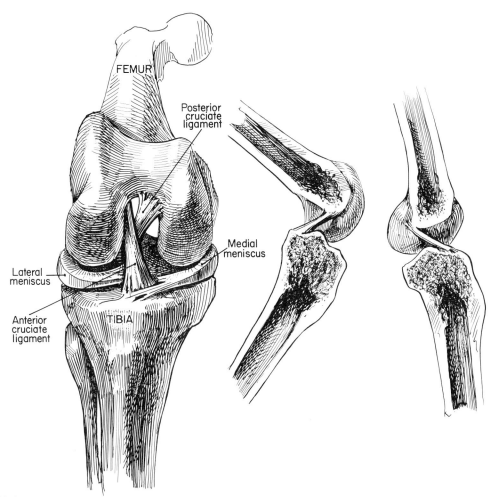

Figure 12-4

The menisci and cruciate ligaments, which help to stabilize the knee: *(left to right)* a flexed knee in anterior view, showing the position of both cruciates and menisci; a flexed knee in sagittal section, showing the posterior cruciate's role; and an extended knee in sagittal section, showing the anterior cruciate's role.

ited degree of medial or lateral rotation occurs also. The knee is not constructed to bend laterally or medially, that is, to abduct or adduct. The forceable production of such movements, as when a football player is tackled from the side, commonly results in serious injury, especially if the player's knee is locked.

Various soft tissues play an important role in the functioning of the

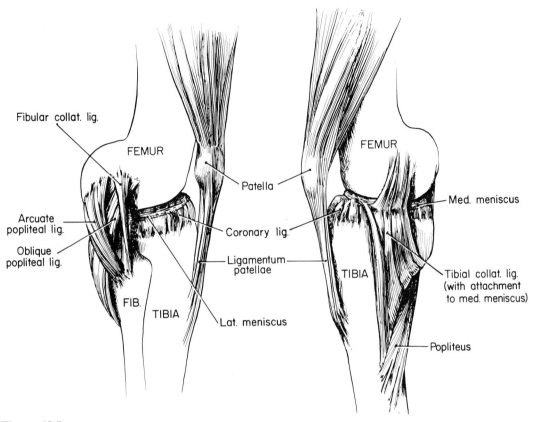

Figure 12-5

Soft tissues of the joint capsule of the knee in *(left)* lateral and *(right)* medial view.

knee. The bony condyles of the femur and tibia are not highly congruent, but in life their congruency is increased by the lateral and medial menisci, the two structures that are attached to the proximal tibia by coronary ligaments and are commonly referred to as the cartilages of the knee (Figure 12-4). In superior view, each meniscus is crescent-shaped in outline; in anterior view, each is wedge-shaped, with the broad part of the wedge toward the edge of the tibial head. The menisci are concave upward, to receive the femoral condyles (Figure 12-5). Their shape is such that the maximum congruency is produced either by a slight medial rotation of the femur on the tibia at the end of extension or — when the tibia is not weight-bearing, as when a seated individual raises a leg and extends a knee — by a lateral rotation of the tibia on the femur. Achieving this position of maximum congruence is

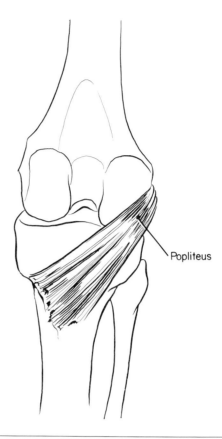

Figure 12-6

The popliteus muscle, which unlocks the knee from the screw home position by rotating the femur laterally on the fixed tibia, in posterior view.

called locking the knee or, more technically, screw home, because of the role of the anterior and posterior cruciate ligaments in this action. The cruciate ligaments work to maintain the integrity of the knee by keeping the tibia and femur close together. The anterior cruciate ligament arises from the anterior intercondylar fossa of the tibia and inserts on the medial side of the intercondylar fossa of the femur. The posterior cruciate ligament arises from the posterior intercondylar fossa of the tibia and inserts on the lateral side of the intercondylar fossa of the femur. In screw home, these two ligaments twist around each other, thus shortening the distance between the tibia and femur and producing a highly stable configuration.

To unlock the knee, a slight lateral rotation of the femur upon the tibia is produced by the action of the popliteus muscle (Figure 12-6). This muscle arises on the proximal end of the posterior tibia, and its tendon inserts on the lateral epicondyle of the femur. A contraction of the popliteus muscle therefore rotates the femur in a lateral direction and unlocks the knee from the screw home position. The cruciate ligaments also perform other important functions. In extension, the anterior cruciate prevents the femur from rotating too far on its condyles and slipping off the tibia in a posterior direction. In flexion, the posterior cruciate prevents the femur from rotating too far and slipping off the tibia in an anterior direction.

Four other ligaments — the tibial, fibular, arcuate, and oblique — play major roles in maintaining the integrity of the knee. The capsule of the knee is reinforced on both lateral and medial sides by the fibular and tibial collateral ligaments. The fibular collateral ligament does not blend with the capsule, being entirely extracapsular, and the tibial collateral ligament is extracapsular except where it attaches to the medial meniscus. These ligaments work to limit abduction or adduction of the leg at the knee. Even in flexion, when the collateral ligaments are more relaxed, abduction or adduction at the knee is very restricted. Appreciable abduction or adduction of the lower limb can be produced only at the hip. Posteriorly, the arcuate and oblique ligaments are thickenings of the joint capsule that increase joint stability. Circumduction at the knee is not possible, in part because these four ligaments limit motion.

The ankle, or talocrural joint, is also primarily a hinge joint at which dorsiflexion and plantarflexion are possible. The axis of movement passes through the malleoli and the talus below the trochlea. The tibia and fibula are tightly bound together by ligaments and thus act as a single unit with respect to the talus. They articulate with the anterior trochlea in dorsiflexion and with the posterior trochlea in plantarflexion. Prolonged, extreme dorsiflexion, as in habitual squatting, creates articular facets, also called squatting facets, for the tibia and fibula on the neck of the talus. A limited amount of eversion, or movement of the foot so that the sole faces laterally, and inversion, or movement of the foot so that the sole faces medially, is possible at the ankle. The capsule of the ankle is reinforced by several ligaments. Medially, the deltoid ligament is attached to the medial malleolus superiorly and to the talus, navicular, and calcaneus inferiorly. Laterally, the joint capsule is reinforced by the anterior talofibular ligament, from the lateral malleolus to the neck of the talus, and the calcaneofibular ligament, from the lateral malleolus to the lateral calcaneus.

The intertarsal joints permit eversion or inversion to occur. In these actions, the talus is fixed within the talocrural joint and moves as if it were a part of the leg. Eversion involves pronation, abduction, and dorsiflexion; inversion is a combination of supination, adduction, and plantarflexion. Many different ligaments connect the tarsals to each other and hold them in position, so that only slight movements are possible at each joint. However, these many small movements work additively to produce important movements of the whole foot. The tarsals and metatarsals, along with the various ligaments that bind them together, collectively function as a spring to absorb some of the stresses of locomotion. The tarsals are arranged so that their plantar surfaces create both a longitudinal or anteroposterior arch and a transverse arch. The anteroposterior arch is maintained in part by the plantar aponeurosis, a strong fibrous band that runs from the inferior calcaneus to the head of the first metatarsal. Several strong ligaments on the plantar surface of the foot also help maintain this arch, including the long plantar ligament which runs from the calcaneal tuberosity to the tuberosity of the cuboid. The transverse arch is formed by the navicular, cuboid, cuneiforms, and metatarsals and is also reinforced by ligaments.

The tarsometatarsal joints are mostly planar and thus permit gliding. As with the intertarsal joints, the range of movement at each tarsometatarsal joint is limited, but these joints collectively impart some flexibility to the anterior foot.

Small intermetatarsal joints occur between each pair of adjacent metatarsals, except for between m/t I and II. These are also planar joints that permit a small amount of gliding. On the whole, however, the metatarsals are so closely bound together by ligaments that, with the exception of m/t I, independent movements are impossible or severely limited.

The metatarsophalangeal joints permit flexion or extension and abduction or adduction. As with the hand, abduction or adduction in the foot occurs relative to a plane through a digit, but the digit involved is the second digit, not the third, because the foot muscles producing abduction and adduction are arranged symmetrically around the second digit. This arrangement of muscles means that the other toes move toward or away from the second toe. The interphalangeal joints are hinge joints, permitting flexion or extension.

MUSCLES OF THE HIP

The muscles of the hip are associated with particular actions, although most movements are produced by a combination of muscles acting together, both to produce and to control movements. Unlike the bones of the shoulder girdle, the elements of the pelvic girdle remain relatively immobile during movements at the hip. Therefore, most of the musculature at the hip is devoted to producing movements of the femur relative to a fixed torso or of the torso relative to a fixed leg. Many of these movements are important in walking.

Extension at the hip is controlled by a set of muscles that arises from the pelvis and posterior femur and inserts on the proximal tibia. The primary extensor of the thigh is a group of three muscles — the biceps femoris, the semimembranosus, and the semitendinosus — known collectively as the hamstrings (Figure 12-7). The biceps femoris arises from two heads, one long and one short. The long head of the biceps femoris, as well as the semitendinosus and semimembranosus, originate from the ischial tuberosity. The belly of the biceps femoris proceeds inferiorly until it is joined by the short head, which arises from the lateral lip of the linea aspera and from the upper part of the lateral supracondylar line. The biceps femoris then crosses behind the knee to insert on the head of the fibula. The semitendinosus arises in common with the biceps and inserts on the upper part of the medial surface of the tibia. The tendons of the biceps femoris and the semitendinosus are readily felt in living humans as strong tendons on the lateral and medial borders of the posterior surface of the knee. The semimembranosus arises more laterally on the ischial tuberosity than the other two muscles and from the adjacent ischiopubic ramus. The semimembranosus inserts on the proximal, medial region of the posterior tibia. All three muscles cross both the hip and the knee. They work to extend the hip and to flex the knee simultaneously.

Another major muscle involved in extension of the hip is the gluteus maximus, the large rounded muscle that gives shape to the buttocks. This muscle arises from the gluteal surface of the ilium medial to the posterior gluteal line and from the posterior surface of the sacrum (Figure 12-8). It passes laterally and inferiorly to insert on the lateral lip of the proximal end of the linea aspera. The gluteus maximus is a powerful extensor of the thigh at the hip or, when the lower limbs are fixed, a powerful extensor of the trunk upon the thigh. Although it is used little during walking or normal standing, it participates in running, climbing, and other locomotor activities involving some force. It

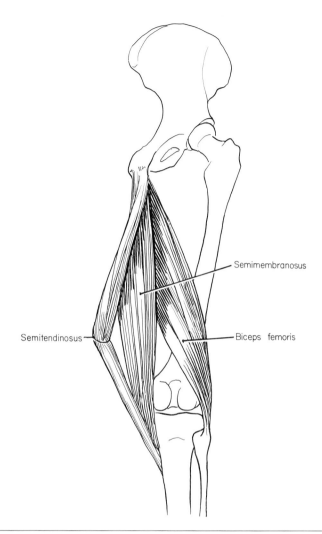

Figure 12-7

Hamstring muscles of the lower limb in posterior view: biceps femoris, semi-membranosus, and semitendinosus. These are the major extensors of the hip and flexors of the knee.

may help to control hip action as the individual moves from standing to sitting or vice versa. A less important action of the gluteus maximus is lateral rotation or abduction of the thigh.

The gluteus medius and gluteus minimus, which arise from the gluteal surface of the ilium underneath the gluteus maximus, work together to produce both abduction of the hip and medial rotation of the thigh. The gluteus medius arises between the posterior and ante-

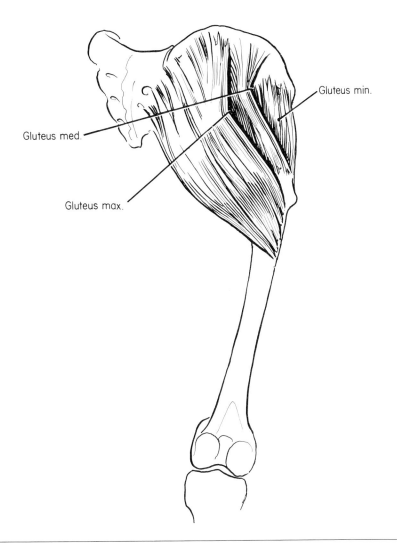

Gluteus min.

Gluteus med.

Gluteus max.

Figure 12-8

Gluteal muscles of the hip in posterior view: gluteus maximus, medius, and minimus. The gluteus maximus is a powerful extensor of the hip. The other two muscles contribute to medial rotation and abduction of the thigh.

rior gluteal lines; the gluteus minimus arises between the anterior and inferior gluteal lines. Both pass anteriorly and laterally to insert on the greater trochanter, with the medius inserting on its lateral aspect and the minimus on its anterior aspect. Contraction of either of these muscles abducts and medially rotates the thigh if it is not weight-bearing. The most important action of these muscles occurs in walking,

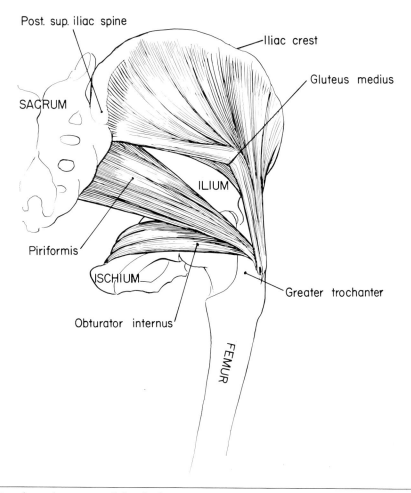

Post. sup. iliac spine

Iliac crest

SACRUM

Gluteus medius

Piriformis

ILIUM

ISCHIUM

Greater trochanter

Obturator internus

FEMUR

Figure 12-9

Two lateral rotators of the thigh in posterior view: piriformis and obturator internus.

when the thigh is weight-bearing. In this situation, the gluteus medius and gluteus minimus act to abduct the pelvis, so as to tilt the opposite side of the pelvis upward and bring or hold the body weight over the leg in question. Medial rotation also helps pivot the body around the supporting or stance leg during walking.

Another important action in locomotion is lateral rotation at the hip. Lateral rotation of one leg on the pelvis occurs when that leg is brought forward to initiate a new step. The effect of this rotation is to keep the feet pointing approximately straight ahead. Six small muscles are responsible for lateral rotation: the piriformis, the obturator in-

ternus, the obturator externus, the superior gemellus, the inferior
gemellus, and the quadratus femoris (Figure 12-9). All six muscles
arise from near the midline on the pelvis and travel anteriorly and
laterally to insert on the proximal femur. The piriformis arises from
the pelvic surface of the sacrum and from the adjacent area on the
medial surface of the ilium. It passes laterally through the greater
sciatic notch and inserts on the upper, posterior border of the greater
trochanter. The obturator internus and obturator externus arise primarily from opposite surfaces of the obturator membrane, which
closes the obturator foramen. The obturator internus passes out of the
pelvis via the lesser sciatic notch and inserts upon the greater trochanter near the piriformis insertion. The obturator externus inserts
on the trochanteric fossa, inferior and posterior to that of the obturator internus. The tendon of the obturator externus lies in a shallow,
horizontal groove on the posterior surface of the femoral neck medial
to its insertion. The ischial tuberosity and spine give origin to the
superior and inferior gemelli respectively. This pair of muscles inserts
onto the obturator internus tendon, which in turn inserts onto the
greater trochanter.

To take a step, flexion at the hip is needed. Flexion, like many other
movements, is produced by a group of muscles. The most important of
these muscles is the iliopsoas, which is comprised of a broad lateral
part, the iliacus, and a narrower, longer, medial part, the psoas major
(Figure 12-10). The iliacus arises from the iliac fossa on the internal
surface of the ilium; the psoas major arises from the intervertebral
discs, their transverse processes and anterior surfaces of the lumbar
vertebrae. The two muscles cross anterior to the hip joint to form a
common tendon that inserts on the lesser trochanter.

Another major flexor of the hip, though of less importance than the
iliopsoas, is a complex muscle called the quadriceps femoris. This
muscle has four separate parts: the rectus femoris, the vastus lateralis,
the vastus intermedius, and the vastus medialis (Figure 12-11). Only
the rectus femoris is directly involved in flexion of the hip. It arises
from the anterior inferior iliac spine and from the rim of the acetabulum. The belly of the rectus forms the large powerful muscle of the
anterior thigh. The belly becomes tendinous near the knee, where it is
joined by the other parts of the quadriceps, and together they insert
onto the superior and anterior patella. The tendon covers the anterior
surface of the patella and continues inferiorly, as the patellar ligament,
to insert on the tibial tuberosity. The vastus lateralis has a long, narrow
origin from the trochanteric line, the greater trochanter, and the lat-

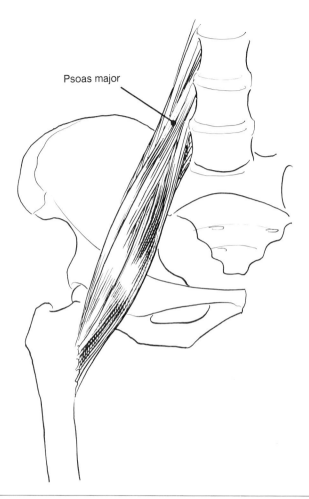

Psoas major

Figure 12-10

A major flexor of the hip, the psoas major muscle, in anterior view. It arises from the transverse processes and intervertebral discs of the lumbar vertebrae.

eral lip of the linea aspera, where it is closely associated with the gluteus maximus. The vastus lateralis provides the muscular bulk on the lateral aspect of the thigh and inserts with the rectus femoris on the patella and, via the patellar ligament, onto the tibia. The vastus medialis occupies the lower part of the medial thigh, although its origin lies higher on the femur. It originates from the intertrochanteric crest and the spiral line, which is the superior, medial branch of the linea aspera. It joins the other parts of the quadriceps femoris in insertion onto the patella and tibia. Finally, the vastus intermedius has a large,

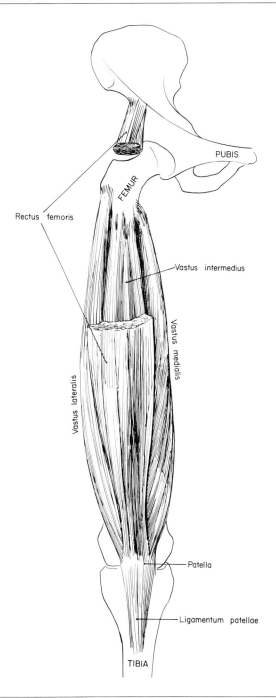

Figure 12-11

Another flexor of the hip and the major extensor of the knee in anterior view: the quadriceps femoris. It has four portions, all of which are extensors of the knee: rectus femoris, the only portion that is also a flexor of the hip; vastus lateralis; vastus medialis; and vastus intermedialis.

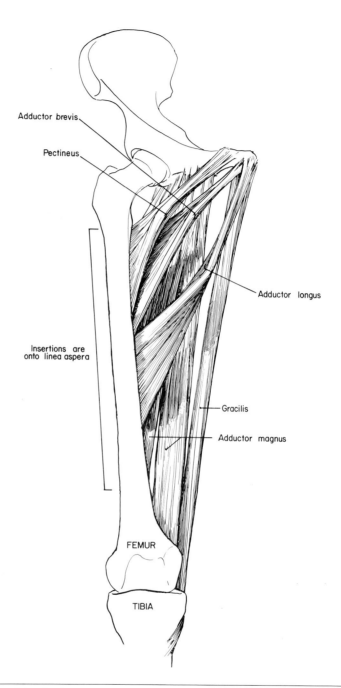

Adductor brevis

Pectineus

Insertions are
onto linea aspera

Adductor longus

Gracilis

Adductor magnus

FEMUR

TIBIA

Figure 12-12

Adductors of the thigh in anterior view: adductor magnus, adductor longus, adductor brevis, pectineus, and gracilis.

fleshy origin from the anterolateral aspect of the upper two-thirds of the femoral shaft. It, too, inserts onto the patella and tibial crest.

Although only the rectus femoris participates in flexing the hip, all four parts of the quadriceps play a major role in extending the knee. As a whole, the quadriceps femoris is one of the most powerful muscles in the body and is used in many movements related to posture and locomotion. Contracting the quadriceps femoris produces an upward and lateral pull on the patella, because of the carrying angle of the femur, which tends to displace the patella laterally from its groove, particularly in individuals with wider hips or lower lateral lips to the patellar groove.

Adduction at the hip is important in pulling the body weight over the supporting leg in walking. Several muscles on the medial surface of the thigh are responsible for adduction (Figure 12-12). The largest and most important of these are the adductor magnus, adductor brevis, and adductor longus. The adductor magnus has two separate origins: one part arises from the body of the pubis and the ischiopubic ramus; the other part arises from the posterior ischial ramus and from the ischial tuberosity. The ischiopubic part of the muscle inserts on the posterior femur, along the linea aspera and medial supracondylar ridge. The portion from the ischial tuberosity inserts via a tendon onto the adductor tubercle on the medial epicondyle of the femur. The adductor brevis originates from the body and inferior ramus of the pubis and inserts onto the upper linea aspera. The adductor longus arises from the pubis near the symphysis and inserts onto the medial lip of the linea aspera. The gracilis and pectineus muscles, both arising from the superior pubic ramus and inserting on the linea aspera, assist in adduction.

MUSCLES OF THE KNEE

The major muscles of the thigh that are responsible for flexion of the knee are the hamstrings. Another important flexor of the knee is the triceps surae, which originates below the knee.

The triceps surae, which is a two-part muscle consisting of the gastrocnemius and the soleus, makes up the fleshy bulk of the calf. The gastrocnemius arises from two heads, one from the medial and the other from the lateral side of the distal femur (Figure 12-13). The two heads fuse at midline behind the proximal tibia and insert via a tendon, called the Achilles tendon, onto the calcaneal tuberosity. The Achilles tendon is shared with the soleus muscle, which lies beneath and anterior to the gastrocnemius. The soleus arises from the posterior aspects

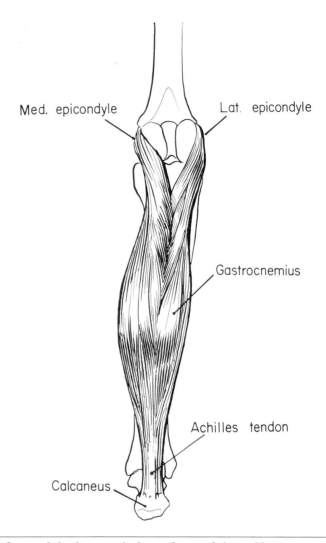

Figure 12-13

A major flexor of the knee and plantarflexor of the ankle, in posterior view: gastrocnemius.

of the head and proximal end of the fibula. The gastrocnemius is both a flexor of the knee and a plantarflexor, whereas the soleus is only a plantarflexor.

The popliteus, like the triceps surae, originates below the knee and inserts above it. The role of the popliteus is to unlock the knee by laterally rotating the femur upon the tibia.

MUSCLES OF THE ANKLE AND FOOT

The major muscles arising in the leg region primarily either produce movements at the ankle or affect the foot per se. Flexion and extension of the toes are produced mostly by the extrinsic foot muscles, which originate in the leg, with assistance from some intrinsic foot muscles.

Muscles arising in the leg produce four different actions at the ankle: plantarflexion, dorsiflexion, inversion, and eversion. The most powerful plantarflexor is the triceps surae, since both the gastrocnemius and the soleus attach to the calcaneal tuberosity. In addition, the peroneus longus muscle plantarflexes the foot (Figure 12-14). This muscle arises from the lateral condyle of the tibia and from the head and upper two-thirds of the lateral side of the fibular shaft. It becomes tendinous near the ankle. The tendon passes posterior to the lateral malleolus, behind and below the peroneal tubercle on the lateral side of the calcaneus, and turns at the cuboid to pass onto the sole of the foot by running through a groove on the cuboid. This tendon inserts on the lateral side of the plantar surface of the first cuneiform and on the adjacent area on the base of m/t I. Contracting the peroneus longus therefore pulls the base of the hallux downward in plantarflexion and the foot outward in eversion.

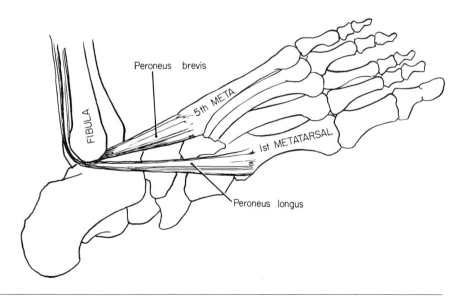

Figure 12-14

Other plantarflexors and evertors of the foot in inferolateral view: peroneus brevis and peroneus longus.

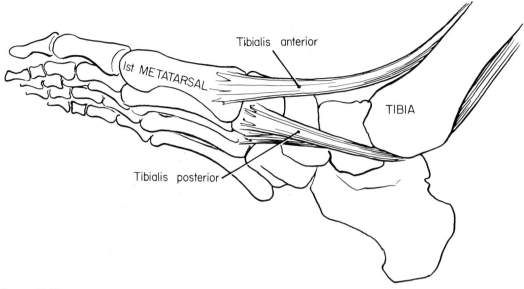

Figure 12-15

Major dorsiflexor and major invertor of the foot in inferomedial view: tibialis anterior and tibialis posterior.

Plantarflexion and eversion are also produced by the peroneus brevis. This muscle lies farther from the leg's surface, or deeper, than the peroneus longus, and arises from the lower two-thirds of the lateral side of the fibular shaft. Its tendon also curves around behind and below the lateral malleolus. It then travels anteriorly along the lateral calcaneus, passing superior to the peroneal tubercle. The peroneous brevis inserts on the base of m/t V.

Both dorsiflexion and inversion are produced by the tibialis anterior (Figure 12-15). This muscle originates from the lateral condyle of the tibia and from the upper two-thirds of the tibial shaft on the lateral side. Its tendon crosses anterior to the ankle, passing under the extensor retinaculum, and inserts on the dorsal surfaces of the base of m/t I and the first cuneiform. Because its insertion is so medially placed, the tibialis anterior both dorsiflexes and inverts the foot.

The principal invertor of the foot, however, is the tibialis posterior. Like the radius and ulna, the tibia and fibula are joined by a strong interosseous membrane that attaches to the interosseous crest or border on the shaft of each bone. The tibialis posterior is a deep muscle arising from the posterior surface of the interosseous membrane, from the posterior fibular shaft, and from the upper tibial shaft lateral and

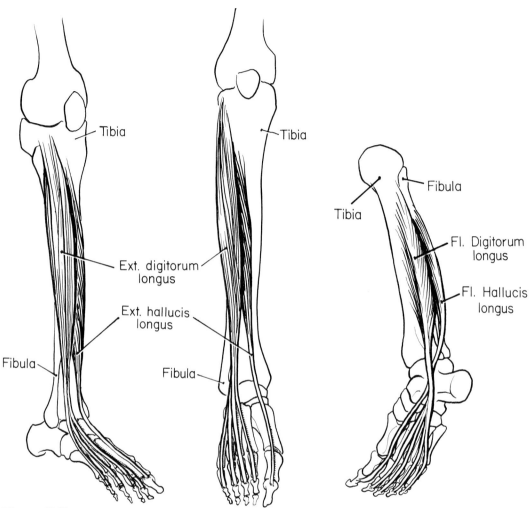

Figure 12-16

Extensors and flexors of the toes in *(left)* anterolateral, *(center)* anterior, and *(right)* posteromedial view: extensor digitorum longus, extensor hallucis longus, flexor digitorum longus, and flexor hallucis longus.

inferior to the popliteal line. Its tendon passes behind and below the medial malleolus, where it is held close to the bone by the flexor retinaculum. It inserts on the large tubercle of the navicular, thus attaching to the medial side of the plantar surface of the foot. Smaller branches of the tendon continue to all three cuneiforms, the cuboid, the tendon sheath of the peroneus longus, and the bases of m/t II–IV.

The leg also gives rise to muscles producing flexion and extension of the toes (Figure 12-16). One muscle, the extensor digitorum longus, extends the second through fifth toes, and another muscle, the extensor hallucis longus, extends the hallux. Similarly, there is a flexor for the second through fifth digits, the flexor digitorum longus, and another flexor for the hallux, the flexor hallucis longus. The flexors arise from the anterior surfaces of the tibia and fibula, and the extensors arise from their posterior surfaces. The axis of dorsiflexion and plantarflexion passes mediolaterally through the malleoli. Therefore, any muscle passing in front of this axis must act as a dorsiflexor, and any muscle passing behind it must act as a plantarflexor. For this reason, flexion of the toes is associated with plantarflexion and extension of the toes is associated with dorsiflexion.

The extensor digitorum longus originates from the interosseous membrane and from most of the anterior shaft of the fibula. The belly of the muscle divides into four tendons at the ankle, where they pass under the extensor retinaculum. One tendon goes to each of the lateral toes. At the metatarsophalangeal joint, the tendon expands and fuses with the joint capsule. Distal to this expansion, the tendon divides into a central portion, which inserts on the base of the middle phalanx, and two collateral portions, which insert on the base of the terminal phalanx.

The extensor hallucis longus also arises from the interosseous membrane and from the middle half of the anterior surface of the fibula. It passes under the flexor retinaculum, forms a dorsal expansion over the metatarsophalangeal joint, and proceeds distally to insert on the base of the terminal phalanx.

The flexor digitorum longus arises from the posterior tibia, below the popliteal line. Its tendon passes behind and beneath the medial malleolus, under the flexor retinaculum, and medial to the sustentaculum tali of the calcaneus. As it passes under the tarsometatarsal joints, the tendon divides into four branches, one for each of the lateral toes. Each tendon inserts on the distal phalanx, running through a fibrous sheath in which it is accompanied by the tendon of the short flexor, called the flexor digitorum brevis, which is an intrinsic muscle of the foot.

The flexor hallucis longus arises from the lower two-thirds of the posterior surface of the fibula. Its tendon passes under the flexor retinaculum, runs through the groove on the posterior talus and then through the groove under the sustentaculum tali, where it lies lateral to the flexor digitorum longus. It crosses superior to the flexor digitorum longus under the tarsals, or closer to the bones, and passes anteriorly, lying between the two sesamoids at the metatarsophalangeal joint, to insert on the distal phalanx of the hallux. Because the flexor digitorum longus passes behind the axis at which the ankle dorsiflexes and plantarflexes, it also acts as a plantarflexor.

INTRINSIC MUSCLES OF THE FOOT

There is only one intrinsic muscle on the dorsum of the foot, the extensor digitorum brevis, the medial part of which is sometimes called the extensor hallucis brevis (Figure 12-17). From an origin on the superior surface of the anterior calcaneus, this muscle passes anteriorly, lying underneath the long extensor muscle, and divides into four tendons. The lateral three tendons insert on the second through fourth digits by joining the extensor expansion and then contributing slips that insert on the base of each middle phalanx. The most medial tendon inserts at the base of the first proximal phalanx, beneath the tendon of the extensor hallucis longus. Unlike the extensor digitorum longus, the extensor digitorum brevis does not send a tendon to the fifth toe. The extensor digitorum brevis thus extends the metatarsophalangeal and the proximal interphalangeal joints of the second through fourth toes and the metatarsophalangeal joint of the hallux. The extensor digitorum longus, in contrast, extends

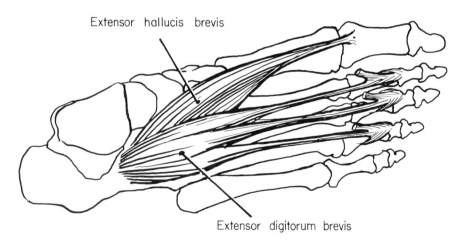

Extensor hallucis brevis

Extensor digitorum brevis

Figure 12-17

Intrinsic muscles of the dorsum of the foot in superior view: extensor digitorum brevis, of which the most medial part, extensor hallucis brevis, can contract independently.

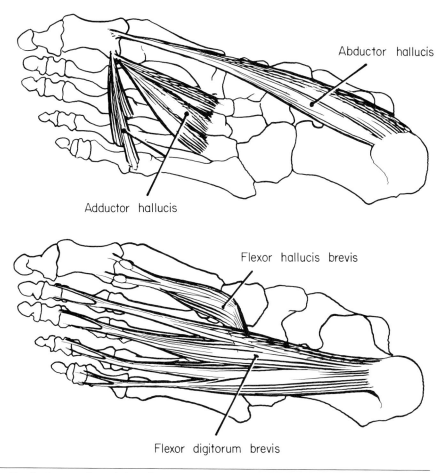

Abductor hallucis

Adductor hallucis

Flexor hallucis brevis

Flexor digitorum brevis

Figure 12-18

Intrinsic muscles of the plantar aspect of the foot: *(top)* abductor hallucis and adductor hallucis, major short muscles of the hallux in the inferior muscle layer, and *(bottom)* flexor hallucis brevis and flexor digitorum brevis, major short flexors of the toes in the superior muscle layer.

only the most distal interphalangeal joints of the second through fifth digits.

The plantar surface of the foot bears many different muscles. The hallux receives three intrinsic muscles: the abductor hallucis, the adductor hallucis, and the flexor hallucis brevis (Figure 12-18). The latter two muscles are deep within the foot, whereas the abductor is in the most superficial layer of muscles. The abductor hallucis arises from the medial side of the plantar surface of the calcaneal tuberosity and inserts into the medial sesamoid lying at the metatarsophalangeal joint and onto the base of the proximal phalanx. Contracting the abductor moves the hallux medially, away from the other digits.

The adductor hallucis has a transverse and an oblique head, which function separately. The transverse head attaches to the joint capsules of the metatarsophalangeal joints of the second through fifth digits, thus tying these digits together and limiting their independent motion. It inserts upon the fibrous sheath surrounding the flexor hallucis longus. The oblique head arises from the long plantar ligament and from the sheath of the peroneus longus. It inserts onto the lateral sesamoid and the base of the first proximal phalanx. Both heads thus work to pull the hallux laterally.

The flexor hallucis brevis arises from a fibrous intermuscular septum on the medial side of the plantar surface of the foot and from the portion of the tibialis posterior that inserts on the metatarsal bases. The flexor hallucis brevis divides into medial and lateral portions, each of which inserts on the corresponding sesamoid and the base of the proximal phalanx on its side.

The second through fifth digits also receive a short flexor muscle, the flexor digitorum brevis. In the foot, this muscle lies superficial to the long flexor muscle. It arises from the medial side of the plantar surface of the calcaneal tuberosity and divides into four tendons, which accompany the long flexor tendons in their sheaths. Each short flexor tendon divides to permit the long flexor tendon to pass between its limbs. The short flexor tendon then inserts along the sides of the middle phalanx. Thus, the long flexor muscle flexes the distal interphalangeal joints, and the short flexes the proximal interphalangeal and the metatarsophalangeal joints.

Like the hand, the foot receives three additional sets of muscles: five lumbricals, three plantar interossei, and four dorsal interossei. Their origins and insertions are similar to the lumbricals and interossei of the hand. The only significant difference is that the pedal lumbricals and interossei abduct and adduct the digits relative to a plane through the second digit, not the third. The lumbricals arise from the long flexor tendons in a complex pattern. The third through fifth lumbricals each arise from two heads, one from the tendon with the same number and one from the next medial tendon. The second lumbrical arises only from the tendon to the second digit. Each lumbrical inserts on the medial side of the base of the appropriate proximal phalanx. The lumbricals help flex the metatarsophalangeal joints and may assist the interossei in abduction and adduction, but this action is limited in most individuals.

The three plantar interossei arise from the bases of m/t III, IV, and V and from the peroneus longus sheath. They insert on the medial side of the base of the proximal phalanx of the digit from which they arise. Their action is to abduct the digits, although a more important function is to maintain the integrity of the metatarsal arch. The four dorsal interossei each arise from the adjacent shafts of two metatarsals and insert on the base of a proximal phalanx. The fifth dorsal interosseous muscle inserts on the lateral side of the base of the fourth proximal phalanx, the fourth inserts on the lateral side of the third proximal phalanx, and the third inserts on the lateral side of the second proximal phalanx. The second dorsal interosseous, however, does not insert on the lateral side of the first proximal phalanx. Instead, it inserts on the medial side of the base of the second proximal phalanx. Because this axis of symmetry passes through the second digit, abduction and adduction in the toes occur around a plane through the second digit, rather than through the third digit as in the hand. The dorsal interossei abduct the toes and strengthen the metatarsal arch. Both lumbricals and interossei are smaller and less important muscles in the foot than in the hand.

An additional muscle in the foot, the abductor digiti minimi, abducts the fifth digit, and the flexor digiti minimi brevis flexes the fifth digit. There is an accessory flexor, the quadratus plantae, which may act to flex the toes, when the ankle is dorsiflexed, by pulling on the long flexor tendon distal to the ankle.

BIPEDAL LOCOMOTION

Walking is a complex, learned behavior. During most of the gait cycle, walking involves balancing the body weight over a single support while controlling forward motion. The walking cycle is divided into units called strides: one stride is defined as the activities between one heel strike, or the onset of a step, and the next heel strike on that side. A stride is in turn divided into two phases: the stance phase, in which the limb in question is supporting the body, and the swing phase, in which that same limb advances forward to initiate a new step.

The actions of the limbs in stance phase and swing phase exhibit the different features and movements involved in walking (Figure 12-19). A stride starts with heel strike, an action in which the heel of the swing leg first comes into contact with the ground or other substrate. To produce heel strike, the foot is moved out and forward by the flexors of the hip

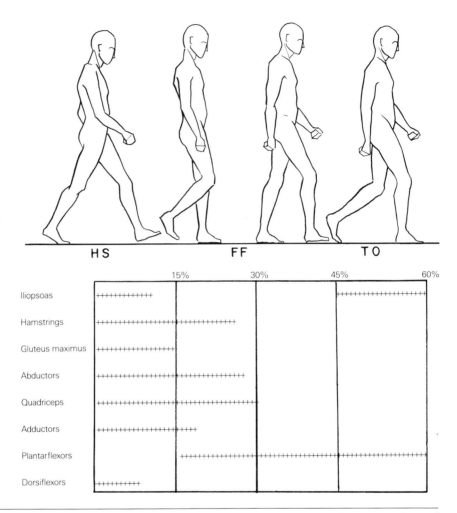

Figure 12-19

Human walking, showing the stance phase of the left limb and the swing phase of the right limb. A full stride is both a stance and swing phase for one limb. *(Top)* The stance phase begins with heel strike *(HS)* with the left foot and continues through flat foot *(FF)* to toe off *(TO)*, which begins the swing phase of the left limb. *(Bottom)* The timing of muscle actions of the left limb during stance phase.

and the lateral rotators. The knee is simultaneously extended. Once that foot has contacted the substrate, the body is pulled over it by means of the adductors. The leg in question is now the stance leg and supports the body. The body weight is shifted from the heel diagonally forward to the lateral side of the ball of the foot and then medially to the ball of the hallux. In this position, known as flat foot, the knee is extended and the long axis of the limb is approximately vertical. The body weight is then shifted forward again, by extending the hip and knee and starting to plantarflex the foot so that weight is transferred onto the hallux. The action known as toe off occurs as the hallux flexes and the foot plantarflexes. At this point, the stance leg becomes the swing leg and vice versa, and the body weight is transferred to the new stance leg. The new swing leg is pulled forward by the hip flexors with the knee in flexed position and the foot dorsiflexed. This knee flexion and foot dorsiflexion, combined with the abduction of the stance leg hip by the gluteus medius and minimus, keep the swing leg foot from dragging on the ground. The body pivots around the stance leg as the swing leg moves forward and rotates laterally to initiate a new step with another heel strike. This heel strike marks the end of the cycle. Only about 25 percent of the stride cycle involves body support by both limbs.

Normal walking thus involves a complex series of muscle actions and postures as well as adaptations in the bony elements, such as the structuring of the femoral head and neck to withstand the high forces transmitted across this joint in walking, or the arrangement of bones and ligaments in the foot to maintain the longitudinal and transverse arches. The contraction of different muscles during a stride and the resulting joint movements help to make walking efficient by minimizing the displacement of the center of gravity or the body weight so that a minimum amount of energy is expended in such displacement.

Theoretically, the most efficient gait would involve absolutely no displacement of the center of gravity: imagine a sphere rolling on a completely straight pathway so that it never moves its center of gravity from side to side or up and down, but only forward. Humans are not, however, spherical, so such locomotion is not possible. The simplest form of bipedal locomotion is the hypothetical compass gait, named after the two-legged instrument used to draw circles (Figure 12-20). In the compass gait, the knee and ankle are fixed in anatomical position and the hip is capable only of flexion and extension. Thus, in walking with a compass gait, the center of gravity is displaced markedly in both a mediolateral and a superoinferior direction. The center of gravity in such a stride follows a scalloped track with respect to the superoinferior motion and a broad sinuous track with repect to the lateral motion.

There are six determinants that make normal human gait different from the compass gait: pelvic rotation; pelvic tilt; knee flexion; two complex adjustments of the knee, ankle, and foot; and lateral pelvic

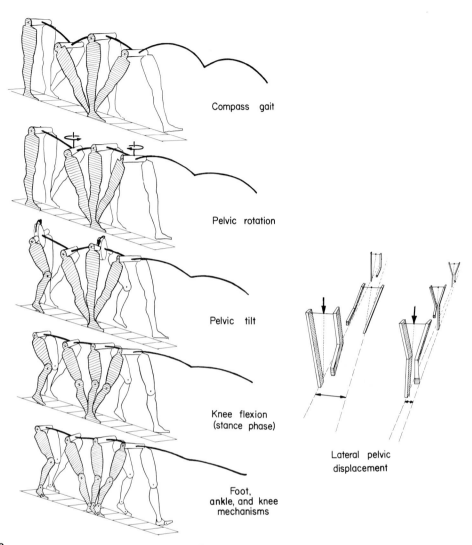

Compass gait

Pelvic rotation

Pelvic tilt

Knee flexion
(stance phase)

Foot,
ankle, and knee
mechanisms

Lateral pelvic
displacement

Figure 12-20

Determinants of normal human gait. Compass gait is a theoretical mode of walking in which the hip, knee, and ankle are fixed and the vertical displacement of the body's weight *(solid line)* is maximal. Pelvic rotation is achieved by the body pivoting about the stance leg, lessening the vertical displacement of the body's weight. Pelvic tilt is produced by abducting the hip of the stance leg, minimizing the drop of the swing leg as weight is transferred to the stance leg. Knee flexion during the stance phase also decreases the up-and-down displacement of the body's weight. Other mechanisms of the knee, ankle, and foot during the stance phase smooth transitions from heel strike to flat foot. Lateral displacement of the body's weight *(dotted line)* is minimized by bringing the knees and feet close to the center of gravity rather than placing them directly under the hip joint.

displacement. These determinants can be used to analyze abnormal gaits, so that the difficulties can be precisely identified and overcome if possible. Knowing which determinant is lacking may pinpoint the problem as paralysis or weakness of a particular group of muscles.

In the first determinant of normal human gait, pelvic rotation, the body pivots around the stance leg and the swing leg rotates laterally to initiate heel strike. Incorporating pelvic rotation in the gait therefore flattens the curvature of the superoinferior track: the center of gravity is displaced less far vertically. This determinant reflects the actions of the lateral rotators of the thigh at the hip.

The second determinant of normal gait, pelvic tilt, is produced by the abduction at the hip of the stance leg. Without abduction of the stance hip, the swing hip drops downward abruptly as weight is transferred to the stance leg. Abduction minimizes this drop by holding the pelvis more nearly horizontal. This action serves to flatten the arc traced on the vertical axis still further, making gait more efficient. Pelvic tilt is lacking in individuals with paralysis of the gluteus medius and minimus, which may occur bilaterally or only on one side. Other conditions inhibiting normal pelvic tilt are a dislocated femoral head and a fracture to the neck of the femur. Clinically, the inability to produce normal pelvic tilt is known as having a positive Trendelenburg sign.

The third determinant of normal gait, knee flexion, is important in the early part of the stance phase, when the center of gravity reaches the highest point on the arc. Bending the knee slightly at such points in the gait cycle flattens the arc still further. Knee flexion is produced by the hamstrings and the gastrocnemius.

The fourth and fifth determinants of gait are a complex series of knee, ankle, and foot mechanisms that operate throughout the stance phase. These mechanisms involve many slight flexions and extensions at these joints to modulate the primary movements. The effect is to smooth the transitions at heel strike, flat foot, and toe off, so that the sharp, lower points of the arcs of the compass gait disappear. Nearly all of the muscles of the lower limb participate in the fourth and fifth determinants.

Finally, the sixth determinant of normal gait involves the minimization of lateral pelvic displacement. If walking is carried out with the feet planted directly below the hip joints, a lurching gait results, in which the torso and center of gravity are thrown from side to side. Such a gait is commonly seen in infants learning to walk, in drunks, or in people with particular gait abnormalities. Both the carrying angle of the femur and the abduction and adduction of the thigh at the hip at various points during walking minimize the lateral displacement of the center of gravity. In normal walking, the feet are kept close to each other and to the body's midline.

13
THE SKULL

The skull is a complex three-dimensional structure. Its shape and structure are intimately involved with eight of the most crucial functions of the human body: thinking, speaking, hearing, seeing, breathing, smelling, eating, and tasting. Perhaps because of these functions, the skull has assumed a special place in symbolism and mythology. For example, the eyes are called the window of the soul, or the size and complexity of the brain are said to distinguish humans from all other animals.

The skull is comprised of two parts, the cranium and the mandible or lower jaw. The cranium also has two major divisions: the splanchnocranium and the neurocranium. The splanchnocranium is the facial region of the cranium, which carries or houses the anatomical apparatus for the senses of taste, sight, and smell. The neurocranium houses the brain and the anatomical apparatus for hearing and provides the exits for the cranial nerves and the spinal cord.

The skull is comprised of thirteen bones, many of which are paired. These are the frontal, nasal, maxilla, zygomatic, lacrimal, ethmoid, vomer, inferior concha, palatine, sphenoid, temporal, parietal, and occipital bones. In addition, there are three ossicles, or tiny bones, in each ear. These are the malleus, incus, and stapes. Additional ossicles, also known as sutural or Wormian bones, may be found in the neurocranium. On each side of the skull, a normal adult has eight maxillary and eight mandibular teeth. The hyoid bone at the root of the tongue, though not technically part of the skull, is generally included with it.

MAJOR LANDMARKS

From superior to inferior, the major bones forming the anterior aspect of the skull are the frontal, paired maxillae, and mandible (Figure 13-1). Within each orbit or bony eye socket are, medially, the lacrimal and the ethmoid and, laterally, parts of the sphenoid. The bridge between the orbits and the roof of the nasal aperture is made up of the paired nasals and a thin process of the paired maxillae. The vomer is a flat, bony sheet at midline. The interior concha is a

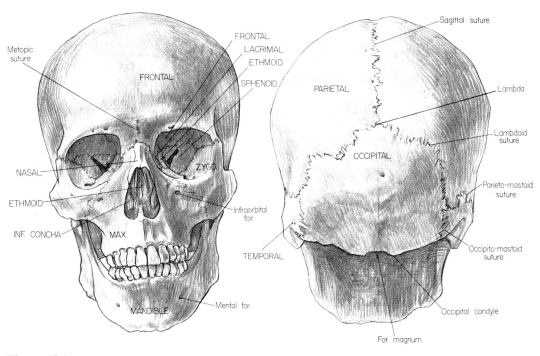

Figure 13-1

The human skull in *(left)* anterior and *(right)* posterior view. To the left of lambda, along the lambdoid suture, is a wormian bone.

thin-walled, hollow structure on the lateral walls of the nasal aperture; this bone is frequently damaged or absent on laboratory skulls. The bodies of the maxillae form the floor of the orbits, surround the nasal aperture, and hold the maxillary dentition. Meeting the maxillae at the inferolateral corners of the orbits are the paired zygomatic bones.

On the lateral aspect of the skull, the frontal bone articulates with the parietal, one on either side of the cranial vault, in an interdigitated suture called the coronal suture (Figure 13-2). The coronal suture lies on the coronal plane. The frontal articulates laterally with a part of the sphenoid that lies just posterior to the orbit on either side. Most of the sphenoid lies at midline deep within the cranium. The zygomatic projects posteriorly in a bony process that is met by one from the temporal, the two processes forming the zygomatic arch. Along its inferior margin, the parietal also articulates with the temporal in the squamous suture, which is continuous posteriorly with the parieto-mastoid suture. At the posterior end of the zygomatic arch, the temporal has a large opening, the external auditory meatus, over which the

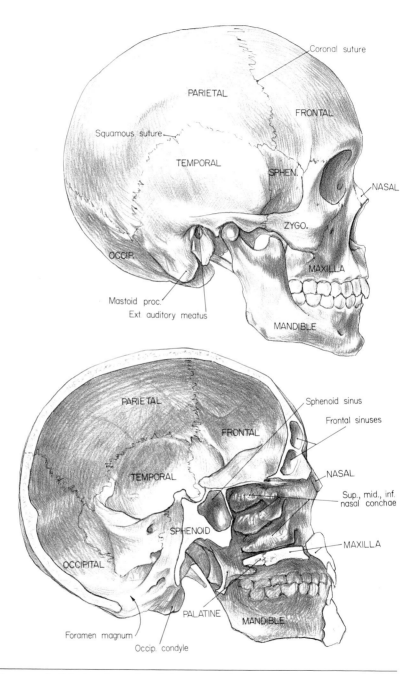

Figure 13-2

The human skull in *(top)* lateral and *(bottom)* medial view of a sagittally sectioned specimen.

fleshy ear lies. The highest point on the external auditory meatus is
called porion. Just anterior to the external auditory meatus, the mandibular or glenoid fossa of the temporal articulates with the condyle of
the mandible. Just posterior to the external auditory meatus is a blunt,
triangular projection from the temporal, the mastoid process. The
posterior edge of the temporal bone articulates with the occipital, the
large bone that makes up the inferior portion of the posterior surface
of the skull.

In posterior view, the cranium is divided into three segments. Inferiorly, the cranium is comprised of the large, roughly triangular occipital
bone. It articulates with a parietal on either side of midline, via the
interdigitated lambdoid suture, so named for the Greek letter lambda
(Λ), which suggests the shape of the suture. Inferiorly, the lambdoid
suture is continuous with the occipito-mastoid suture. The two parietals meet each other at midline in another interdigitated suture, the
sagittal suture.

The inferior aspect of the cranium reveals a large, circular opening
within the occipital bone, which is the foramen magnum, the hole
through which the spinal cord passes out of the cranium (Figure 13-3).
Many smaller openings appear anterior or lateral to the foramen magnum. Anterior to the foramen magnum and lying to each side of midline are the occipital condyles, for articulation with the superior articular facets of the atlas. Anterior to these, the occipital articulates with
the sphenoid at the basilar suture. The pterygoid processes of the
sphenoid project inferiorly from the cranium just posterior to the palate. The palate itself is comprised of the two maxillae anteriorly and the
two palatines, which meet at midline and articulate with each other
and the posterior edge of the palatine processes of the maxillae.

Internally, the base of the cranium is divided into three fossae:
anterior, middle, and posterior. At midline, the right and left anterior
fossae are separated from each other by the lacy cribriform plate and
its accompanying bony ridge, the crista galli. Both these features are
part of the ethmoid bone. In life, the anterior fossae house the frontal
lobe of each cerebral hemisphere, a part of the brain that is generally
associated with abstract thinking and emotions. The floor of the anterior fossa is comprised of parts of the ethmoid, frontal, and sphenoid.
On a lower level and posterior to the anterior fossa is the middle cranial
fossa, which houses the temporal lobe of each cerebral hemisphere.
The temporal lobe houses the speech centers of the brain and stores
visual memories. Several large foramina are on the floor of the middle
cranial fossa. At midline, the complex structures of the body of the

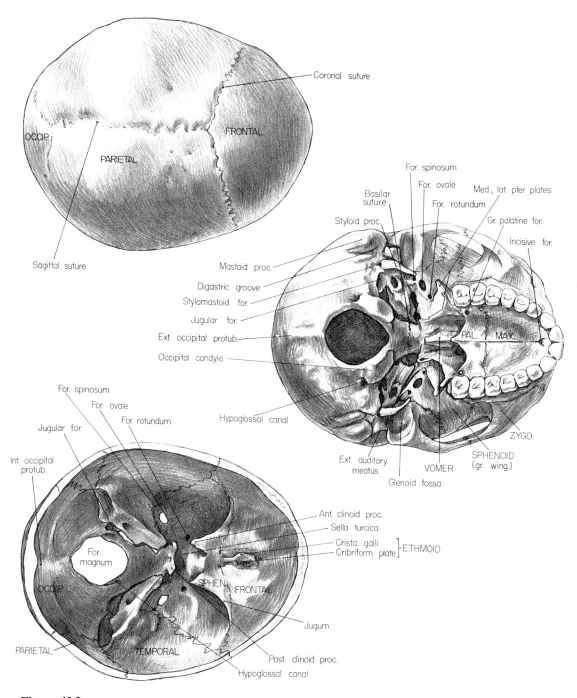

Figure 13-3

The human cranium: *(top to bottom)* superior view, inferior view, and internal surface of the base of a transversely sectioned specimen.

sphenoid are visible. Among these is a depression, bounded by anterior and posterior protrusions, called the sella turcica or Turk's saddle. It houses the hypophysis, or pituitary gland, which secretes hormones that help regulate growth. The sella turcica is part of the sphenoid. The temporals and parietals also contribute to the middle cranial fossa. The posterior cranial fossa is the largest, lowest, and most posterior. It is made up of the temporal and occipital bones and houses the occipital lobe superiorly and the cerebellar hemisphere inferiorly. The occipital lobe is closely linked with the processing of visual information. The cerebellum is important in the regulation and coordination of motor activities, in both complex endeavors, such as walking, and simple actions. At the anterior edge of the posterior fossa is the large sigmoid sulcus or groove for the sigmoid sinus, a channel that participates in draining blood from the brain. At midline, leading inferiorly from the posterior wall of the posterior cranial fossa, is the continuation of the sagittal sulcus, which houses the superior sagittal sinus that also drains the brain. The sagittal sulcus meets the large transverse sulcus at a point marked by a bony bump, the internal occipital protuberance. The transverse sulcus carries the transverse sinus, another large channel draining the brain, and is continuous with the sigmoid sulcus.

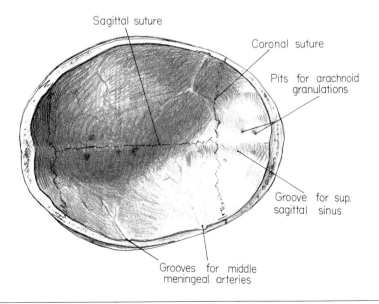

Figure 13-4

The calvaria in a transversely sectioned cranium. Anterior is to the right.

The superior portion of the cranium is the skullcap or calvaria (Figure 13-4). From anterior to posterior, the calvaria is comprised of the frontal, parietal, and occipital bones. The frontal crest projects posteriorly at midline from the anterior end of the calvaria. Along the midline run the sagittal suture and the sagittal sulcus. Near the posterior limit of the calvaria, the sagittal suture divides to form the two limbs of the lambdoid suture, between the parietals and the occipital. The sagittal sulcus continues at midline past this point down onto the posterior, internal wall of the base of the cranium until it meets the transverse sulcus. Small, circular pits near the sagittal sulcus mark the location of arachnoid granulations, which are tiny protrusions of one of the meninges surrounding the brain.

The hyoid is a small, U-shaped bone in the anterior throat. In the skeleton, it lies anterior to the body of the third cervical vertebra. It anchors the muscles of the tongue and is suspended from the cranium by the stylohyoid ligaments. It does not articulate with other bones.

THE SPLANCHNO-CRANIUM

The most superior bone of the splanchnocranium is the frontal, an unpaired bone of which the vertical portion forms the forehead and the horizontal portion forms the roof of the orbits (Figure 13-5). The vertical portion of the frontal has two surfaces, an external and an internal. The external surface shows, to variable degree, two lateral eminences, or bosses, that indicate the location of the original centers of ossification. The inferior edge of the vertical portion is marked by the supraorbital margins, above which lie the superciliary arches, or brow ridges. Each superciliary arch usually bears a superciliary notch or foramen, through which runs a sensory branch of the fifth cranial nerve on its way from the orbit to the forehead. Lateral to each superciliary arch is a bony ridge, the temporal line, for the attachment of the temporalis muscle. The temporal line arches slightly and passes posteriorly along the frontal onto the parietal. The frontal has two processes, the zygomatic and nasal. Each zygomatic process hangs down at the lateral side of the supraorbital margin to articulate with the zygomatic bone. The nasal process is the part of the frontal at midline, for articulation with the nasals and the maxillae. The inverted V in the external bone at midline is called the nasal notch. The articular portion of the nasal process is longer than the external surface, and a bony spike, the nasal spine, protrudes inferiorly.

The internal surface of the entire frontal bone houses the frontal

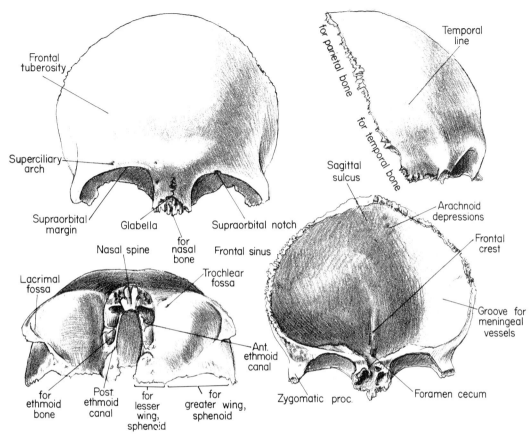

Figure 13-5

The frontal: *(clockwise from top left)* anterior view, lateral view, internal surface in posterior view, and inferior view.

lobes of the brain. The pars orbitalis, the horizontal portion that covers the orbits, has a rippled superior surface to receive the anterior lobes of the brain. The vertical portion of the frontal curves upward from the horizontal portion, and its left and right sides are separated by the distinct frontal crest that protrudes between the right and left frontal lobes of the brain. At the base or inferior end of the crest is a small hole, the foramen cecum. The crest diminishes as it proceeds posteriorly and superiorly, to be replaced by a midline depression, the sagittal sulcus, that continues on the interior surfaces of the parietals. On either side of the sulcus are a variable number of arachnoid granulations or depressions. Lateral and superior to the orbital roof on each side are small, branching grooves for the meningeal blood vessels. These are better defined on the adjacent surfaces of the parietals.

The thin bone of the horizontal portion of the frontal forms the roof of the bony orbits. Its superior surface is rippled, but its inferior surface is smoothly concave. Laterally on the inferior surface of each orbit is a depression for the lacrimal gland, called the lacrimal fossa. Medially, the two orbits are separated by a broad slit, the ethmoidal notch, into which the superior surface of the ethmoid fits. An irregular series of bony cells, the anterior and posterior ethmoidal canals, occur along the lateral margins of the opening for the ethmoid. There is an opening into the frontal sinus, a space lined with mucous membrane in life. The frontal sinus is of variable extent in different individuals and ethnic groups. There are rough articular surfaces for the zygomatic bone at the anterolateral edge of each orbit and for the sphenoid at the postero-lateral edge.

The frontal bone has twelve articulations with other bones. The largest area, the entire posterior edge of the vertical portion of the frontal, is taken up by the coronal suture for the two parietal bones. At the inferior end of coronal suture on each side and posterior to the orbit, the frontal articulates with the sphenoid. The horizontal portion of the frontal also articulates with the sphenoid along its entire posterior edge. Anteriorly at midline, the frontal articulates with two nasals, and just posteriorly it articulates with the ethmoid. To either side of the nasals, the frontal articulates with the frontal processes of the two maxillae. The medial side of each orbit articulates with the lacrimal and, more posteriorly, with the lateral side of the ethmoid. The zygomatic processes at the lateral side of the vertical portion of the frontal articulate with the zygomatic bone on each side.

The frontal bone grows from two centers of intramembranous ossification, one on each side, starting in the eighth week of fetal life. In young individuals a midline suture, the metopic suture, may still be visible. Fusion of the metopic suture at midline occurs in early childhood, at 1–7 years, although the suture itself may remain visible in some individuals.

The nasals are small, nearly rectangular bones that articulate with the frontal at midline between the orbits (Figure 13-6). They have an external surface, which is smooth and concave superoinferiorly, and an internal surface, which bears several elongate grooves. The medial portion of the nasal has a triangular-shaped, roughened articular surface for its partner. Superiorly, the nasal has another roughened surface for articulation with the frontal. In anterior view, the nasal is

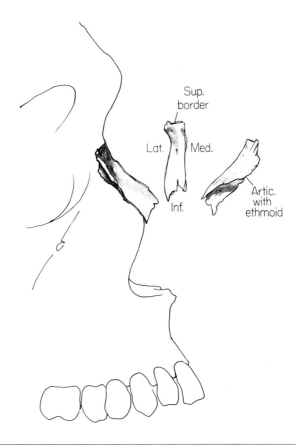

Figure 13-6

The nasal: *(left to right)* placement in the cranium, anterior view, and medial view.

broadest inferiorly, narrower in the middle, and broader again superiorly. The inferior end of the nasal, which participates in defining the apex of the nasal aperture, is thin and flattened. The lateral edge of the nasal is thin but roughened for articulation with the frontal process of the maxilla. The nasal ossifies in membrane beginning in the third fetal month.

The maxillae are large, paired bones that comprise most of the anterior surface of the midfacial region (Figure 13-7). The major portion of the maxilla is the body, which houses the large maxillary sinus. The body has four surfaces: the anterior or facial surface, the infratemporal surface, the orbital surface, and the nasal surface. These face anteriorly, posteriorly, superiorly, and medially respectively. The most obvious feature of the anterior surface is the nasal notch, which defines the nasal aperture when the maxilla is articulated with its

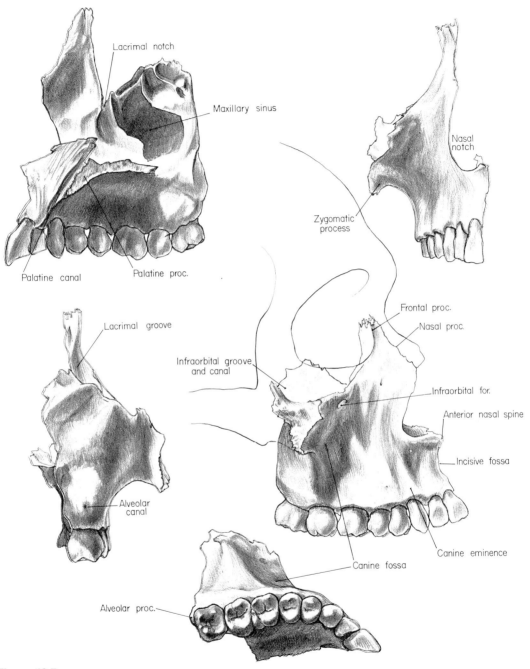

Figure 13-7

The maxilla: *(clockwise from top left)* medial view, anterior view, placement in the cranium, inferior view, and posterior view.

partner and the nasals. In humans, the margin of the nasal notch is thin and sharp. At midline, the inferior margin of the notch protrudes anteriorly in the anterior nasal spine. Lateral to the notch and just inferior to the orbital surface is the large infraorbital foramen, which transmits a sensory branch of the fifth cranial nerve to the midfacial region.

Inferiorly, the alveolar processes hold the teeth. In adult humans there are thirty-two teeth, divided into eight upper and eight lower teeth on each side. Proceeding distally from midline, these teeth are the central incisor, the lateral incisor, the canine, the first premolar, the second premolar, the first molar, the second molar, and the third molar. Each tooth is commonly designated by the first letter of its type (I for incisor, C for canine, P for premolar, or M for molar) and a number. The placement of the number reveals whether the tooth is maxillary, in which case the number is a superscript, or mandibular, in which case it is a subscript. If the number is placed neither as a superscript nor as a subscript, both uppers and lowers are being referred to. Because there is only one canine on each side, upper and lower canines are distinguished by the placement of a tick (') rather than a number. Human premolars are designated P3 and P4, not P1 and P2, for evolutionary reasons. Whereas primitive mammals have four premolars (P1–4), humans in the course of evolutionary history have lost the first two premolars, leaving only P3 and P4. In a complete dental formula, the letters are dropped and the number of upper and lower teeth of each type is separated from its fellows by periods. The formula for upper teeth is placed above a horizontal line, and that for lower teeth is placed below the line. Thus, the formula for a normal adult human with two incisors, one canine, two premolars, and three molars is $\frac{2.1.2.3}{2.1.2.3}$.

The roots of the teeth cause bulges and depressions on the anterior surface of the maxilla. Inferior to the nasal notch and between the roots of the central and lateral incisor is a depression called the incisive fossa. Lateral to this depression and overlying the long canine root, the bone bulges outward in the canine eminence. Still farther laterally and inferior to the infraorbital foramen is a large depression called the canine fossa.

The frontal process is the portion of the maxilla that extends superiorly to articulate with the frontal superiorly, the nasal medially, and the lacrimal laterally. The nasal border is sharp and thin compared to the thicker, more rounded border for the lacrimal. In posterior view, the frontal process and the adjacent orbital surface show a pronounced groove, the lacrimal groove, running superoinferiorly. With the lacrimal in place, this area forms the anterior wall of the bony passage for the nasolacrimal duct. The medial surface of the frontal process is smooth and concave and forms the lateral wall of the nasal aperture.

The orbital surface of the maxilla faces superiorly and forms the floor of the bony orbit and the roof of the maxillary sinus. The bone is very thin and translucent here. Crossing the orbital surface from posterior to anterior is the infraorbital groove, which dives into the bone anteriorly as a canal of the same name and comes out on the facial surface as the infraorbital foramen. The groove, canal, and foramen transmit a branch of the fifth cranial nerve. Medially, the orbital surface participates in the lacrimal notch, into which the lacrimal bone fits. Posterior to the lacrimal notch, the orbital surface articulates with the ethmoid, which forms most of the medial wall of the orbit.

The zygomatic process protrudes laterally between the anterior and infratemporal surfaces of the maxilla. It bears a large, triangular-shaped, roughened surface for articulation with the zygomatic bone. Like many other sutures in the cranium, the bone of this articular surface interdigitates with the opposing bone.

The infratemporal surface faces almost directly posteriorly. The alveolar process terminates posteriorly in the maxillary tuberosity. The palatine process of the maxilla is visible medially as a horizontal shelf of bone extending to midline. Just below the level of the palatine process on the infratemporal surface is a roughened area for articulation with the pyramidal process of the palatine bone. Lateral to the articulation are several openings, most often two in number, to the alveolar canals.

The nasal or medial surface of the maxillary body is dominated by a large opening into the maxillary sinus. The inferior concha articulates with the maxilla along the inferior edge of this opening. Anteriorly, the nasal surface is marked by the lacrimal groove for the nasolacrimal duct. Posteriorly, the greater palatine groove, also called the pterygopalatine canal, travels diagonally downward and forward. This canal carries the greater palatine nerve and its accompanying vessels to the palate. When the maxilla is articulated with the palatine bone, the greater palatine canal terminates in the greater palatine foramen. Superiorly, the nasal surface meets the orbital surface; inferiorly, it is bounded by the palatine process of the maxilla.

The palatine process is a nearly horizontal shelf of bone extending medially from the anterior two-thirds of the nasal surface of the maxilla. The medial edge of the palatine process is irregular for articulation with the other maxilla. Just posterior to the alveolus for the central incisor, the palatine or incisive canal plunges anteroinferiorly from the superior surface of the palatine process, to terminate in the incisive foramen which lies between the two maxillae. The superior surface of the palatine process is smooth and concave. Along the suture between the two maxillae is the articulation for the vomer. The posterior edge of the palatine process is roughened for articulation with the palatine bone, the body of which extends the bony palate posteriorly. The inferior surface of the palatine process is marked by many small vascular foramina.

The maxilla articulates with nine other bones. The two maxillae meet at midline below the nasal aperture and along the palatine process. Thus, the maxillae define the lateral and inferior edges of the nasal aperture; they also form the floor of the orbits. The anterior surface of the maxilla articulates with the frontal superiorly, with the nasal and the other maxilla medially, and with the zygomatic laterally. In the medial wall of the orbit, the maxilla articulates with the lacrimal anteriorly and the ethmoid posteriorly. Within the nasal aperture, the maxilla articulates with the vomer and the inferior concha. The palatine process and infratemporal surface of the maxilla each articulate with the palatine bone posteriorly.

The maxilla grows in membrane from two centers, one center for the premaxillary region, which is inferior to the nasal aperture and extends laterally to just distal to I^2, and one center for the rest of the bone. The center for the maxillary body appears first, during the sixth fetal week, followed in the eighth week by the premaxillary center.

The lateral margin of the orbit is formed by the zygomatic bone (Figure 13-8). The zygomatic has a malar, or cheek, surface that faces anteriorly and a temporal surface that faces posterolaterally. The malar surface bears one or more small zygomaticofacial foramina but is otherwise smooth and convex. The temporal surface is concave mediolaterally. Four projections are found on the zygomatic, of which three—the frontosphenoidal, maxillary, and temporal processes—are in the plane of the malar surface. The frontosphenoidal process projects superiorly, to articulate with the frontal at the lateral, superior corner of the orbit. The maxillary process projects medially, to articulate with the maxilla along the zygomaxillary suture that starts in the middle of the inferior orbital margin and proceeds diagonally downward and laterally across the cheek region. The temporal process

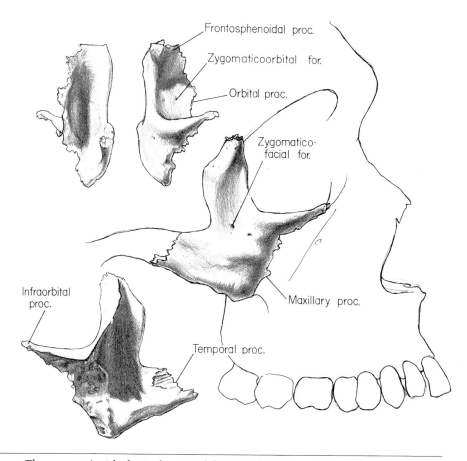

Figure 13-8

The zygomatic: *(clockwise from top left)* posterior view, anterior view, placement in the cranium, and medial view.

projects laterally and slightly posteriorly. It forms the anterior half of the zygomatic arch, while the zygomatic process of the temporal forms the posterior half of the arch. The fourth projection, the orbital process, projects posteriorly and slightly medially from the lateral margin of the orbit to form its lateral wall. Here, the sphenoid joins the zygomatic to complete the lateral wall of the orbit. The articulation for the sphenoid is continuous superiorly with that for the frontal and medially with that for the maxilla.

Three borders of the zygomatic are not articular: the one forming the lateral margin of the orbit, the one between the frontosphenoidal process and the temporal process, and the one between the temporal and maxillary processes. This last border is rounded and reinforced

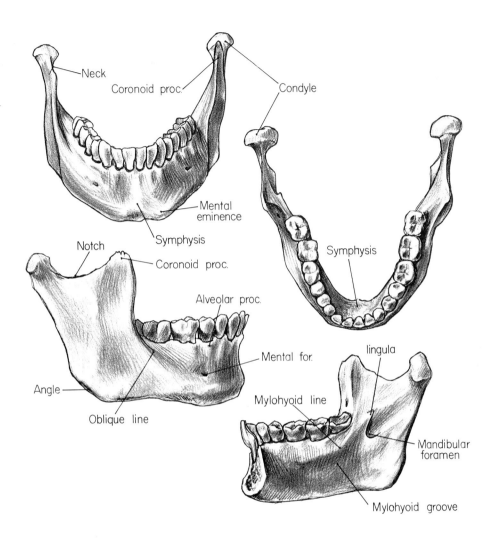

Figure 13-9

The mandible: *(clockwise from upper left)* anterior view, superior view, medial view in a sagittally sectioned specimen, and lateral view.

because it is the origin of the masseter, one of the major muscles of mastication. The membranous center of ossification for the zygomatic appears during the eighth week of fetal life.

The mandible is the bone of the lower jaw and holds the lower dentition (Figure 13-9). It consists of a U-shaped, horizontal body or corpus and a flattened, vertical extension called the ramus. The ramus carries the mandibular condyle, for articulation with the glenoid fossa of the temporal bone, and the coronoid process. The body is flattened buccolingually and has a rounded inferior margin. The mental protuberance appears on the external surface of the mandible at midline; it corresponds to the chin. To either side of it on the external surface lie the two mental eminences. Farther laterally, the external surface is perforated by the two mental foramina, which lie inferior to the left and right P_4. The internal surface of the mandibular body at midline may show several genial, or chin, tubercles, which often occur in one or two pairs. Lateral to these tubercles on each side is a small depression near the inferior margin of the body called the digastric fossa. Leading diagonally upward and posteriorly from this fossa is a small, bony ridge called the mylohyoid line. Below this line is a depression known as the submandibular fossa, and above the anterior portion of the line is the sublingual fossa; both fossae house salivary glands in life. Posteriorly, the body of the mandible terminates in the gonial angle, where the bone turns upward to form the ramus. In muscular individuals, the inferior margin and the lingual face of the gonial angle may be reinforced by extra bone.

The ramus is more flattened buccolingually and less rounded than the body. It rises nearly vertically, approximately perpendicular to the body, at about the level of M_3, although it may take off somewhat anterior or posterior to this tooth. The external surface of the ramus is smooth and gently convex. Its internal surface is mildly concave. At about the level of the tooth row, the internal surface of the ramus is marked by a large hole, the mandibular foramen, that leads into the mandibular canal within the body. This canal is continuous with the mental foramen on the anterior, external body. A small flattened, bony projection, the lingula, is found on the anterior edge of the mandibular foramen. The posterior end of the mylohyoid line is close to the mandibular foramen. The superior, anterior corner of the ramus is prolonged in a pointed projection called the coronoid process. Posterior to the coronoid process, the superior margin of the ramus dips to form the mandibular notch. The posterior corner of the ramus is occupied by the mandibular condyle. Its articular surface is a mediolaterally elongated oval in superior view. It is attached to the ramus by its neck.

Most of the mandible ossifies in membrane from two centers, one for each side. Small regions at the symphysis, coronoid process, and condyle ossify in cartilage starting during the sixth fetal week. At birth

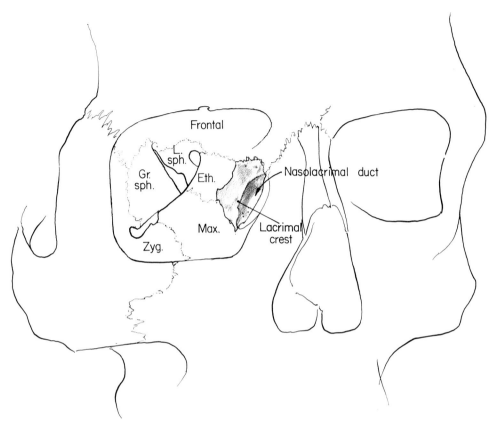

Figure 13-10

The lacrimal and bones of the orbit in anterolateral view: ethmoid, maxilla, zygomatic, greater wing of the sphenoid, and lesser wing of the sphenoid.

the two halves of the mandible are joined at the symphysis by fibrous tissue, and fusion is completed by the end of the first year. The remnants of the mandibular fusion are found at midline.

Immediately posterior to the most anterior bones of the splanchnocranium is another set of bones. These are the lacrimal, ethmoid, inferior concha, vomer, and palatine bones. All of them are fragile and thus are often fragmented or absent in archaeological or fossil specimens.

The lacrimal is a small, thin bone situated at the medial, anterior corner of the orbit (Figure 13-10). Laboratory skulls often do not have lacrimals because these bones are so readily broken when people pick up the skull by putting a finger in each orbit. The lacrimal is quadrilateral in outline and compressed mediolaterally. The anterior margin of the lacrimal is grooved from top to bottom. This groove, together with the corresponding groove on the frontal process of the maxilla, forms the bony canal for the nasolacrimal duct that drains tears from the eye into the nose and throat. Superiorly, the lacrimal articulates with the frontal; posteriorly, it articulates with the ethmoid; and inferiorly, it articulates with the orbital process of the maxilla. The lacrimal ossifies in membrane starting in the twelfth fetal week.

The ethmoid is another delicate, thin-walled bone located between the orbits (Figure 13-11). At midline on the ethmoid is the perpendicular plate, which hangs down vertically from the horizontal cribriform plate. The cribriform plate is a lacy network of bone through which the olfactory nerves pass from the inferior surface of the brain to the nose. The cribriform plate and its bony projection, the crista galli, lie in the ethmoidal notch of the frontal. Attached to the lateral edges of the cribriform plate is an elaborate series of sinuses surrounded by thin bony walls, known as the labyrinth. Many of the surfaces of these sinuses are open; others are closed only by articulation with adjacent bones. Laterally, the labyrinth shows a closed surface, the orbital plate, that completes the medial wall of the orbit. Medially, the labyrinth bears the superior and middle conchae that are on the lateral wall of the nasal aperture. The ethmoid articulates with the frontal above and the orbital surface of the maxilla below. Anteriorly, the ethmoid articulates with the frontal and the lacrimal. Posteriorly and superiorly, it articulates with the sphenoid at the back of the orbit.

Each labyrinth of the ethmoid ossifies from its own cartilaginous center, as does the perpendicular plate. The onset of ossification is during the fourth fetal month for the labyrinth and during the first year of postnatal life for the perpendicular plate. The three centers fuse to each other during the second year.

The inferior concha is a thin-walled, fragile bone that closely resembles the superior and middle conchae of the ethmoid (Figure 13-12). Both lateral and medial surfaces are irregular and perforated by many tiny foramina, but the lateral surface is concave and the medial is convex. The superior border of the inferior concha is thin and irregular for articulation with the maxilla anteriorly, the lacrimal in the middle, and the perpendicular plate of the ethmoid posteriorly. On the lateral surface, posterior to the midpoint between its anterior and posterior edges, the maxillary process projects downward and laterally. This process articulates with the lower border of the opening for the maxillary sinus. The cartilaginous precursor of the inferior concha begins to ossify during the fifth fetal month.

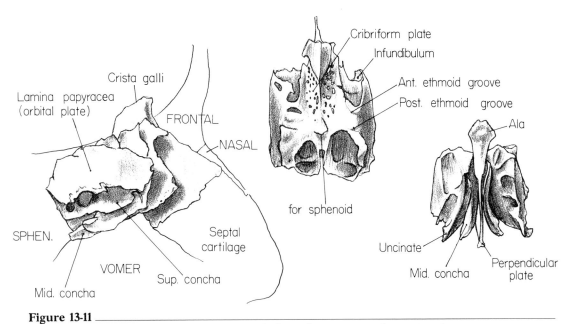

Figure 13-11

The ethmoid: *(left to right)* lateral, superior, and anterior view.

The vomer is a flattened plate of bone that lies at midline within the nasal aperture (Figure 13-13). It forms the posterior portion of the nasal septum, the anterior portion of which is formed by cartilage. In outline, the vomer is roughly diamond-shaped. Anteriorly, it meets the cartilage of the nasal septum. Its inferior margin articulates with the palatine processes of the maxillae at midline, and its posterior margin is free. The superior margin articulates anteriorly with the perpendicular plate of the ethmoid. Posteriorly, the vomer divides into two alae, or wings, which articulate with the vaginal or sheath-like processes on the inferior surface of the sphenoid. The vomer ossifies in membrane from two centers starting in the eighth fetal week.

The palatine is divided into a perpendicular and a horizontal plate (Figure 13-14). The horizontal plate extends the bony palate posteriorly from the palatine process of the maxilla. The posterior margin of its inferior surface carries a projection which, with its counterpart from the other palatine, makes up the posterior nasal spine. Its medial and anterior margins are irregular for articulation with the other palatine and the maxilla respectively. The perpendicular plate runs vertically from the lateral edge of the horizontal plate; it lies medial to the medial surface of the maxilla. The medial surface of the perpendicular plate is crossed horizontally by two crests. The inferior one is the

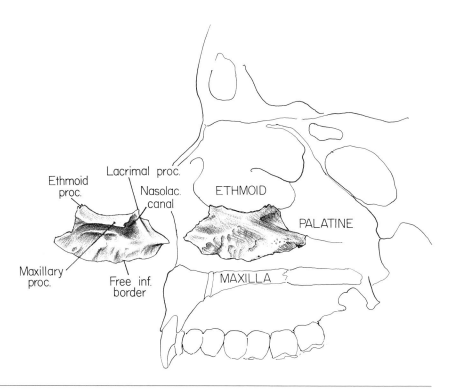

Figure 13-12

The inferior concha: *(left)* lateral view and *(right)* medial view and placement in the cranium.

conchal crest, for articulation with the inferior concha, and the superior one is the ethmoidal crest, for articulation with that bone. At the superior end of the perpendicular plate are two processes. The small orbital process passes anteriorly to participate in the floor of the orbit; the sphenoidal process passes posteriorly to articulate with the sphenoid. Between these two small processes lies the sphenopalatine foramen. At the junction of the horizontal and perpendicular plates, the pyramidal process extends laterally and inferiorly on the diagonal, to articulate with the infratemporal surface of the maxilla. The lateral surface of the perpendicular plate is grooved for the pterygopalatine or greater palatine canal. In about the eighth fetal week, the palatine begins to ossify in membrane.

The sphenoid, the most posterior bone in the splanchnocranium, is the most important to the cranium. Centrally placed in the cranium, it joins the splanchnocranium to the neurocranium. While some parts of the sphenoid are delicate, others are strong, and these parts frequently survive in archaeological or fossil specimens.

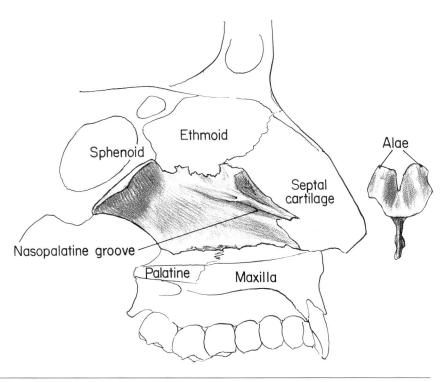

Figure 13-13

The vomer: *(left)* medial view and placement in the cranium and *(right)* posterior view.

The sphenoid consists of a central body and three paired sets of projections: the greater wings, the lesser wings, and the pterygoid plates (Figure 13-15). The greater and lesser wings project laterally, and the pterygoid plates project inferiorly from the body. The body itself is a hexahedron surrounding and enclosing the sphenoidal air sinuses. Its superior surface forms part of the floor of the interior surface of the cranium. From anterior to posterior, the superior surface of the body is marked by several features. Its anterior margin is thin and serrated, protruding anteriorly in the ethmoidal spine, for articulation with the posterior ethmoid. The lesser wings are the two superoinferiorly flattened, triangular-shaped flanges of bone that extend laterally from the anterosuperior aspect of the body. Posterior to the origin of the lesser wings is a smooth, mediolaterally oriented groove across the superior surface of the body; this is the optic or chiasmatic groove. Anteriorly, each lateral end of the groove terminates in a large, rounded hole, the optic foramen. In life, the optic foramina carry the optic nerves posteriorly from the eyes; these two

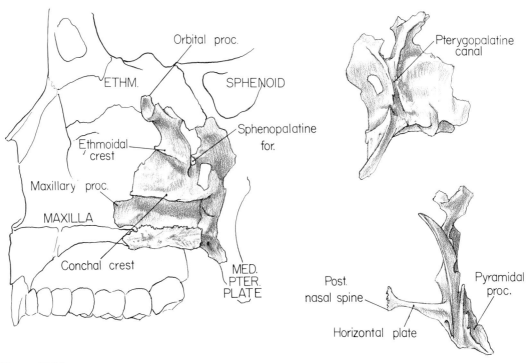

Figure 13-14

The palatine: *(clockwise from left)* placement in the cranium, lateral view, and anterior view.

large nerves then cross each other in the optic groove, the right optic nerve crossing to the left side of the brain and vice versa. The posterior margin of the optic groove is a raised ridge, the tuberculum sellae. The lateral ends of the tuberculum sellae are demarcated by two bony bumps, the middle clinoid processes. Posterior to those and to the tuberculum sellae is a smooth, concave surface bounded posteriorly by a large bony projection that protrudes anteriorly and superiorly. The concave surface is the sella turcica, so named for its fancied resemblance to a Turkish saddle. The posterior margin of the sella turcica is a large, upward protuberance, called the dorsum sellae or "back of the saddle." The lateral edges of the anterior margin of the dorsum sellae extend anteriorly as two bony knobs, called the posterior clinoid processes.

The lateral surfaces of the body of the sphenoid are smooth. Each bears a large carotid groove that runs anteroposteriorly for the artery

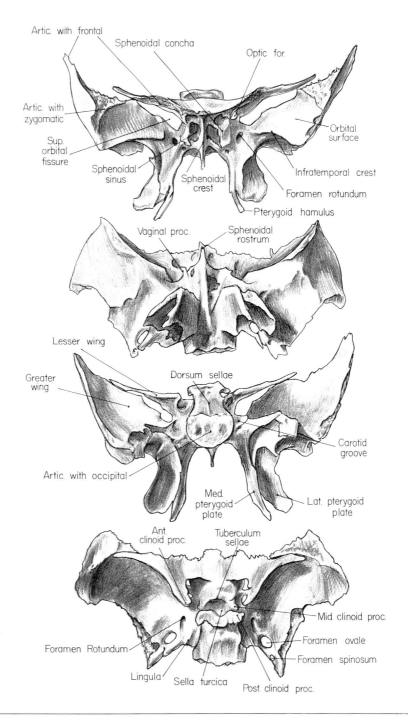

Figure 13-15

The sphenoid: *(clockwise from left)* anterior, inferior, posterior, and superior view.

of that name. The lateral lip of the carotid groove may be extended in a lingula.

The posterior surface of the sphenoidal body fuses to the basilar portion of the occipital just anterior to the foramen magnum. The cartilage interposed between the occipital and the sphenoid begins to diminish at about 18 years, and the suture is usually closed by age 25. Prior to fusion, the surface of the posterior surface of the sphenoidal body is irregular and ridged, as are many metaphyseal surfaces.

The anterior surface of the sphenoidal body bears at midline a distinct, vertically oriented ridge, called the sphenoidal crest, for articulation with the perpendicular plate of the ethmoid. To either side of the crest are thin plates of bone that cover over the large, sphenoidal air sinus that occupies most of the volume of the body.

The inferior surface of the body is divided at midline by a large crest, the sphenoidal rostrum, which fits into the V-shaped cavity between the alae of the vomer. Laterally, each ala of the vomer also articulates with a slit called the vaginal process of the sphenoid. Lateral to the vaginal processes, the pterygoid plates hang downward from either side of the body.

The lesser wings of the sphenoid are paired, flat, triangular-shaped plates of bone that extend laterally from the anterior aspect of the superior surface of the body. They roof the optic foramina on either side and articulate with the posterior margin of the horizontal part of the frontal. Lateral and posterior to the region that covers the optic foramen, each lesser wing bears a rounded feature that protrudes posteriorly and medially, the anterior clinoid process. It points toward and nearly touches the posterior clinoid process that extends forward from the dorsum sella. The lesser wings make up a small part of the posterior region of the medial wall of the orbit.

The greater wings of the sphenoid depart from the middle and posterior parts of the lateral sphenoidal body. In superior view, the greater wing is a large, smooth-surfaced, concave structure that resembles a butterfly's wing in outline. The greater wing meets the lesser wing on its inferior surface near its most lateral extent. Inferior to the lesser wing and superomedial to the greater wing is an elongated slit, the superior orbital fissure, that runs laterally and superiorly from just inferior to the optic foramen. The superior surface of the greater wing contributes to the middle cranial fossa that houses the temporal lobes of the brain. Two large foramina are visible on the superior surface of the greater wing. The foramen rotundum is more medially placed, lying just lateral to the body. The foramen ovale, the opening of which is oval rather than round, lies in the posterolateral region of the greater wing. A third, smaller foramen, the foramen spinosum, lies at the posterolateral corner of the greater wing. The anterior and lateral borders of the greater wing are roughened for articulation with the frontal anteriorly and the parietal and temporal laterally.

Anteriorly, the greater wing of the sphenoid presents an orbital surface, which is smooth, flat, and nearly vertically oriented. The orbital surface faces anteromedially. It forms the posterolateral portion of the orbit, articulating with the horizontal portion of the frontal superiorly and with the zygomatic anteriorly. Both articular surfaces are roughened for interdigitating sutures. Inferior to the orbital surface of the sphenoid in an intact cranium is an elongated slit, the inferior orbital fissure, bounded superiorly by the orbital surface of the sphenoid and inferiorly by the orbital surface of the maxilla. Medial and inferior to the orbital surface, the sphenoid is perforated by two holes. The larger and more lateral of these is the foramen rotundum, which comes out on the superior surface of the greater wing. The more medial foramen is the pterygoid canal, which continues horizontally through the sphenoid just superior to the attachment of the pterygoid plates and exits on the posterior surface.

The greater wing of the sphenoid also presents a lateral surface, which is found on the external surface of the cranium just posterior to the orbit. The lower margin of this surface is marked by the infratemporal crest, a strong, horizontally oriented ridge of bone. Inferior to the infratemporal crest, the sphenoid runs horizontally toward midline and then gives rise to the pterygoid plates.

Two pterygoid plates, designated as medial and lateral, hang downward on either side of the body of the sphenoid. Anteriorly, the two plates are joined along their superoinferior borders, but posteriorly they deviate from each other as separate plates. Between the two plates lies the pterygoid fossa. The plates are separated from each other inferiorly by the pterygoid fissure. The sloping inferior end of each plate articulates with a part of the palatine. This part of the lateral pterygoid plate articulates with the sphenoidal process of the palatine, while the end of the medial plate articulates with the perpendicular plate of the palatine. The lower end of the medial plate is prolonged into a hooked structure that swings laterally, to form the pterygoid hamulus.

The sphenoid, because of its complex shape and central location, articulates with eight other bones of the cranium: the frontal, vomer, ethmoid, palatine, zygomatic, parietal, temporal, and occipital.

It meets, but does not articulate with, the orbital surface of the maxilla.

The sphenoid ossifies from several centers. The greater wings and pterygoid plates ossify in membrane, starting between the eighth and tenth weeks of fetal life. The anterior body and lesser wings begin to ossify in cartilage at about the same time. At birth, the sphenoid is in three major pieces, one piece consisting of the body and lesser wings, and each of the other two pieces consisting of a greater wing with attached pterygoids. The parts of the sphenoid fuse to each other during the first year of life.

THE NEUROCRANIUM

From superior to inferior, the bones of the neurocranium are the parietals, temporals, and occipital. The small, irregularly shaped ossicles known as sutural or Wormian bones are found occasionally along the various sutures of the cranium. The frequency of such bones differs in different populations, depending on genetic factors. As a result, their presence or absence serves as a genetic marker that indicates the degree of relatedness within and between skeletal populations.

The parietal forms most of the lateral wall of the cranial vault (Figure 13-16). It is nearly square in outline, with a strongly convex external surface and a strongly concave internal surface. All four margins are shaped for articulation with adjacent bones. Anteriorly, the parietal articulates with the frontal along the coronal suture and, at the anteroinferior corner, with the lateral surface of the greater wing of the sphenoid. Medially, the two parietals articulate with each other along the sagittal suture. Posteriorly, the parietal articulates with the occipital in the lambdoid suture. All three of these sutures—the coronal, sagittal, and lambdoid—are strongly interdigitating. In contrast, the squamous suture, where the inferior margin of the parietal articulates with the temporal, is beveled. The articular surface of the temporal overlaps that of the parietal and lies lateral to it. This arrangement gives a characteristically striated appearance to the inferior margin of the parietal that differs markedly from the texture of the other margins. The inferior margin is also curved, with the concavity facing downward. Crossing from anterior to posterior on the external surface are the superior and inferior temporal lines, between which lies the origin of the temporalis muscle that inserts upon the coronoid process of the mandible. The parietal eminence or boss is the region where the convexity of the external surface is most marked. It occurs at the site of the earliest center of ossification.

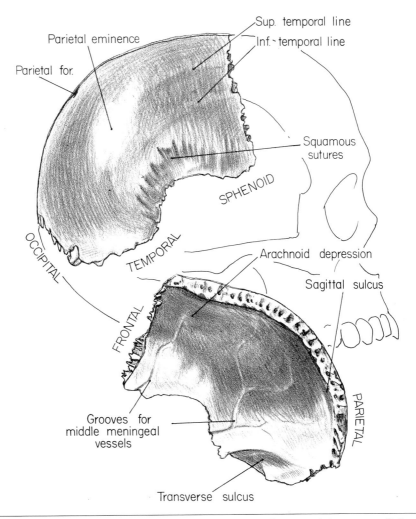

Figure 13-16

The parietal: *(top)* placement in the cranium in lateral view and *(bottom)* medial or internal view.

The internal surface of the parietal has a corresponding region of greatest concavity called the parietal fossa. A major feature of this surface is the series of dendritic grooves for the middle meningeal vessels. There are usually two sets of grooves, both of which run superiorly and posteriorly across the internal surface. One set commonly arises from the anteroinferior corner, which is sometimes called the sphenoidal angle, and the other commonly arises along the posterior third of the inferior margin. The angle and positioning of these grooves distinguish right and left parietals. When one of the

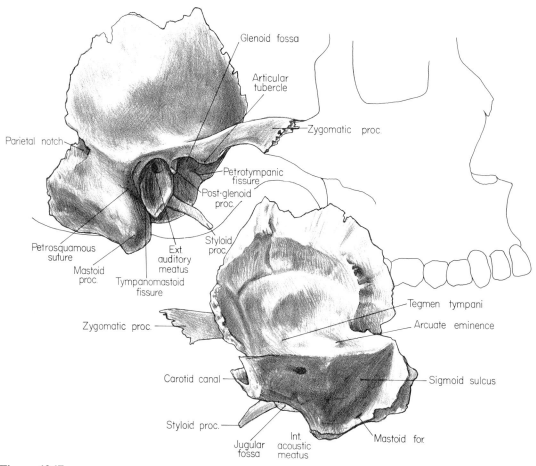

Figure 13-17

The temporal: *(top)* placement in the cranium in lateral view and *(bottom)* postero-medial view.

grooves is covered by a roof of bone, it is known as a sylvian crest. Along the superior margin of the parietal, just inferior to the serrations for the sagittal suture, is a longitudinal depression, the sagittal sulcus. In life, this sulcus houses a large vein, the superior sagittal sinus. One or more parietal foramina for small emissary veins are found along the sagittal suture, as are a variable number of pits for arachnoid granulations. At the posteroinferior corner the parietal overlaps the temporal in a reverse beveling, for articulation with the mastoid region of the temporal. The internal surface of this corner bears a large, curved groove, the transverse sulcus, which houses the transverse sinus. The parietal is ossified in membrane from two centers that appear at about the eighth week of fetal life and fuse to each other shortly thereafter.

The temporal forms the inferior portion of the lateral wall of the cranium and also contributes significantly to its base (Figure 13-17). There are four major portions of the temporal bone: the squamous, which is the tabular, vertical portion; the mastoid, which bears the mastoid process; the petrous, a dense region that houses the apparatus for hearing; and the tympanic, which forms the inferior tube of bone demarcating the external auditory meatus.

The most anterior part of the temporal is the squamous. Projecting anteriorly from its external surface is the zygomatic process, which articulates with its counterpart from the zygomatic bone to form a complete zygomatic arch. Continuing posteriorly from the zygomatic process is the suprameatal crest, a ridge of bone superior to the external auditory meatus, the large hole over which the fleshy, external ear sits and within which the tympanic membrane or ear drum lies in life. The superior margin of the squamous is beveled to overlie the inferior margin of the parietal. The beveling changes abruptly to serration at the parietal notch, a pronounced indentation in the superior margin of the temporal that marks the posterior extent of the squamous. The anterior margin is serrated for articulation with the lateral surface of the greater wing of the sphenoid. Inferior to the anterior root of the zygomatic process is the articular tubercle. This tubercle bounds the anterior end of the mandibular or glenoid fossa, which articulates with the condyle of the mandible. The glenoid fossa itself is oval in shape, with the long axis arranged mediolaterally. It is concave and bounded posteriorly by the post-glenoid process. Both the articular tubercle and the post-glenoid process help define the temporomandibular joint (TMJ) between the mandibular condyle and the glenoid fossa. The internal surface of the squamous portion shows the distinctive beveling of the squamous suture. Crossing the internal surface diagonally upward and backward is a groove for the middle meningeal vessels which then continues across the internal surface of the parietal.

From the lateral view, the segment of the temporal that is posterior to the parietal notch comprises the mastoid. The most prominent feature of its external surface is the mastoid process, which is triangular in outline and has a roughened external surface for the origin of the sternocleidomastoid muscle. Generally, the external surface of the mastoid process is perforated by the mastoid foramen. Although dense in appearance, the mastoid process is not solid bone; typically it is filled with air cells that may be exposed on the surface of mildly damaged specimens. The mastoid process is an indicator of sex, since it is usually larger in males. In inferior view, a strong channel, the digastric groove, runs medial and posterior to the mastoid process. The groove's posterior opening is the mastoid notch. On its interior surface the mastoid carries a deep, broad groove, the sigmoid sulcus, which carries the sinus of the same name and terminates in the jugular fossa on the petrous portion.

The petrous portion of the temporal protrudes medially and anteriorly from the mastoid region. It is named for its dense, rocklike bone, since *Peter* means "rock" in Latin. In archaeological and fossil specimens the petrous is often the only part of the temporal that is preserved. The petrous is roughly triangular in section, having an anterior, a posterior, and an inferior surface. Its anterior surface meets the squamous at the petrosquamous suture, which remains visible in young adults. Laterally, the petrous shows a slight depression, called the tegmen tympani. Medial to this depression is a bony protrusion, the arcuate eminence. More medial still, the hiatus of the facial canal is a groove leading laterally to a small foramen. The medial end of the petrous articulates with the body of the sphenoid and forms the lateral edge of the foramen lacerum, a lacerated or jagged hole.

In life, the foramen lacerum is closed by membrane. Its superior surface is crossed by the carotid artery, which travels a complicated course through and across the cranial bones. The carotid artery enters the cranium via the carotid canal on the inferior surface of the petrous. This canal runs superiorly for a few millimeters, about one-quarter of an inch, and turns at almost a right angle within the petrous. It proceeds medially and anteriorly toward the body of the sphenoid, where the artery leaves the enclosed canal and runs in the carotid groove. This close spatial association of the carotid artery and the hearing apparatus within the petrous accounts for the familiar sensation of hearing one's pulse when lying in a quiet room with one's ear against a pillow.

The inferior surface of the petrous bears four major features: the carotid canal, the jugular fossa, the stylomastoid foramen, and the styloid process, which is often missing. The carotid canal opens in a large, medially placed foramen. Medial to the carotid canal, the inferior surface of the petrous is roughened for articulation with the sphenoid. Posterolateral to the carotid canal is an even larger, spherical depression known as the jugular fossa. With the corresponding notch on the occipital, this fossa forms the jugular foramen, through which the jugular vein exits from the cranium. The stylomastoid foramen, a small, deep hole, lies posterolateral to the jugular fossa. Anterior to this foramen lies the styloid process, a fragile, elongated spine of bone that angles forward and downward from the petrous. From the styloid process comes the stylohyoid ligament that supports the hyoid bone in life. Because the hyoid anchors the muscles of the tongue, the presence of a styloid process has been linked with the capacity for speech. However, this process is often absent in crania of modern humans of perfectly normal speech capabilities. In fact, the styloid process may remain mostly cartilaginous until the age of about 40.

The posterior surface of the petrous shows two major features: the internal auditory meatus, also called the internal acoustic meatus, and part of the sigmoid sulcus. The internal auditory meatus is the large opening on this surface. Although it lies almost directly medial to the external auditory meatus and transmits several vessels and nerves from the internal ear to the brain, there is no patent, bony canal between the two. Lateral to the internal auditory meatus is a deep, broad groove that is part of the sigmoid sulcus that provides venous drainage for the brain.

The tympanic portion of the temporal bone, best seen in inferior view, is a small, curved sheet of bone that provides the inferior and posterior margins of the external auditory meatus. Anteriorly, the tympanic is separated from the squamous by the squamotympanic fissure. Medially, this fissure becomes the petrotympanic fissure. Posteriorly, the tympanomastoid fissure sets off the tympanic from the mastoid.

The temporal bone articulates with five other bones: the occipital posteriorly, the parietal superiorly, the sphenoid superoanteriorly, the zygomatic anteriorly, and the mandible inferiorly. The temporal ossifies from eight different centers. The squamous portion ossifies in membrane, like other tabular bones, from a single center that appears in the eighth week of fetal life. The petrous and mastoid portions ossify cartilaginously from four different centers that appear later, in the fifth and sixth fetal months; these fuse to each other to form the petromastoid region. The tympanic part is again membranous, its center beginning to ossify in about the third fetal month. The styloid process ossifies from two separate centers, which appear just before and just after birth. The upper part fuses to the petromastoid region during the first year of life; the lower portion fuses to the upper during adulthood.

The occipital is a large, dense bone that makes up both the posterior part of the cranium and most of its base (Figure 13-18). It consists of three major parts; the squamous, which comprises the back of the

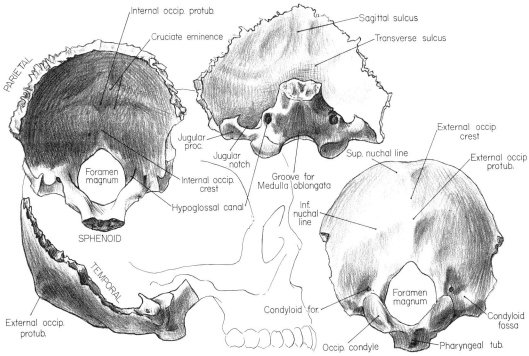

Figure 13-18

The occipital: *(clockwise from top left)* internal surface in superior view, internal surface in anteroinferior view, external surface in posteroinferior view, and lateral view and placement in the cranium.

cranium; the lateral or condylar, which lies lateral to the foramen magnum on the base of the cranium; and the basilar, which lies anterior to the foramen magnum on the base of the cranium.

The squamous part resembles the other vault bones in being tabular. Superiorly, the squamous part articulates with the two parietals along the lambdoid suture; the angle between the two parietals causes its distinctive triangular shape. The convex, external surface bears most superiorly the lambdoid suture, which is strongly interdigitated with the parietals and may include one or more small, irregular sutural bones. The lower third of the lambdoid suture, sometimes called the occipito-mastoid suture, articulates with the mastoid portion of the temporal, and this region of the suture is less deeply serrated than the upper two-thirds. Lying at midline about 5 cm (2 in) below the apex of the lambdoid suture is the external occipital protuberance. It is more pronounced in males than in females and may be somewhat hooked in populations of European descent. On either side of the external occipital protuberance is an arching, bony crest known as the superior nuchal line. Several important muscles of the neck and back, including the trapezius, attach to the superior nuchal line. Directly inferior to the external occipital protuberance is a bony ridge, the external occipital crest. About 4–5 cm (1.5–2″) inferior to the external occipital protuberance is the inferior nuchal line, which intersects the external occipital crest at a right angle. The point of intersection is often a raised, bony bump. Between the superior and inferior nuchal lines and along the lower margin of the inferior line a number of muscles attach to the cranium; these are important in maintaining the position and movement of the head and neck.

The internal surface of the squamous part of the occipital is also strongly marked, but by grooves for blood vessels and fossae for the brain rather than by muscle attachments. The internal surface is concave, to receive the posterior portions of the brain. A large, cross-shaped structure, the cruciate eminence, is apparent along the midline of the internal surface. The transverse members of the cruciate eminence are the transverse sulcus, which holds the transverse sinus in life. Its superior, vertical portion is comprised of the continuation of the sagittal sulcus that is also on the parietals. The inferior, vertical part of the cruciate eminence is a bony ridge, the internal occipital crest. At the point of intersection of the transverse and vertical members of the cruciate eminence is the internal occipital protuberance. Although the internal and external occipital crests correspond to each other in location, the internal occipital protuberance is often inferior to the external occipital protuberance. The cruciate eminence effectively divides the concave, internal surface of the squamous part into four fossae. The inferior two fossae are for the cerebellum, while the superior two fossae hold the occipital lobes of the cerebral hemisphere. This part of the occipital forms the posterior margin of the foramen magnum.

The lateral part of the occipital provides the lateral margin of the foramen magnum. Immediately lateral to the foramen magnum, and most readily observed on the external surface, is the condyloid foramen, which lies in a small depression called the condyloid fossa. On either side of the foramen, anterior to this fossa, is the occipital condyle. It bears an articular facet for the atlas that is approximately oval in outline. The long axis of each condyle runs from anteromedial to posterolateral. The articular surface is strongly convex along its long axis. Running anterolaterally within the bone just superior to each condyle is the hypoglossal canal, which carries the twelfth cranial nerve that controls movement of the tongue. Lateral to each condyle is a jugular process, anterior to which is a concavity known as the jugular notch. Together with the corresponding structure on the temporal, the jugular notch participates in forming the jugular foramen, through which the jugular vein exits the brain.

The basilar part of the occipital passes anteriorly to articulate with the sphenoid in the basilar suture. Its superior surface forms a broad, smooth groove for the medulla oblongata, a part of the brain stem. The inferior surface of the basilar part shows the pharyngeal tubercle at midline, to which some of the soft structures associated with speech and swallowing are attached.

The occipital bone, forming the entire posterior portion of the cranium, articulates with three other bones. Its squamous part articulates with the parietal along the superior portion of the lambdoid suture and with the temporal along the inferior portion of that suture. The lateral or condylar part meets the temporal in the petro-occipital suture. The basilar part articulates with the sphenoid anteriorly in the basilar suture. The occipital ossifies from three pairs of centers and from one center located at midline. All centers of ossification first appear at about the eighth fetal week. The squamous part superior to the highest nuchal line ossifies from one pair of centers; the squamous part inferior to that line ossifies from a separate pair of centers. Each condylar part ossifies from its own center, as does the basilar part. The two pairs of centers for the squamous part fuse to each other by the twelfth fetal week. The seven centers of ossification fuse to each other at 3–6 years; the basilar suture closes at 18–25 years.

THE BONY EAR

In life, each temporal bone also houses three ossicles: the malleus, incus, and stapes (Figure 13-19). Although the ear ossicles are so small that they are rarely found in fossil or archaeological sites, they are occasionally recovered from dirt or matrix that has filled the external auditory meatus of a skull.

The placement of these bones within the temporal is closely related to their function in transmitting sound waves. In life, the tympanic membrane lies within the auditory tube, the opening to which is the external auditory meatus. The tympanic membrane is angled within

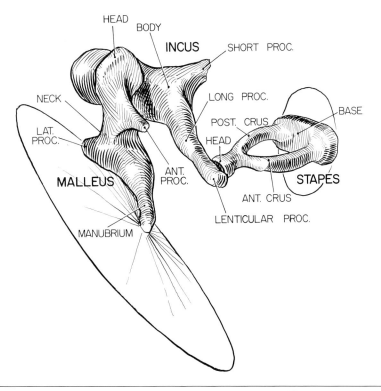

Figure 13-19

Bones of the ear in anterolateral view: the malleus embedded in the tympanic membrane, incus, and stapes.

the tube, so that its superior edge is lateral to its inferior edge. Sound waves coming down the tube cause the tympanic membrane to vibrate and transmit those vibrations mechanically to the ossicles.

The malleus, or hammer, is the first ear ossicle that receives these vibrations. It has a bulbous head at its superior end, set off by a constricted region called the neck. Projecting anteriorly from the neck is a small, pointed anterior process. Projecting from a point just inferior to the origin of the anterior process is a lateral or short process. The malleus continues inferiorly as the manubrium or handle, an elongated process that angles posteromedially. Both the manubrium and the lateral process are embedded in the tympanic membrane and thus directly receive any vibrations of that membrane. The posterior surface of the head of the malleus has a saddle-shaped articular surface for the incus, with which it forms the incudomallear joint.

The incus, or anvil, has a body and two processes, also called crura. The anterior surface of the body bears the articular surface for the malleus. The short process, or crus, is a thick, blunt-tipped pyramid that protrudes posteriorly from the body. The long process or crus projects inferiorly from the body and lies approximately parallel in course to the manubrium. At the tip of the long crus is the lenticular process, which projects medially and bears a rounded articular surface for the stapes.

The stapes is named for its resemblance to a stirrup. Its head, which lies lateral to the rest of the bone, bears a concave articular surface that participates in the ball-and-socket incudostapedial joint. Medial to the head is a constricted neck, from which arise the anterior and posterior crura. Each crus is curved, so that in medial view the head and two crura outline a semicircle. The crura are attached to the base or foot-plate, which is flat mediolaterally and has a kidney-shaped outline in medial view.

All three ear ossicles lie within a chamber, the tympanic cavity or middle ear, which is defined on five sides—anterior, posterior, superior, inferior, and medial—by the bone of the petrous portion of the temporal. On the sixth side the tympanic cavity is bounded by the tympanic membrane. Within the medial wall of the tympanic cavity is an opening, the fenestra vestibuli or oval window, that is closed by the base of the stapes. On the other side of the fenestra vestibuli lies the inner ear, which contains the fluid-filled membranes of both the cochlea, a spiral canal, and three semicircular canals. Only the cochlea is involved in hearing; the semicircular canals are involved in balance and sense of position.

As sound waves reach the tympanic membrane, they cause it to vibrate. These vibrations are transmitted directly to the malleus via the manubrium and lateral process. The chain of the three ossicles acts as a mechanical lever system. The elongated manubrium of the malleus and the long process of the incus increase the magnitude of the vibrations as they pass from malleus to incus to stapes. As the stapes moves in the fenestra vestibuli, it pushes on the incompressible fluid within the membrane-lined cochlea, creating waves of motion. The waves created by the stapes' movements bend tiny hairs projecting from hair cells within the cochlea, and the nervous impulse resulting from the bending of these hair cells is perceived as sound by the brain. Because the fluid in the cochlea is incompressible, each push of the stapes must be compensated for elsewhere in the system. This compensation is the role of another membrane-covered hole, the fenestra cochlea, which leads from the cochlea back into the tympanic cavity. Each push of the stapes terminates in a bulge of the membrane of the fenestra cochlea.

THE HYOID

The hyoid is the small, U-shaped bone found suspended in life from the stylohyoid ligaments. These ligaments run anteriorly and inferiorly from the styloid processes of the temporals on either side of the hyoid. The hyoid consists of an anteriorly convex body, two greater horns or cornua that project posterolaterally from the body, and two lesser horns that project superiorly at the junction of the greater horns and the body (Figure 13-20). The body is flattened anteroposteriorly. Its anterior surface is marked by a pair of bony ridges, one horizontal and one vertical, which form a cross at midline. At the center of the cross lies the median tubercle. Superior to the horizontal ridge is a large, depressed area of attachment for the geniohyoid muscle; inferior to it lie linear, horizontally oriented attachments for three other muscles of the tongue — the omohyoid, mylohyoid, and sternohyoid. The lesser horn projects superiorly and somewhat posteriorly from the superior edge of the body. The tip of the lesser horn bears the attachment of the stylohyoid ligament from the skull. The greater horns project posterolaterally and superiorly from the body. Along their lateral and superior surfaces the greater horns give attachment to many other muscles of the pharynx and tongue.

The hyoid undergoes cartilaginous ossification from six centers: two centers for the body and one for each horn. The centers for the greater horns appear first, ossifying just before birth. The centers for the body

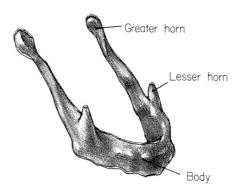

Figure 13-20

The hyoid in anterolateral view.

ossify shortly after birth, and those for the lesser horns ossify at puberty. Fusion of the different centers of the hyoid to each other occurs in middle life or later.

METRIC COMPARISONS

To describe and compare skulls metrically, both a standardized plane and a set of standardized points are used. The standardized plane, called the Frankfurt horizontal, is the position of the skull or cranium in which a line drawn from the lowest point on the inferior orbital margin (orbitale) to the most superior point of the external auditory meatus (porion) is horizontal. There are many standardized osteometric points on the skull, which are best observed from different aspects (Figure 13-21).

In anterior view, there are five osteometric points along the midline of the cranium: bregma, glabella, nasion, nasospinale, and alveolare. Bregma occurs at the intersection of the coronal and sagittal sutures. Glabella is the most anteriorly placed point between the superciliary arches. Nasion lies at the intersection of the frontal suture and the suture between the two nasal bones. Nasospinale is at the intersection of an imaginary line joining the two most inferior points of the nasal aperture margin with midline. Alveolare is the most inferior point of the alveolar margin between the upper central incisors.

The mandible's midline bears two other osteometric points in anterior view: infradentale and gnathion. Infradentale, the equivalent of alveolare, is the most superior point of the alveolar margin between the lower central incisors. Gnathion lies at the lower margin of the mandible at midline.

Lateral to the midline and still in anterior view, there are seven paired osteometric points: frontotemporale, dacryon, ectoconchion, orbitale, zygomaxillare, alare, and mentale. Frontotemporale is the most medial point of the temporal line. Dacryon is the conjunction of the frontal, maxillary, and lacrimal bones on the medial wall of the orbit. Ectoconchion is the most lateral point of the lateral orbital margin. Orbitale is the lowest point of the inferior orbital margin. Zygomaxillare is the most inferior point of the zygomaticomaxillary suture. Alare is the most lateral point of the nasal margin. Mentale occurs at the most anterior point on the margin of the mental foramen.

In lateral view, there are six osteometric points: vertex, apex, porion, asterion, mastoidale, and gonion. The most superior point along the mid-sagittal plane, with the skull in the Frankfurt horizontal, is vertex, which may or may not coincide with bregma. Apex is the point on the

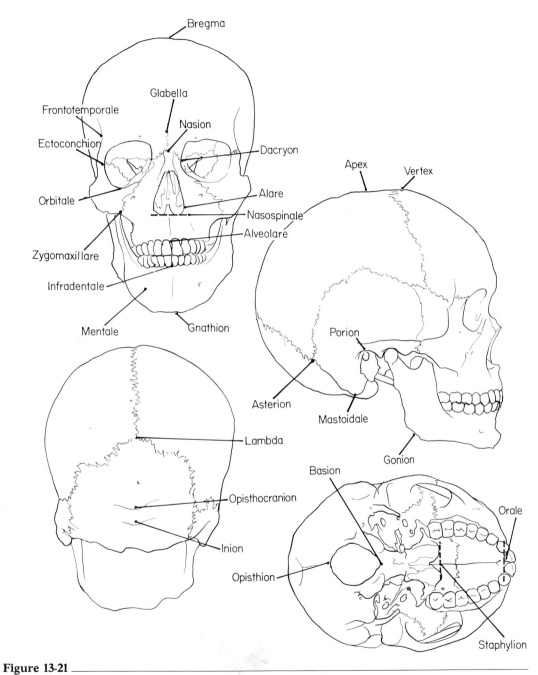

Figure 13-21

Osteometric landmarks on the skull: *(clockwise from top left)* anterior, lateral, inferior, and posterior view.

sagittal suture that lies directly superior to porion when the skull is in the Frankfurt horizontal. Porion, one of the points that define the Frankfurt horizontal, is the highest point on the margin of the external auditory meatus. Asterion occurs at the junction of the sutures between the temporal, parietal, and occipital bones. Mastoidale is the most inferior point on the mastoid process. Gonion is the most lateral point on the gonial angle, at the end of an imaginary line that bisects the angle formed by a tangent to the posterior margin of the mandibular ramus and a tangent to the inferior margin of the mandibular corpus.

In posterior view there are three osteometric points: lambda, opisthocranion, and inion. Lambda is the junction of the sagittal and lambdoid sutures. Opisthocranion is the most posterior point on the cranium, excepting the external occipital protuberance. This point is defined not by anatomical landmarks but by measurement. Inion is at the base of the external occipital protuberance at midline.

In inferior view, there are four osteometric points: orale, staphylion, basion, and opisthion. Orale is the most anterior, lying on the midpoint of an imaginary line joining the most posterior points on the alveoli on the upper central incisors. Staphylion occurs at the intersection of midline with an imaginary line joining the most anterior points in the curvature of the posterior margin of the bony palate. Basion is the midpoint of the anterior margin of the foramen magnum. Opisthion is the midline of the posterior margin of the foramen magnum.

Some of the more common cranial measurements are (after Brothwell, 1981:82):

Maximum cranial length	Glabella to opisthocranion, taken in median sagittal plane
Maximum breadth or width	Greatest breadth from parietal to parietal, taken perpendicular to sagittal plane and avoiding supramastoid crest
Basion-bregmatic height	Basion to bregma
Basion-nasal length	Basion to nasion
Upper facial height	Nasion to alveolare
Bimaxillary breadth	Zygomaxillare to zygomaxillare
Bizygomatic breadth	Maximum breadth between outer surfaces of zygomatic arches
Nasal height	Nasion to nasospinale
Nasal breadth	Alare to alare
Orbital breadth	Dacryon to ectoconchion
Palatal length	Staphylion to orale
Palatal breadth	Middle of lingual alveolar margin of M^2 on one side to same point on other side

14
CHEWING

Although chewing, or mastication, is not the only important function involving the bones of the skull, it is the one most closely related to the size and placement of the major muscles of the skull. These muscles, which leave distinct markings on the bones of the skull, are involved in moving the mandible relative to the fixed cranium in a controlled and regular pattern. Although the cranium also moves relative to a fixed mandible during mastication, this action is of a lesser magnitude than its converse. Similar movements of the mandible and cranium are undertaken during speech. Speech is a function that developed more recently in human evolution than chewing; apparently, it usurped the actions and patterns of movement of the older system.

THE TEMPORO-MANDIBULAR JOINT

The temporomandibular joint (TMJ) is a synovial joint between the convex condyle of the mandible and the concave glenoid fossa of the temporal (Figure 14-1). The articular tubercle and post-glenoid tubercle of the temporal also participate in the TMJ. A fibrous articular disc is interposed between the glenoid and the condyle, dividing the TMJ into a superior and an inferior joint compartment. Because there are two separate compartments in the TMJ, separate movements can occur simultaneously. The disc is attached along its circumference to the articular capsule. The capsule is loose but is reinforced by several extracapsular ligaments. Dislocation of the mandible is almost always bilateral and occurs in an anterior direction, when the condyle passes the apex of the articular tubercle and comes to rest anterior to it.

The curvature of the glenoid and reciprocal curvature of the condyle dictate that the major movement of the mandible is a hinging action that occurs along a transverse, horizontal axis passing through both condyles. This hinging movement results in elevation and depression of the mandible. However, these are not the only movements at the TMJ. The mandible may also be protruded or moved anteriorly and retracted or moved posteriorly, both of which actions involve a gliding motion. Finally, lateral movements are possible, in which the mandible is

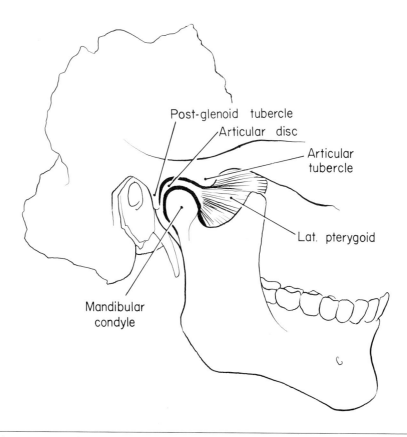

Figure 14-1

The temporomandibular joint, with the lateral wall of the joint capsule removed and the mandible in resting position. The articular disc divides the joint into two compartments, one superior *(black area inferior to glenoid)* and the other inferior *(black area superior to mandibular condyle)*, in which separate movements can occur.

skewed to one side or the other. Such movements are also accomplished by gliding movements. In life, these different actions — elevation or depression, protrusion or retraction, and lateral movements — are often combined.

MUSCLES OF MASTICATION

Five muscles are primarily responsible for producing movements of the mandible: the temporalis, masseter, lateral pterygoid, medial pterygoid, and digastric. The origin and insertion of each muscle determine its action on the mandible. Each of

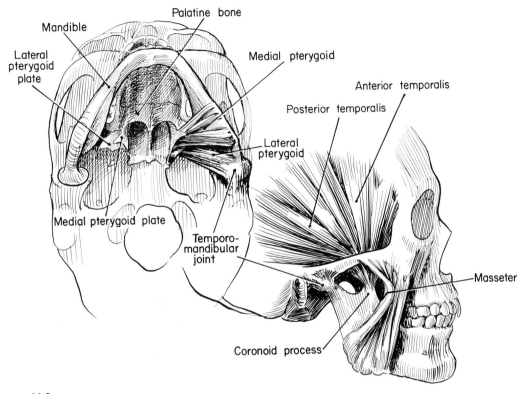

Figure 14-2 ———————————————————————————————————

The muscles of mastication: *(left)* lateral and medial pterygoid muscles in inferior view and *(right)* temporalis and masseter muscles in lateral view.

these muscles is paired and can be found on both the right and left sides of the skull.

Elevation and retraction are produced by the temporalis, a large, fan-shaped muscle that lies on the lateral side of the cranium (Figure 14-2). Its origin is from a large oval outlined in part by the temporal line along the frontal, the sphenoid, and occasionally parts of the zygomatic. The muscle fibers converge on an anteriorly placed apex that passes medial to the zygomatic arch. The temporalis inserts upon the coronoid process of the mandible, and some fibers from the anterior temporalis insert on the anterior margin of the ramus. Thus, the posterior fibers of the temporalis exert an upward and backward pull upon the coronoid when contracted, while the anterior fibers pull directly upward. Since the condyle cannot move inferiorly to any great extent because of the strength of the TMJ capsule, elevation of the mandible actually constitutes pivoting the corpus of the mandible upward around an axis that passes through the TMJ. If both temporalis muscles are contracted simultaneously, this pivoting action occurs without displacing the mandible laterally. However, if only one temporalis is contracted, the mandible is displaced slightly to that side. Although the temporalis muscle as a whole elevates the mandible from a depressed position, the posterior fibers, when contracted alone, move the mandible in a posterior direction.

The masseter is also an elevator of the mandible. It arises from the inferior margin and medial surface of both the zygomatic and temporal portions of the zygomatic arch. The thick, quadrilateral muscle belly passes inferiorly and posteriorly to insert on the lateral surface of the gonial angle and adjacent areas of the ramus. Because of the orientation of its fibers, the masseter tends to pull the mandible upward and forward when contracted. Like the temporalis, contraction of the masseter may be symmetrical or asymmetrical, and the asymmetrical action tends to skew the mandible to one side.

The lateral and medial pterygoid muscles are responsible for protrusion. The lateral pterygoid arises from two heads, an upper and an inferior. The upper head arises from the lateral surface and the infratemporal crest of the greater wing of the sphenoid. The inferior head, which is larger, originates from the lateral side of the lateral pterygoid plate of the sphenoid. The fibers from both heads run posteriorly and laterally to insert on the capsule of the TMJ, the articular disc of the condyle, and the neck of the condyle. The primary action of the lateral pterygoid is to protrude the mandible by pulling the condyle forward toward the pterygoid plates. Contraction of only one of the lateral pterygoids results in a combination of protrusion and lateral movement, toward the side that the muscle is on.

The medial pterygoid is the most effective muscle for producing lateral movements of the mandible. It also arises from two heads, one deep and the other superficial. The deep head is larger and originates from the medial side of the lateral pterygoid plate; thus, the inferior head of the lateral pterygoid and the deep head of the medial pterygoid arise from opposite surfaces of the lateral plate. The superficial head arises from the pyramidal process of the palatine and from the tuberosity on the infratemporal surface of the maxilla. The medial pterygoid passes almost directly laterally and somewhat downward to insert on the medial, or internal, surface of the gonial angle and adjacent part of the ramus. Thus, the insertion of the medial pterygoid lies on the

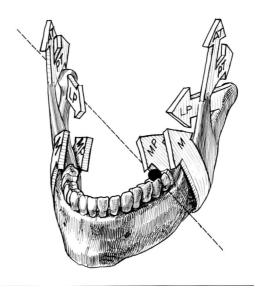

Figure 14-3 Action of the major muscles of the mandible in molar chewing: the anterior temporalis *(AT)*, posterior temporalis *(PT)*, lateral pterygoid *(LP)*, medial pterygoid *(MP)*, and masseter *(M)*. The axis of movement *(dotted line)* passes through the right condyle on the balancing side and the left M_1, where the food *(black dot)* lies at the bite point.

opposite surface of the mandible from the masseter. When the cranium is fixed relative to the mandible, the result of contracting one medial pterygoid is to pull that side of the mandible upward and toward midline, thereby laterally displacing the opposite side of the mandible. Contraction of both medial pterygoids resists lateral movement of the mandible but contributes to elevation of the posterior portions of the mandible.

These four muscles—the temporalis, masseter, lateral pterygoid, and medial pterygoid—move the mandible upward, forward, backward, and from side to side (Figure 14-3). The mandible moves downward mostly as a result of the action of gravity. That is, the temporalis is in almost constant, mild contraction to keep the mandible elevated and the mouth closed. Cessation of this contraction results in depression of the mandible. In addition, two muscles participate in depression, the lateral pterygoid and the digastric. Because the origin of the lateral pterygoid is inferior to its insertion, it produces depression of the mandible to a limited extent. Forceful depression, as in opening the mouth widely, is produced by the digastric.

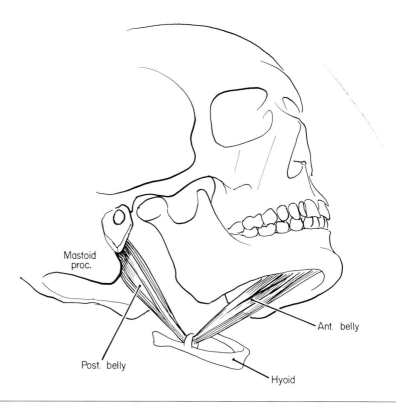

Figure 14-4 _____

The digastric muscle in inferolateral view. It depresses the mandible.

The digastric muscle follows a complicated course (Figure 14-4). It has two fleshy bellies, the posterior and anterior, joined together by a tendon. Unlike some muscles, the digastric muscle does not have a terminal tendon at its insertion but rather has its tendon in the middle. The posterior belly of the digastric arises from the digastric groove that lies just medial to the mastoid process. This belly passes medially, anteriorly, and inferiorly beneath the cranium, toward the hyoid. The posterior belly of the digastric lies just lateral to the greater horn of the hyoid, where it becomes tendinous. The tendon passes through a loop of fibers that hold it close to the greater horn but permit it to slide forward and backward. The anterior belly of the digastric begins anterior to this loop and runs anteriorly to attach to the digastric fossa near midline on the posterior, internal surface of the mandible. When the digastric contracts, the symphyseal region of the mandible is pulled strongly downward and backward, toward the hyoid.

MASTICATION

These muscles combine to produce the regular patterns of mandibular movement that characterize chewing. Chewing occurs in two different modes, incisal and molar, which are named according to the location of the food or other item being processed.

Incisal chewing is a symmetrical action in which the incisors are used to nip or bite off a piece of food (Figure 14-5). Muscles on both sides of the skull act with their partners. The masticatory cycle begins from the resting position, in which the mouth is shut with the molars held lightly in occlusion, or in contact with each other. The lower incisors are typically placed posterior to the upper incisors, and the condyles are centered within the glenoid fossae. Opening the mouth is the first action.

The chewing cycle involves three motions: an opening stroke, power stroke, and closing stroke. In the opening stroke, the mandible is protruded so that the condyles slide forward onto the articular eminences. This action is accomplished by relaxing the temporalis and masseter, to let the mandible drop passively downward, and contracting both lateral pterygoids simultaneously. Because protruding the mandible brings the condyles forward and downward onto the articular eminences, the molars, which were formerly in occlusion, are disengaged.

The power stroke, which brings the upper and lower incisors together edge-to-edge, involves maintaining the protrusion of the mandible while elevating its anterior portion. The lateral and medial pterygoids thus continue to contract while the temporalis and masseter on each side are also contracted. This series of contractions brings the incisors together, slicing through the food, but keeps the molars from engaging.

The closing stroke brings the mandible back to resting position. This involves a relaxation of the masseter and the two pairs of pterygoids. The mandible is retracted by contracting the posterior temporalis fibers. The three strokes blend into a continuous movement. In mastication, as in other muscular activities, muscles fire not only as the action for which they are responsible is produced but also as the opposite action is initiated. An important function of any muscle is to act as an antagonist during the transfer from one action to its opposite, so as to prevent abrupt or jerky movements.

Molar chewing differs from incisal biting in that it is asymmetrical. That is, most people chew their food in a discrete bolus, or lump, that is processed on only one side of the mouth at a time. People often have a preferred side for chewing, which may reflect differences in occlusion.

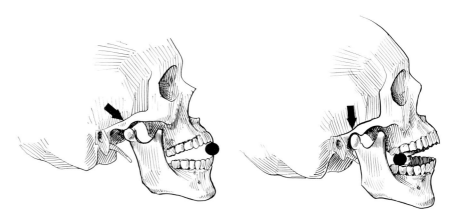

Figure 14-5

Incisal and molar chewing. *(Left)* Incisal chewing is a symmetrical action. The food *(black dot)* lies between the incisors; both condyles are held forward on the articular eminences to absorb the reaction force of biting. *(Right)* Molar chewing is asymmetrical. The food *(black dot)* lies between the right molars, so the right condyle is in the mandibular fossa. The right side is thus the working side. Arrows highlight the change in condyle position.

As a result, in any chewing cycle, there is a working side and a balancing side. The working side is where the food is located; it is also the side upon which the bite force, which deforms the food, is applied. The balancing side has little or no food between its upper and lower molars. Instead, it absorbs the resultant force of the bite, or balances the bite force.

A force that needs balancing is created because the mandible is held in a muscular sling beneath the cranium. If one side, the working side, is pulled forward and downward onto the articular eminence, the other side must in reaction move backward and upward to dissipate the force. This phenomenon expresses the basic physical principle that every force must be balanced by an equal and opposite force. The resultant force is not taken on the glenoid fossa, for the simple reason that the bone of the glenoid both lies directly below the brain and is so thin as to be translucent in anatomical specimens. Such an area is not appropriate for absorbing forces of any magnitude, and bite forces on first molars have been measured at over 100 kg (220 lbs).

The molar chewing cycle illustrates the position of the balancing side condyle during the power stroke, when the resultant force must be absorbed. The initial part of the opening stroke is identical to that in incisal chewing. As the mandible is depressed and protruded, both condyles slide forward onto their articular eminences. Once the mouth is open, however, the working and balancing sides undergo different actions. The working side lateral pterygoid is relaxed, which brings its condyle back into the glenoid fossa and skews the mandible slightly to that side. The balancing side lateral pterygoid continues to contract, holding that condyle forward on the articular eminence. In addition, the medial pterygoid of the balancing side contracts, displacing the mandible even farther toward the working side

The power stroke begins with the contraction of the medial pterygoid on the working side; this action brings the mandible back toward midline. At the same time, the masseters and temporalis muscles on both sides are contracted. The result is that the mandible moves medially and upward simultaneously in a movement that shears and crushes the food between the working side molars. During this stroke, the balancing side condyle remains forward on the dense, articular eminence which absorbs the resultant force.

In the closing stroke, the lateral pterygoid on the balancing side relaxes, allowing that condyle to return to the glenoid fossa. Both masseters and the working side medial pterygoid also relax. The mandible is in the resting position once again, maintained by a slight action of the temporalis.

Molar chewing has two characteristic features. First, the resultant force is taken by the balancing side condyle while it is held forward on the dense bone of the articular eminence. This fact satisfies logic, which dictates that the area absorbing a resultant force will build up extra bone. It also explains why people who have broken the neck of their mandibular condyle chew on the broken side, whereas those with abscessed teeth chew on the healthy side. In the former case, the person makes the injured side the working side, since no force is transmitted through that condyle. In the latter case, the person makes the injured side the balancing side, since no force is transmitted through the teeth on that side. The second characteristic of molar chewing is that the power stroke both shears and crushes the food, due to the asymmetrical contraction of the masticatory muscles. This fact explains how food particles are reduced to an acceptable size for swallowing.

PART THREE
INTERPRETING
BONES

15
AGE, SEX, RACE, AND STATURE

One of the chief reasons for studying skeletal materials is that they present a wealth of biological information about the individuals and populations from which they were drawn. Skeletal remains make it possible to trace patterns of disease and nutrition, evaluate the effects of social or economic changes, and deduce patterns of reproduction and mortality. Such study relies on four basic points of information about the individuals represented in a sample: age, sex, race, and height.

To estimate age and height or to identify sex and race from skeletal remains, statistical procedures must be used. Any deduction about age, sex, race, or stature is in reality a probability statement, based on comparing the unknown skeletal remains with a set of known individuals. The accuracy of the deduction depends upon the size and appropriateness of the reference population used. Human variability is enormous, as can be verified in any public place, and there are no simple, certain criteria for positively determining the age, sex, race, or height of an individual from skeletal remains. However, painstaking work with large collections of individuals of known attributes has revealed guidelines and clues that are statistically diagnostic. Thus, for example, it is possible to say that the maximum stature of an American female with a 348-mm long femur is about 140 cm tall (55 in), or that individuals with an ischium-pubis index greater than 100 are almost certainly female.

Two consequences follow from the use of statistical procedures. One is that large skeletal populations are more readily diagnosed than individual skeletons. As a general rule, males have more robust skeletons than females, although males of one population may be lighter, shorter, and less heavily muscled than females of another population with a different lifestyle. Population variability in a skeletal population can be intuitively appreciated by setting out the same bone, such as the femur, from a large number of individuals before beginning a detailed, bone-by-bone analysis. The overall accuracy of estimating age and size or determining sex and race is improved by a thorough knowledge of the general population from which the skeletal remains are drawn. Seriation, or arranging individuals in order of increasing relative age, greatly facilitates accurate estimation of individual ages within a population.

The other consequence of statistical procedures is that the accuracy of such identifications improves dramatically if whole or nearly whole skeletons are available for study rather than isolated bones. That is, the sex of an individual can be determined with high accuracy from an entire skeleton and with considerably less accuracy from a single bone. In general, the more complete is the skeletal material, the more reliable are the inferences drawn from that material.

Furthermore, as a result of biological reality more than of statistics, particular bones or regions of the skeleton are extremely reliable indicators of a given trait or attribute, while others are effectively useless. For example, the pelvis contains the most useful bones in determining sex, because the demands of childbirth have placed major constraints on female pelvic form and shape, whereas the vertebrae are considerably less useful. Similarly, because humans have two sets of teeth, deciduous and permanent, and because individual teeth erupt or break through the gum at different ages, mandibles and maxillae can be especially useful in estimating age if the individual in question was dentally immature.

Age at death can be estimated with variable accuracy according to the general age range into which the individual falls. Age can be estimated more accurately in young individuals, in whom not all epiphyses are fused and not all teeth are erupted, than in older individuals. Although age in young people and even in middle-aged adults can be estimated with a reasonable degree of accuracy, it is very difficult to determine age in individuals older than about 50. The problem of determining age in older individuals may distort demographic patterns and conclusions drawn from such data.

The different attributes of age, sex, race, and stature have a tremendous influence on each other. For example, age affects indicators of sex, so that determining the sex of skeletons of prepubescent individuals is notoriously difficult, because the hormonal spurt responsible for both puberty and sexual differentiation in the skeleton has yet to occur. Similarly, race affects indicators of age, in that skeletal maturation may be accelerated or retarded by genetic factors that vary in different ethnic groups. These distinctions in maturation rates are blurred both by the extent of racial admixture and by differences in nutritional and health status.

The determination of race poses a special problem because of the difficulty of defining the term. Biologically, a race is viewed as a morphologically recognizable subset of a species. By implication, races represent imperfectly isolated breeding populations in which particular complexes of genes, and hence of phenotypic characters, co-occur in higher frequencies than elsewhere. The human species contains a small number of biological races, among them the Caucasoid, Negroid, and Mongoloid stocks, which were originally associated with particular geographic areas. Less technically, the term *race* applies to small cultural groups, such as tribes. These local races are difficult to identify, although biological "distances," or degrees of relatedness, among skeletal populations from a single region and time period have been estimated by using multivariate statistics. Racial designations based on skeletal morphology and geography, however, have little to do with the self-identified race of individuals. In common usage, race is defined primarily on the basis of social or ethnic affiliation and, secondarily, on the basis of details of appearance, such as color and texture of hair or skin, and of recent ancestry. But in fact, siblings of the same parents may differ widely in the expression of these soft-tissue attributes, even though they have identical ethnic backgrounds.

Neither ethnicity nor soft-tissue attributes are useful modes of racial identification in dealing with skeletal material. There are no skeletal attributes that are population-specific or reliably correlate with soft-tissue or cultural traits; there are only skeletal attributes that occur more commonly, but not exclusively, in particular groups. Both metric and nonmetric traits of skeletons are associated with different races, which enable probability statements to be made about ancestry. However, many skeletons possess features "typical" of two or more racial groups. The limitations of racial determination are illustrated by the studies on skeletal attributes of Negroid populations that have been conducted on Americans designated as "black" during their lifetime. The vast majority of blacks in the United States are descended from slave populations shipped to the New World from Africa. But members of different African tribes, Caucasoid or "white" inhabitants of the New World, and American Indians indigenous to the New World all interbred extensively. The result is that "American blacks" are an admixture of several different racial stocks and are skeletally difficult to differentiate. Often they are morphologically distinct from Africans in areas subjected to less admixture. The crux of the problem is that determining the ancestry or race of skeletal remains is likely to be important only in areas that historically have been subjected to a high degree of racial admixture. In areas with no radical admixture, the race of skeletal remains is a moot point.

Finally, the comparative skeletal data that are available for estimating age or size and for determining race of sex pose a problem. Some populations are better-known and hence better-documented than others. In most cases, data on males are more numerous than data on females. This bias occurs because some of the largest skeletal studies have been performed on individuals killed in war, most of whom are male. Other biases relate to the availability of material. American whites and American blacks, who are more correctly considered ethnic rather than racial groups, are better known than European Caucasoids, Africans, or any of a wide variety of other peoples. The use of standards derived from a different group should be avoided whenever possible. However, in many cases, if skeletal materials are to be analyzed at all, a pragmatic decision must be made to use the most nearly appropriate standards, because no suitable data on the most appropriate population are available.

Once skeletal remains have been encountered, the process of identifying and analyzing them begins. This process involves two tasks. The first task is to remove the remains to an appropriate location for study without either damaging them or losing important contextual and spatial information. The second task is to sort mixed skeletal remains into individuals. This sorting is often performed first on the basis of skeletal maturity. Other criteria for sorting individuals out of a mixed collection of bones are spatial association, color, state of preservation, general size, robustness, congruency of articulations and occlusal surfaces, and individual anomalies. Only after removal and sorting are complete can the appropriate, detailed analysis be performed. Whether skeletons are whole or highly fragmented, it is possible to estimate the minimum number of individuals represented and to record evidence of age, sex, race, and stature.

ESTIMATION OF AGE

There are three broad categories of information from which to estimate age: the amount of growth, the stage of development, and the extent of degeneration (Stewart, 1979). The first category, the amount of growth in different skeletal elements, is a useful indicator of age during the fetal period and the first few years after birth.

Fetal and infant remains are infrequently recovered from forensic, archaeological, or paleontological contexts, but when found, they can be assigned ages based on the length of the diaphyses of the major long bones (Figure 15-1). This procedure is accomplished in two steps. First, fetal stature is estimated from the maximum diaphyseal length by using regression equations derived from individuals of known stature. The mathematical relationship between stature and diaphyseal length of the femur is shown as a regression line that best describes the distribution of points. For the other major long bones, the equations used to estimate fetal stature are (Olivier and Pineau, 1960):

Fetal stature = (7.92) × (diaphyseal length of the humerus)
    − 0.32 ± 1.8cm

Fetal stature = (13.8) × (diaphyseal length of the radius)
    − 2.85 ± 1.62cm

Fetal stature = (8.73) × (diaphyseal length of the ulna)
    − 1.07 ± 1.59cm

Fetal stature = (7.39) × (diaphyseal length of the tibia)
    + 3.55 ± 1.92cm

Fetal stature = (7.85) × (diaphyseal length of the fibula)
    + 2.78 ± 1.65cm

In the second step, estimated fetal stature is used to estimate fetal age in lunar months since conception. Each lunar month is defined as 28 days long. This step is also based upon data from individuals of known age (Olivier and Pineau, 1958).

Fetal stature	Age in lunar months	Fetal stature	Age in lunar months
17.65	4.25	37.85	7.25
19.81	4.5	39.13	7.5
21.88	4.75	40.37	7.75
23.8	5.0	41.58	8.0
25.64	5.25	42.74	8.25
27.4	5.5	43.84	8.5
29.08	5.75	44.97	8.75
30.60	6.0	46.03	9.0
32.23	6.25	47.07	9.25
33.72	6.5	48.08	9.5
35.15	6.75	49.06	9.75
36.52	7.0	50.02	10.0

Although diaphyseal length correlates well and linearly with stature, and stature correlates well and linearly with age, the accuracy of the estimation of age is much less than the accuracy of either of the individual steps in the calculations. This difficulty arises because the accu-

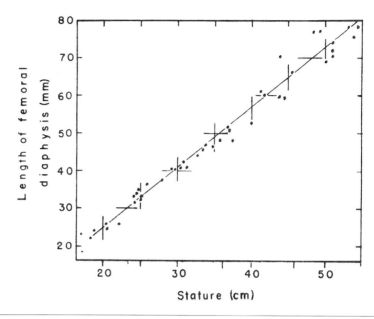

Stature and crown-rump length plotted against length of fetal femoral diaphyses. The horizontal and vertical lines show 10-cm increments in stature. The regression line shows the relationship between stature and femoral diaphysis length.

racy of two sequential calculations is equal to the product of the accuracy of each of those calculations. For example, if each step is 80% accurate, the combination of the two steps is only 64% accurate.

Growth curves have been constructed from protohistoric American Indian remains by plotting maximum diaphyseal lengths of major long bones against age at death as estimated from dental remains of subadults, or individuals who have not yet reached skeletal adulthood. Although such a procedure lacks an external verification of the absolute ages of the individuals involved, it provides a useful means of establishing relative ages within an extinct population. Similarly, modern dental eruption sequences of humans and apes have been applied to extinct hominoid species to provide relative age estimates for subadult individuals. The resulting estimates, such as "individual X is judged to have been 6 years old at death," mean simply that individual X had reached a state of skeletal maturity best matched in modern six-year-olds, however long it may have taken individual X to arrive at that state.

The stage of development exhibited by a set of skeletal remains from one individual provides another good indication of age at death. Both teeth and various long bones are commonly used to estimate age, because different teeth erupt and various epiphyses fuse at different times during an individual's life. Lovejoy and colleagues show that age estimates are significantly more accurate if the results of many different age indicators are combined.

Because teeth are usually well-preserved, dental remains are extremely useful in estimating age. In this regard, it is fortunate that humans normally have two sets of teeth in their lifetime: a deciduous or milk dentition and a permanent or adult dentition. Deciduous dentitions have fewer teeth than adults (5 on each side, upper and lower, versus 8 in adults); this fact correlates with the smaller size of the mandible and maxilla in children. A complete deciduous dentition has the formula $\frac{2.1.0.2.}{2.1.0.2}$. Only incisors, canines, and molars are present in deciduous dentitions; premolars are absent. This reflects the anatomical reality that the milk teeth resemble the adult incisors, canines, and molars, not the premolars. However, deciduous molars are replaced not by permanent molars but by permanent premolars; permanent molars erupt distal to the premolars. The standard notation system is modified to describe deciduous teeth. The letter designating a deciduous tooth is lower case, not capitalized, and it is preceded by a "d." Thus, for example, di_1 indicates a deciduous lower central incisor.

Deciduous teeth can be distinguished from permanent teeth by several features. They are usually smaller than permanent teeth, since enamel does not grow after eruption. They often have thinner enamel, which makes them appear translucent and yellower in color. Finally, deciduous teeth often lack roots or have open roots, because these are dissolved away as the permanent tooth moves toward the occlusal plane to erupt.

Not all teeth erupt simultaneously. The timing of the formation and eruption of each set varies from individual to individual, but it usually follows a standard sequence (Figure 15-2). Although tooth germs begin to form in the maxilla and mandible in utero, humans are born without any visible teeth. Between 6 and 9 months after birth the first teeth break through the gums; these are almost invariably the central incisors. For each tooth there is a time lag between eruption and the onset of wear, that is, when it comes into occlusion.

Eruption of di1 is followed by the eruption of di2 at about one year, dm1 and dc at about 18 months, and dm2 at two years. Starting at about age 6, the first permanent tooth appears; this is the first molar,

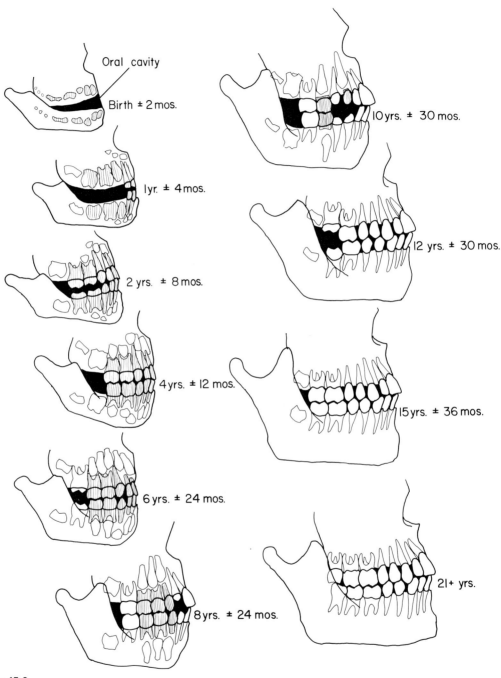

Figure 15-2

Dental eruption sequence from birth to adulthood. Shaded teeth are deciduous.

which erupts distal to dm2. Between the age of 6 and dental adulthood, at about age 18, permanent teeth erupt in the sequence: M1, I1, I2, P3, P4, C, M2, M3. The variation in eruption time provides a key to estimating age from dental remains, although there is a long time lag between the eruption of M2 at about 12 years and the eruption of M3 at 18–21 years.

The identification of individual, isolated teeth is equally important to the estimation of age. But whereas it is relatively easy to "count" teeth emplaced in a mandible or maxilla and to identify them, it is more difficult to recognize isolated teeth. The basic classes of teeth—incisors, canines, premolars, and molars—have distinctive traits that can be used to identify them, whether in adult or in deciduous dentitions.

Anatomically, all teeth share common features (Figure 15-3). Each has a crown, the portion of the tooth that is visible in life and actually does the chewing or cutting, and one or more roots, the elongated projections that hold the tooth in the alveolus. The neck of the tooth is the constricted region at the junction of the crown and the root. The pulp cavity is a chamber within the tooth that contains nerves and vessels in life. At the base of each root is a small hole through which those nerves and vessels enter the tooth.

All teeth are comprised of two basic substances: enamel and dentin. Enamel is the shiny, hard, white material that covers the crown. It is formed of many elongated, calcified prisms stacked in a geometrically complex pattern and covered externally by an amorphous layer called the cuticle. The prisms are separated from each other by interprismatic substance. Dentin is the softer, yellowish material that underlies the enamel in the crown and forms the root. The surface of dentin, when magnified, shows many tubules surrounded by a ring of peritubular matrix; between these sets of rings lies the intertubular matrix. A third tissue, cementum, which is related to bone, cements the root to the surrounding alveolar bone.

Teeth do not enlarge in size once they have been formed. In fact, no more enamel can be laid down, once formation is complete, although dentin formation can continue throughout life. New dentin formed during life does not and cannot enlarge the structure underlying the crown; it grows within the pulp cavity, slowly diminishing the cavity's size and repairing damage due to caries or trauma. Primary dentin, the dentin laid down during tooth formation, is chemically different from secondary dentin, the dentin formed later in life.

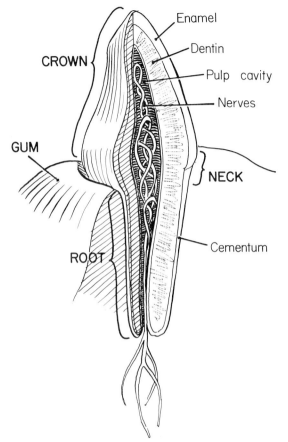

CROWN

GUM

ROOT

Enamel
Dentin
Pulp cavity
Nerves
NECK
Cementum

Figure 15-3

Parts of the tooth in a sectioned incisor.

The fact that more dentin can be formed and more enamel cannot is due to differences between amelogenesis, or enamel formation, and odontogenesis, or dentin formation. Dental tissues, like bone, are formed by specialized cells, called ameloblasts and odontoblasts. These cells secrete the organic matrix of enamel and dentin respectively. In the developing tooth bud, these cells appear in two adjacent layers. The cell layer closest to the surface gives rise to ameloblasts, and the layer farthest from the surface gives rise to odontoblasts. Once the tooth is formed, this junction is known as the dentinoenamel junction (DEJ). The two types of cells then proceed to grow away or migrate from their shared junction, laying down organic material as they go.

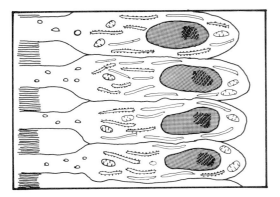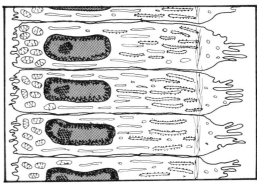

Figure 15-4

Dental cells. Nuclei are darkly hatched structures; short oval structures are mitochondria; and elongate oval structures are rough endoplasmic reticulum *(studded
perimeters)* or Golgi apparati *(plain perimeters)*. The DEJ is in the middle. *(Left)*
Odontoblasts are responsible for producing dentin. Dentin's organic matrix is
secreted by the Tomes' fiber located at the opposite end of the cell from the
nucleus. *(Right)* Ameloblasts are responsible for producing enamel. Enamel's organic matrix is secreted by the conical Tomes' process located at the opposite end
of the cell from the nucleus.

Ameloblasts are long, narrow, roughly rectangular cells derived
from epithelium (Figure 15-4). The large nucleus and many mitochondria tend to cluster at the end nearest the surface; at the other end, the
elongated Tomes' process is found, along with many secretion granules containing material that appears opaque under the electron microscope. The Tomes' process is cylindrical in shape. As ameloblasts
migrate away from the DEJ toward the tooth surface, the Tomes'
processes release the organic matrix of enamel from their surfaces.
Mineralization involves the deposition of apatite crystallites within the
organic matrix, at right angles to their bodies. The adjacent areas
between the Tomes' processes secrete the interprismatic substance.
Amelogenesis stops when the ameloblasts arrive at what will be the
outside of the tooth, at which point they lay down an amorphous layer
of enamel and then die. Thus, no more enamel can be made in a
formed tooth because no more ameloblasts are present.

In contrast, odontoblasts migrate away from the DEJ toward the
pulp cavity, where their cell bodies remain throughout life. An odontoblast is also an elongate, narrow cell with a long, narrow process,
called the Tomes' fiber, protruding from the end closest to the DEJ.
The Tomes' fiber also has smaller, lateral branches protruding from it

in all directions. The large nucleus of the odontoblast resides in its base. Each Tomes' fiber secretes a peritubular matrix around itself, so that it comes to lie within a dentinal tubule. Its lateral branches also apparently secrete the intertubular matrix. Calcification occurs along a calcifying front that typically shows a surface covered with calcospherites, or microscopic balls of mineral. Normally the peritubular matrix is more heavily calcified than the intertubular matrix. Thus, as the odontoblast moves away from the junction and toward the pulp cavity, the Tomes' fiber trails after it like a tail, secreting matrix as it goes, which forms primary dentin. This action slows down after tooth formation is complete, but the formation of secondary dentin can continue throughout life because odontoblasts remain alive within the pulp cavity and can seal it off if, for example, the tooth is broken and the cavity exposed.

The processes of amelogenesis and odontogenesis are basically similar in all mammals and in all teeth. What distinguishes one tooth from another is the genetic programing for shape and size, not the material of which it is made or the cells that make it. Thus, shape and size can be used to identify which tooth and which species are represented by a specimen. The teeth of other mammals that are frequently confused with those of humans are the incisors and molars of suids and the incisors of carnivores and herbivores.

Both central and lateral incisors in humans are simple, single-rooted teeth used primarily for cutting in an edge-to-edge bite (Figure 15-5). The flat, occlusal surface of an incisor is typically long mesiodistally and narrow labiolingually. The labial surface of an incisor is mildly convex, while the lingual surface is concave, sometimes strikingly so. Particular human populations of Mongoloid descent show a high incidence (>80%) of shovel-shaped incisors, in which the lingual surface is surrounded by a raised rim on its mesial and lateral edges, producing a shape like the blade of a shovel. Shovel-shaped incisors are relatively rare (10–15%) in European populations that lack Mongoloid ancestry.

The different incisors—upper, lower, central, and lateral—are distinguished from each other by their features. Upper incisors have broader crowns than lower incisors and more often show a cingulum, a shelf of enamel at the neck of the lingual surface. They also have roots that are roughly triangular in cross-section, and they more commonly show shoveling. Lower incisors have narrower crowns and roughly oval roots in cross-section, with the long axis of the oval

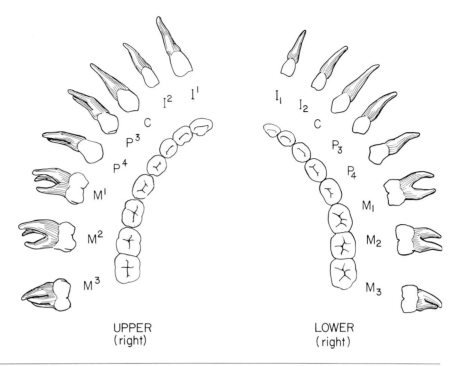

UPPER
(right)

LOWER
(right)

Figure 15-5

The teeth of an adult human: molars *(M)*, premolars *(P)*, canines *(C)*, and incisors *(I)*, in *(far left)* lingual, *(center)* occlusal, and *(far right)* buccal view.

oriented labiolingually. Lower incisors infrequently show cingula or shoveling. Of the incisors, the central uppers are the easiest to identify because they are much broader than the others. In contrast, central lower incisors are the smallest incisors. Both upper and lower central incisors are also recognizable by the angle formed by the mesial and occlusal surfaces. In anterior view, this angle is well-defined and the two surfaces are nearly perpendicular to each other, whereas the angle between the distal and occlusal surfaces is more rounded. These facts can be used to determine the side of the central incisors as well as to distinguish between central lower incisors and upper or lower lateral incisors. Lateral incisors are small teeth. Upper lateral incisors often show a pit at the base of the cingulum. Lower lateral incisors have a broader occlusal surface than either central lower or upper lateral incisors.

Canines, which are also single-rooted teeth, are readily distinguished from incisors by their shape. In labial view the crown of a canine is not triangular, like the incisors, but diamond-shaped, because of its single, pointed cusp. Canines also have longer, larger roots relative to their crown size than do incisors. An upper canine is larger, having a broader crown and more pointed cusp than a lower. Upper canines also have a cingulum, which is absent in lower canines. The distal side of the canine root is more strongly grooved than the mesial, enabling side identification. The tip of the canine cusp lies closer to the mesial than to the distal edge of the tooth.

Premolars are distinguished from canines in that they usually have two cusps, rather than one, and the buccal cusp is less sharp. Premolars may have one root, two separate roots, buccal and lingual, or two fused roots. The roots are often concave on their distal surface. Most premolars with two roots, whether separate or fused, are uppers. Two separate roots are more common in P^3's than in P^4's. Upper premolars also have cusps of more nearly equal size, whereas the buccal cusp is larger in lower premolars. P^3's are distinguished from P^4's by their greater frequency of double roots and by the concavity of their mesial surface. Lower premolars have larger buccal cusps and single roots. P_3's have a more marked discrepancy in the size of their buccal and lingual cusps and have a grooved mesial root surface. P_4's have more equal cusps, sometimes show a double lingual cusp, and lack the groove on the mesial surface of the root.

Molars are readily distinguished from incisors, canines, and premolars because they are larger teeth with more cusps, having a rectangular outline in occlusal view and two or three roots. Upper molars have three roots, whether fused or separate, whereas lowers have only two. Upper molars often have fewer cusps and are wider buccolingually than lower molars, which makes the occlusal outline of the upper molar nearly square, whereas that of the lower molar is clearly rectangular, with the long axis arranged mesiodistally. Different populations show a different incidence of accessory cusps and various minor dental anomalies, but these facts are not often useful in attributing race.

M^1's usually have four cusps and a large, widely divergent lingual root; facets for the P^4 and M^2 are visible in M^1's of adults. M^2's show a large lingual root, though not so strongly splayed as the roots of M^1, and contact facets for M^1 and M^3. M^3's are the smallest upper molars and most commonly have fused roots; they show no contact facet distally, where there is normally no tooth. In upper molars, the position of the roots denotes the side. They have a lingual, a mesiobuccal, and a distobuccal root; the lingual is the largest and the most divergent from the others.

The lower molars are all elongated mesiodistally; their roots tend to be concave distally. M_1's commonly show five cusps, rather than four, and have two separate roots. Contact facets are present both mesially and distally. M_2's have four cusps. Their two roots may be fused and are more strongly curved than those of M_1. M_3's are often smaller molars and most often have fused roots. The side of lower molars is shown by both the curvature of their roots, which is concave distally, and the features of the crown. When there are five cusps on a lower molar, three of them are aligned along the buccal edge and two along the lingual. When only four cusps are present — a condition common in M_2's and M_3's — the buccal surface of the crown is more strongly convex than the lingual; this feature is most clearly seen in either mesial or distal view of the molars.

Like teeth, bones can indicate the stage of development reached by an individual at death because the different epiphyses of the bones appear and then fuse at different ages. Although many bones bear epiphyses, the smaller bones are less frequently recovered from archaeological, forensic, or paleontological sites, so that the times of appearance and fusion of epiphyses of the major long bones have assumed greater importance in age estimation. Sex has a major impact on fusion times, girls being advanced in skeletal maturity over boys by as much as two years on average. A range of about four years from the onset of fusion in early-maturing individuals to the completion of fusion in late-maturing individuals is normal, according to osteological studies. Radiological studies give even earlier dates for the onset of fusion, owing to the fact that fusion often begins at the center of the epiphysis, which is not apparent from gross observation. Thus, fusion of epiphyses is viewed more properly as a process, which occurs over time, than as an event.

The major epiphyses of the long bones fuse at about 13.5–18 years (Table 15-1). The earliest epiphyses to appear and fuse are those of the distal humerus. The first of these, the capitulum, appears at about 3 months in both males and females; the last, the lateral epicondyle, appears at 8–11 years in females and 10–12 years in males. The lateral three centers of the distal humerus begin to fuse to each other at 13–14 years and fuse to the shaft at about 16 years, to be followed within a year or two by the epiphysis of the medial epicondyle. Fusion in the rest of the skeleton then occurs sequentially in the proximal radius and ulna, hip, ankle, knee, wrist, and shoulder (Figure 15-6). Often the last postcranial epiphysis to fuse is the one at the medial end of the clavicle, which has been documented as incompletely fused in some 30-year-old males.

By studying cranial suture fusion in individuals of known age, Meindl and Lovejoy have developed a new method of estimating age. Ten one-centimeter long sites along the external surface of the cranial sutures are scored on a 0–3 scale which ranges from fully open to obliterated by closure. Scores for the different groups of sites are summed, yielding composite scores. Age is estimated from these composite scores by referring to the control population. Cranial suture fusion is a useful indicator of age, especially if it is used in conjunction with other indicators.

The extent of degenerative change in skeletal remains is the last indicator of age at death. Dental remains undergo degenerative change primarily in terms of wear or attrition of occlusal surfaces. As a rule, older individuals show more extensive wear than younger ones, and this effect is more pronounced in populations that incorporate a

Table 15-1		Age at Onset of Fusion of Major Postcranial Epiphyses	
Epiphysis		Female Age Range	Male Age Range
Humerus			
	Proximal	15 yrs 8 mos – 18 yrs 2 mos	16 yrs – 18 yrs 2 mos
	Distal	13 yrs 4 mos – 16 yrs 4 mos	14 yrs – 16 yrs 4 mos
	Medial epicondyle	10 yrs – 14 yrs	12 yrs – 14 yrs
Ulna			
	Proximal	13 yrs 10 mos – 15 yrs	14 yrs – 15 yrs
Femur			
	Head	13 yrs 4 mos – 16 yrs 4 mos	14 yrs – 16 yrs 4 mos
	Distal	14 yrs – 17 yrs	16 yrs – 17 yrs
Tibia			
	Proximal	14 yrs – 18 yrs	15 yrs – 18 yrs
	Distal	13 yrs – 18 yrs	14 yrs 9 mos – 18 yrs
Fibula			
	Proximal	14 yrs – 18 yrs	16 yrs – 18 yrs

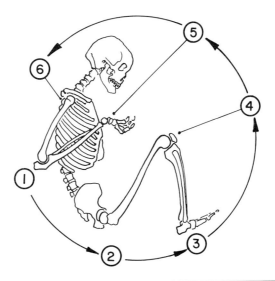

Figure 15-6

Sequence of epiphyseal fusion in humans. *(1)* elbow, *(2)* hip, *(3)* ankle, *(4)* knee, *(5)* wrist, and *(6)* shoulder.

greater amount of grit or other abrasive substance in their food than is common today in urban societies. The rate of wear is directly related to the diet consumed and to the preparation of that diet, since these influence the abrasiveness of the substances chewed. Thus, the technique of estimating age on the basis of dental attrition is primarily useful for within-population studies and not for between-population comparisons, unless there are extrinsic reasons to suppose that diet and food preparation were the same in both populations. In some populations diet may also vary by sex. As a result, dental attrition studies are most profitably undertaken in conjunction with studies of bony remains. Moreover, many individuals use their teeth for functions other than eating, such as nail-biting and bruxism, or tooth-grinding, or as tools of various sorts. Such activities affect tooth wear, sometimes considerably. In order to assess dental attrition, the extent and location of dentin exposure on molars are compared to a standard for each tooth, and that standard is linked to an age estimate based on bony remains (Figure 15-7).

Another means of estimating age is based on the changes in the surface of the pubic symphysis that occur between the ages of about 18 and 60. Todd's original technique involved identifying ten different

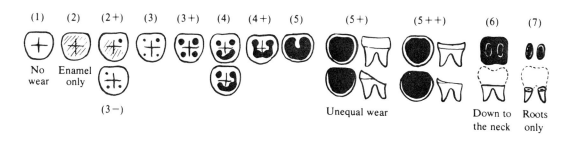

Age period (years)	About 17–25			25–35			33–45			About 45+		
Molar number	M1	M2	M3	M1	M2	M3	M1	M2	M3	M1	M2	M3
Wear pattern												

Figure 15-7

Age estimation based on dental attrition at time of death. *(Top)* Molar wear is classified into numerical stages by comparing the amount of enamel wear and dentin exposure *(black)* with these standards. *(Bottom)* Associated skeletons that are sufficiently complete to provide information on both dental attrition and age at death, as shown by osteological indicators, are used to establish the stage of dental attrition that characterizes different age periods. The table can be used to estimate age on individuals known only from teeth in that population.

morphological stages in the appearance of the entire articular surface of the pubis. In a revision by McKern and Stewart, the pubic symphysis is divided into three components: the dorsal demiface, the ventral demiface, and the entire articular surface. Each component goes through six sequential morphological stages, which are represented by scores of 0–5 (Figure 15-8). The scores for the individual components are summed to provide a total score. Because this technique was developed by studying a skeletal population of known age at death, the range and mean of individuals obtaining particular total scores are known (Table 15-2). Therefore, summed scores can be used to estimate age at death of unknown individuals of other populations. One problem with this technique is that it is much less reliable for females

Component I

Component II

Component III

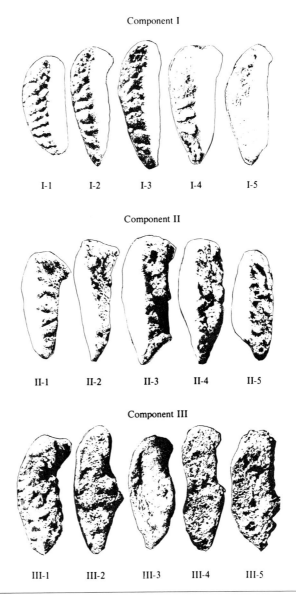

I-1   I-2   I-3   I-4   I-5

II-1   II-2   II-3   II-4   II-5

III-1   III-2   III-3   III-4   III-5

Figure 15-8

Morphological criteria for age estimation based on male pubic symphyses (McKern and Stewart, 1957). Unknowns are scored on each of three components by comparison with these standards. The scores appear below each pubis, following the component number. Areas of the pubis not included in a particular component are not shown. Anterior is to the right. Component I is the dorsal demiface of the pubic symphysis. A score of 0 is given to specimens lacking a dorsal margin. Component II is the ventral demiface of the pubic symphysis. A score of 0 is given to specimens lacking ventral beveling. Component III is the entire symphyseal surface. A score of 0 is given to specimens lacking a distinct elevated rim.

than for males, for unexplained reasons. A further revision by Meindl and coworkers has greatly improved the accuracy of this technique for both sexes.

The degeneration of various load-bearing joints may also give information about age in adults. Osteoarthritis is observed as the loss of bone from articular surfaces and the build-up of new bony ridges or spikes, called osteophytes, around the joint margins (Figure 15-9). Such changes are typically seen at the shoulder, elbow, hip, knee, and intervertebral joints. The severity of these changes and their frequency at various joints increases with age. As a rule, osteoarthritic changes may begin to be visible in individuals in their twenties. At about age 40, the rate at which such changes occur increases in terms of both the extent of lipping and osteophyte formation and the number of joints involved. Differences in the physical rigors of different lifestyles may cause an earlier or later onset of osteoarthritis or may change the pattern of joints affected. Care must be taken to distinguish between osteoarthritis and degenerative changes that have occurred as a result of trauma. Traumatic changes are likely to be confined to a single anatomical region of the body rather than occurring in several widely separated joints.

The microscopic structure of cortical bone is also used to estimate age in adults. Since remodeling is a function of the time elapsed since deposition, the density of osteons in cortical bone reflects the age at death. In this technique, thin sections of major long bones, usually femora or tibiae, are taken at midshaft and inspected under a microscope. Different variants of this technique involve obtaining slightly

Table 15-2   Scores of Individuals of Known Age, Based on Pubic-Aging Technique

Total Score	Number of Individuals	Age Range	Mean Age	Standard Deviation
0	7	17	17.29	0.49
1–2	76	17–20	19.04	0.79
3	43	18–21	19.79	0.85
4–5	51	18–23	20.84	1.13
6–7	26	20–24	22.42	0.99
8–9	36	22–28	24.14	1.93
10	19	23–28	26.05	1.87
11–13	56	23–39	29.18	3.33
14	31	29+	35.84	3.89
15	4	36+	41.00	6.22

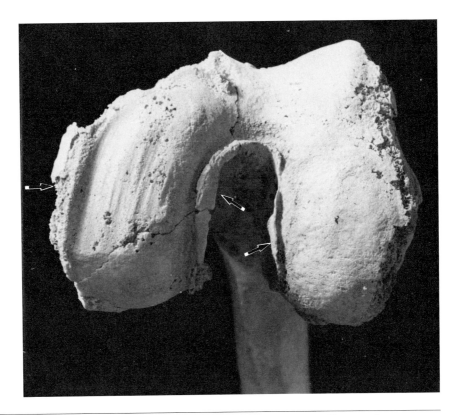

Figure 15-9

Effect of osteoarthritis on the femur. It causes a build-up of bony spikes or osteo-phytes *(arrows)* around the joint margins. This femur also shows a more severe degeneration of the joint, where the loss of hyaline cartilage has led to eburnation or polishing of the subchondral bone by bone-on-bone wear.

different data: counting the frequency of osteons, osteon fragments, and non-Haversian canals and the percentage of lamellar bone in a microscopic field that measures 1.62 mm in diameter; establishing the number of squares, out of 100 squares in a 1-mm² grid, that are more than half-filled by osteons or osteon fragments; and counting the total number of osteons, the average number of lamellae per osteon, and the average minimum diameter of the Haversian canals in two randomly selected fields near the periosteum, using a 10x objective and a 10x widefield ocular. Data indicative of the extent of remodeling yield an estimated age when they are substituted into a regression equation that describes the mathematical relationship between similar data on bones from individuals of known age.

One problem in using microscopic techniques to estimate age is that they involve the destruction of skeletal material, and such actions are often neither permissible, as on many museum specimens, nor justifiable. An equally serious problem is that the extent of remodeling is directly related to the degree of physical stress to which a bone is exposed. Thus, a highly active individual's bones may be extensively remodeled and thus appear older than they are, while a relatively inactive individual's bone may undergo so little remodeling as to appear substantially younger than they are.

Microscopic techniques can also be applied to teeth. In Gustafson's technique, the degree of attrition, cementum formation, root resorption, periodontosis, secondary dentin formation, transparency of root, and degree of root closure are scored on thin sections of teeth. Summed scores for individual teeth are substituted into a regression equation derived from summed scores of individuals of known age. The accuracy of this technique is open to debate. Although information about age is clearly encoded in dental microanatomy, the use of different teeth, the incidence of pathologies, and dietary abrasion all seem to affect the resultant estimate, as do minor technical variations in preparation. Maples revised this technique to omit root closure as being the least reliably correlated with age. When Maples' estimates of ages are compared to the known ages of the same individuals, his estimates are accurate within plus or minus 9–13 years of the actual age, depending upon which tooth is used. Microscopic inspection of dental remains is promising but inexact. This technique also requires the destruction of material.

Any attempts to estimate age should use as many different indicators as are available and seem warranted. The best result that can be obtained is an estimate based on several different types of evidence. Even so, the age thus obtained actually represents the mean in a range of possible ages. When skeletal remains from populations are available, these age estimates can then be used as the basis of demographic studies and reconstructions.

ATTRIBUTION OF SEX

Skeletal differences between males and females are well documented. The most reliable attributions of sex, some of which approach 100% accuracy, involve several skeletal elements rather than just one (Table 15-3). In archaeological, forensic, or paleontological studies, however, entire or even partial skeletons are not always available, and the accuracy of sex attribution falls accord-

Table 15-3 Accuracy of Different Techniques for Determining Sex of Adult Skeletal Remains

Element	Type of Analysis	Collection or Population Used in Study	Accuracy (%)	Primary Description of Technique or Results
Whole skeleton	Morphological	Todd Collection	90/95–100	Krogman 1962, Stewart 1948, 1951
Cranium	Morphological	Todd Collection	82/87–92	Krogman 1962
			80	Stewart 1948, 1951
			80 (90 with mandible)	Hrdlicka (in Stewart 1948)
	Morphological & univariate statistics	Cape colored	85	Keen 1950
	Discriminant function analysis	Todd & Terry Collections	82–89	Giles & Eliot 1963
	Discriminant function analysis	Forensic cases	88	Snow et al. 1979
Skull	Discriminant function analysis	Japanese	89	Hanihara 1958a
Mandible	Discriminant function analysis	Todd & Terry Collections	85	Giles & Eliot 1963
Sternum	Penrose size/shape statistic	Portuguese	89	Pons 1955
Clavicle	Parson's 1912 formula	Modern English	88	Parson 1916
	Parson's 1912 formula	St. Bride's series	91	Steel 1967
	Discriminant function analysis	Modern English	88	Steel 1967
		St. Bride's series	96	Steel 1967
Humerus, ulna, radius, femur, tibia	Discriminant function analysis	Japanese	97	Hanihara 1958b
Pelvis	Morphological	Todd Collection	85/90–95	Krogman 1962
			90–95	Stewart 1948, 1951
	Morphological	Terry Collection	96	Phenice 1969
	Ischiopubic index	Terry Collection blacks	93.5	Thieme & Schull 1967
			82–94	Richman et al. 1979
	Ischiopubic index	Terry Collection whites	91–95	Richman et al. 1979
		Howard University blacks	95.8	Richman et al. 1979

Table 15-3 continued

Element	Type of Analysis	Collection or Population Used in Study	Accuracy (%)	Primary Description of Technique or Results
	Ischiopubic index & sciatic notch width	Bantu	98	Washburn 1948
	Ratio of sciatic notch width to vertical diameter of acetabulum	Todd Collection	90	Kelley 1978
	Acetabulum-pubis ratio	Terry Collection blacks	92	Schulter-Ellis et al. 1983
	Morphological on ischiopubic ramus	Terry Collection	92	Phenice 1969
Pelvis/femur	Ischiopubic index & femoral dimensions	Terry Collection blacks	99	Thieme & Schull 1957
		Terry Collections blacks & whites & Howard University blacks	92–99	Richman et al. 1979
	Acetabulum-pubis index & femoral dimensions	Terry Collection blacks	96	Schulter-Ellis et al. 1983
	Discriminant function analysis & femoral dimensions	Terry Collection blacks	97	Schulter-Ellis et al. 1983
Femur	Discriminant function analysis	Portuguese	94	Pons 1955
	Shaft diameter & stepwise discriminant function analysis	North American whites (American Museum of Natural History)	82	DiBennardo & Taylor 1979
		Terry Collection blacks	76.4	DiBennardo & Taylor 1979
Tooth crown	Discriminant function analysis	American whites	65–81	Owsley & Webb 1983

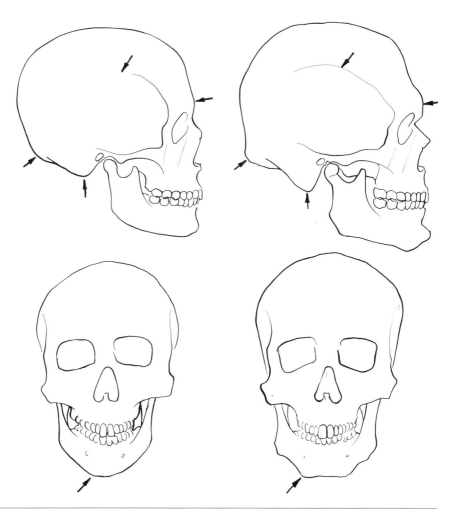

Figure 15-10

Sexual differences in the skull: *(left)* female and *(right)* male. Males have a more pronounced supraorbital torus, larger mastoid process, squarer chin, and stronger muscle markings on the temporal line and nuchal crest.

ingly. As a general rule, all skeletal elements of males are larger and show more robust muscle markings than those of females. Three skeletal elements are more reliable predictors of sex than other elements: the skull, pelvis, and appendicular bones.

A number of features of the skull distinguish males from females, although not all of these differences characterize all populations (Figure 15-10). Male skulls generally are larger and more robust. In addition, they have stronger and more pronounced muscle markings, as on temporal ridges, nuchal crests, and masseter origins and insertions; larger mastoid processes and thicker zygomatic arches; more rounded superior margins of the orbits; longer palates and larger teeth; square chins, versus pointed or rounded chins in females; larger frontal sinuses and supraorbital ridges; and longer suprameatal crests that may extend posterior to the external auditory meatus.

The most reliable assessment of sex based on cranial remains involves comparing a score derived from a set of measurements with a similarly derived set of scores from individuals of known sex. The cranial measurements most widely used to determine sex are basion-nasion length, maximum bizygomatic breadth, basion-prosthion length, prosthion-nasion height, maximum cranial height (bregma-basion), mastoid length, maximum cranial vault length (glabella-occipitale), and maximum cranial width on the coronal plane but avoiding the suprameatal crests. Since the values for these measurements also vary with racial ancestry, it is necessary to identify the race of a specimen before attributing sex. The most useful statistical technique for deriving and comparing the scores is discriminant function analysis. Giles and Elliot first applied discriminant function analysis to the problem of sexing cranial remains. In their approach, each measurement is given a weighting factor, which roughly corresponds to its power to describe crucial shape differences, based on analysis of individuals of known sex. The value of each measurement is then multiplied by its weight factor, and the results are summed to yield a score. Scores of both unknowns and individuals of known sex from the appropriate racial group are plotted. Next, a sectioning point, which divides the known males from the known females on the plot with the fewest errors, is determined. Finally, the individuals of unknown sex that fall on the same side of the sectioning point as known males are judged to be male, and those falling with known females are judged to be female.

The pelvis is the most useful part of the skeleton for determining sex. Qualitative and quantitative differences exist between male and female pelves, due to the demands of childbirth on the female pelvis. The qualitative differences of the female pelvis include a shallower, broader, and less acutely flared shape; a deeper (longer) pubic symphysis; a more rectangular pubis, as opposed to a more triangular pubis in males; a concave inferior pubic ramus, versus a convex one in males; a larger subpubic angle formed by the inferior rami of the two articulated pubes, usually more than 90°; smaller, more triangular obturator foramina, whereas those in males are more oval; an acetabulum that is both smaller in diameter and shallower; a more raised

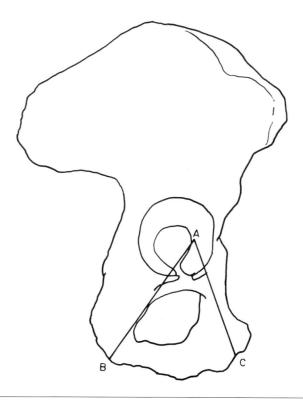

Figure 15-11

The ischiopubic index, used to sex innominates. The ischium, ilium, and pubis meet at point A. The index equals the length of the pubis *(AC)* × 100, divided by the length of the ischium *(AB)*.

auricular surface for articulation with the sacrum; a wider greater sciatic notch, sometimes approaching 90°; and sometimes scars of parturition, which are small pits on the internal posterior pubis near the symphysis or on the ilium lateral to the interior margin of the sacroiliac joint, although there are cases of "scars of parturition" on male pelves as well.

Of the quantitative differences between male and female pelves, the most useful one involves the ischium-pubis index. This index is calculated from the maximum lengths of the pubis and ischium, starting from the point at which the ischium, pubis, and ilium unite to form the innominate. The length of the pubis is multiplied by 100, and the result is divided by the length of the ischium (Figure 15-11).

In American populations, both "white" and "black" males show means of 84 or lower on this index, while females show means of

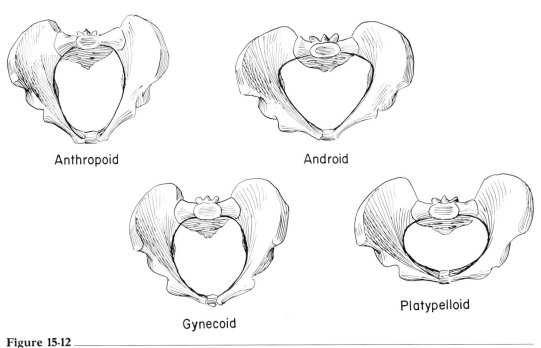

Anthropoid   Android

Gynecoid

Platypelloid

Figure 15-12

Gynecological classification of female pelvic shapes.

95–100. Some males and females yield ambivalent values of 90–95 in whites and 84–88 in blacks. Such ambivalent values occur in 5–25% of individuals, depending on the population.

The variability of pelvic shape and size in females has crucial implications for the ease and success of childbirth. Female pelvic shapes are classified according to the shape of the pelvic inlet, which is the roughly circular plane defined by the pubic symphysis anteriorly, the superior pubic ramus and linea terminalis medially, and the sacral promontory posteriorly. The fetal head enters the pelvic inlet facing laterally, then turns to face obliquely within the pelvic cavity, and is delivered facing either anteriorly or posteriorly. The pelvic outlet, through which delivery occurs, is a roughly diamond-shaped opening formed by the ischiopubic rami, the ischial tuberosities, the sacrotuberous ligaments, and the tip of the coccyx. The shape of the pelvic inlet determines its transverse diameter and hence the ease of delivery.

There are four main pelvic shapes: gynecoid, android, anthropoid, and platypelloid (Figure 15-12). Gynecoid pelves are rounded; this shape is found in about half of all females. A pelvic inlet that is broad posteriorly and narrower anteriorly, with a heart shape, is called android. An oval pelvic inlet, with its long axis oriented anteroposteriorly, is called anthropoid, because of its resemblance to the pelvic inlet shape of higher, nonhuman primates. Males often have anthropoid pelvic inlets. A platypelloid pelvic inlet is unusually broad transversely and narrow anteroposteriorly; this shape is uncommon.

Appendicular bones show few simple morphological features that discriminate between the sexes. Statistical studies using a combination of metrical features on the clavicle, humerus, radius, ulna, femur, and tibia have proven excellent predictors of sex in particular populations. Further, as a general rule, males' bones are larger and more robust than females'. Therefore, when the size of joint surfaces or the widths and lengths of major limb bones from a skeletal population reveal a bimodal distribution, it can be reasonably assumed that the smaller group probably represents females, even if detailed statistical studies of individuals of known sex are unavailable.

ATTRIBUTION OF RACE

Despite the difficulty of determining race or geographic ancestry in modern populations, the attribution of race in whatever sense is important in forensic cases as well as in studies of prehistoric populations which seek to find links between recent and ancient groups. Certain features of the skull can be used to identify the racial group to which skeletal remains belong.

Various qualitative features of the skull are useful in determining race, although assessing these subtle differences requires experience (Figure 15-13). In general, individuals of Negroid stock have rectangular-shaped orbits placed somewhat lower on the narrow cranium, a wider interorbital distance, less prominent nasal bones, a wider nasal aperture, and a more marked prognathism of the alveolar region and lower face. Negroid individuals also lack sharply defined inferior margins to the nasal aperture. Individuals of Caucasoid stock, on the other hand, have angular orbits placed higher on the narrow cranium, more prominent nasal bones and midfacial region, a narrower nasal aperture, and an orthognathous lower face. Individuals of Mongoloid descent have broader skulls with rounded orbits of intermediate location, nasal bones of intermediate prominence, an intermediate nasal aperture, and an intermediate degree of alveolar prognathism. Mongoloids also most commonly show shoveling of the incisors and extreme breadth of the zygomatic arches.

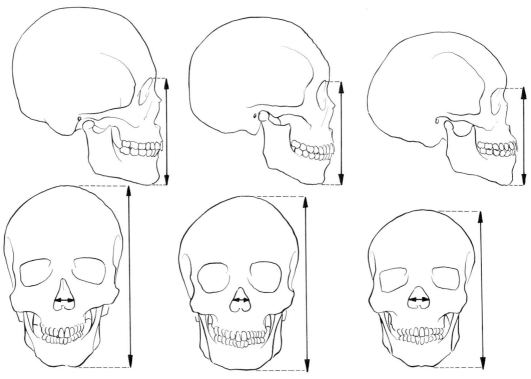

Figure 15-13

Racial differences in the skull: *(left to right)* male Mongoloid, male Caucasoid, and male Negroid. The differences involve nasal aperture breadth, orbital placement and shape, and alveolar prognathism.

Perhaps the most successful and objective means of attributing race involves discriminant function analysis of metrical measurements taken on crania. The measurements used are nearly identical to those used in sexing crania: basion-prosthion length, glabella-occipitale length, maximum width, basion-bregma length, basion-nasion length, maximum bizygomatic breadth, prosthion-nasion length, and nasal breadth (alare-alare). Since such methods yield a high degree of accuracy (80 – 95%) in tests of known individuals, they can be employed when attribution of race is an important issue. The statistical distance between the scores of different skeletal populations is probably a measure of genetic relatedness between those groups. Racial differences in postcranial bones are less pronounced than the cranial differences and are not often useful in attributing race.

ESTIMATION OF STATURE

Stature can be more reliably estimated from skeletal remains than can weight, the other component of body size, probably because stature is less variable than weight throughout adult life. Once adult stature has been attained, it is relatively impervious to change, except for changes related to trauma or serious injury.

Standards for estimating stature from the length of long bones were developed by Trotter and Gleser by studying the remains of over 5,000 known individuals (Table 15-4). These individuals were males and females of Caucasoid, Negroid, and Mongoloid ancestry. Later, Genovés conducted comparable studies of original Mexican males, although the numbers of whites and blacks upon which the original formulae are based are much greater than the numbers of Mongoloids or Mexicans. The studies show that lower limb bones are better predictors of stature than upper limb bones. The combination of femoral and tibial lengths often yields the most accurate estimates. Stature is an attribute particularly sensitive to nutritional status during childhood. Few, if any, prehistoric populations show mean statures comparable to those documented for modern humans.

Table 15-4 Maximum Stature Expected from Maximum Long Bone Lengths in American Individuals[a]

Hum. (mm)	Rad. (mm)	Ulna (mm)	Stature		Fem. (mm)	Tib. (mm)	Fib. (mm)	Fem. + Tib. (mm)
			(cm)	(in)[b]				
				White American Males				
265	193	211	152	59^7	381	291	299	685
268	196	213	153	60^2	385	295	303	693
271	198	216	154	60^5	389	299	307	701
275	201	219	155	61	393	303	311	708
278	204	222	156	61^3	398	307	314	716
281	206	224	157	61^6	402	311	318	723
284	209	227	158	62^2	406	315	322	731
288	212	230	159	62^5	410	319	326	738
291	214	232	160	63	414	323	329	746
294	217	235	161	63^3	419	327	333	753
297	220	238	162	63^6	423	331	337	761
301	222	240	163	64^1	427	335	340	769
304	225	243	164	64^5	431	339	344	776
307	228	246	165	65	435	343	348	784
310	230	249	166	65^3	440	347	352	791
314	233	251	167	65^6	444	351	355	799
317	235	254	168	66^1	448	355	359	806

Table 15-4 continued

Hum. (mm)	Rad. (mm)	Ulna (mm)	Stature (cm)	(in)[b]	Fem. (mm)	Tib. (mm)	Fib. (mm)	Fem. + Tib. (mm)
320	238	257	169	66[4]	452	359	363	814
323	241	259	170	66[7]	456	363	367	821
327	243	262	171	67[3]	461	367	370	829
330	246	265	172	67[6]	465	371	374	837
333	249	267	173	68[1]	469	375	378	844
336	251	270	174	68[4]	473	379	381	852
339	254	273	175	68[7]	477	383	385	859
343	257	276	176	69[2]	482	386	389	867
346	259	278	177	69[5]	486	390	393	874
349	262	281	178	70[1]	490	394	396	882
352	265	284	179	70[4]	494	398	400	889
356	267	286	180	70[7]	498	402	404	897
359	270	289	181	71[2]	503	406	408	905
362	272	292	182	71[5]	507	410	411	912
365	275	294	183	72	511	414	415	920
369	278	297	184	72[4]	515	418	419	927
372	280	300	185	72[7]	519	422	422	935
375	283	303	186	73[2]	524	426	426	942
378	286	305	187	73[5]	528	430	430	950
382	288	308	188	74	532	434	434	957
385	291	311	189	74[3]	536	438	437	965
388	294	313	190	74[6]	540	442	441	973
391	296	316	191	75[2]	545	446	445	980
395	299	319	192	75[5]	549	450	449	988
398	302	321	193	76	553	454	452	995
401	304	324	194	76[3]	557	458	456	1003
404	307	327	195	76[6]	561	462	460	1010
408	309	330	196	77[1]	566	466	463	1018
411	312	332	197	77[4]	570	470	467	1026
414	315	335	198	78	574	474	471	1033
			Black American Males					
276	206	223	152	59[7]	387	301	303	704
279	209	226	153	60[2]	391	306	308	713
282	212	229	154	60[5]	396	310	312	721
285	215	232	155	61	401	315	317	730
288	218	235	156	61[3]	406	320	321	739
291	221	238	157	61[6]	410	324	326	747
294	224	242	158	62[2]	415	329	330	756
297	226	245	159	62[5]	420	333	335	765

Table 15-4 continued

Hum. (mm)	Rad. (mm)	Ulna (mm)	Stature (cm)	Stature (in)[b]	Fem. (mm)	Tib. (mm)	Fib. (mm)	Fem. + Tib. (mm)
300	229	248	160	63	425	338	339	774
303	232	251	161	63^3	430	342	344	782
306	235	254	162	63^6	434	347	349	791
310	238	257	163	64^1	439	352	353	800
313	241	260	164	64^5	444	356	358	808
316	244	263	165	65	449	361	362	817
319	247	266	166	65^3	453	365	367	826
322	250	269	167	65^6	458	370	371	834
325	253	272	168	66^1	463	374	376	843
328	256	275	169	66^4	468	379	381	852
331	259	278	170	66^7	472	383	385	861
334	262	281	171	67^3	477	388	390	869
337	264	284	172	67^6	482	393	394	878
340	267	287	173	68^1	487	397	399	887
343	270	291	174	68^4	491	402	403	895
346	273	294	175	68^7	496	406	408	904
349	276	297	176	69^2	501	411	413	913
352	279	300	177	69^5	506	415	417	921
356	282	303	178	70	510	420	422	930
359	285	306	179	70^1	515	425	426	939
362	288	309	180	70^7	520	429	431	947
365	291	312	181	71^2	525	434	435	956
368	294	315	182	71^5	529	438	440	965
371	297	318	183	72	534	443	445	974
374	300	321	184	72^4	539	447	449	982
377	302	324	185	72^7	544	452	454	991
380	305	327	186	73^2	548	456	458	1000
383	308	330	187	73^5	553	461	463	1008
386	311	333	188	74	558	466	467	1017
389	314	336	189	74^3	563	470	472	1026
392	317	340	190	74^6	567	475	476	1034
395	320	343	191	75^2	572	479	481	1043
398	323	346	192	75^5	577	484	486	1052
401	326	349	193	76	582	488	490	1061
405	329	352	194	76^3	586	493	495	1069
408	332	355	195	76^6	591	498	499	1078
411	335	358	196	77^1	596	502	504	1087
414	337	361	197	77^4	601	507	508	1095
417	340	364	198	78	605	511	513	1104

Table 15-4 continued

Hum. (mm)	Rad. (mm)	Ulna (mm)	Stature (cm)	(in)[b]	Fem. (mm)	Tib. (mm)	Fib. (mm)	Fem. + Tib. (mm)
			White American Females					
244	179	193	140	55[1]	348	271	274	624
247	182	195	141	55[4]	352	274	278	632
250	184	197	142	55[7]	356	277	281	639
253	186	200	143	56[2]	360	281	285	646
256	188	202	144	56[6]	364	284	288	653
259	190	204	145	57[1]	368	288	291	660
262	192	207	146	57[4]	372	291	295	668
265	194	209	147	57[7]	376	295	298	675
268	196	211	148	58[2]	380	298	302	682
271	198	214	149	58[5]	384	302	305	689
274	201	216	150	59	388	305	309	696
277	203	218	151	59[4]	392	309	312	704
280	205	221	152	59[7]	396	312	315	711
283	207	223	153	60[2]	400	315	319	718
286	209	225	154	60[5]	404	319	322	725
289	211	228	155	61	409	322	326	732
292	213	230	156	61[3]	413	326	329	740
295	215	232	157	61[6]	417	329	332	747
298	217	235	158	62[2]	421	333	336	754
301	220	237	159	62[5]	425	336	340	761
304	222	239	160	63	429	340	343	768
307	224	242	161	63[3]	433	343	346	776
310	226	244	162	63[6]	437	346	349	783
313	228	246	163	64[1]	441	350	353	790
316	230	249	164	64[5]	445	353	356	797
319	232	251	165	65	449	357	360	804
322	234	253	166	65[3]	453	360	363	812
324	236	256	167	65[6]	457	364	366	819
327	239	258	168	66[1]	461	367	370	826
330	241	261	169	66[4]	465	371	373	833
333	243	263	170	66[7]	469	374	377	840
336	245	265	171	67[3]	473	377	380	847
339	247	268	172	67[6]	477	381	384	855
342	249	270	173	68[1]	481	384	387	862
345	251	272	174	68[4]	485	388	390	869
348	253	275	175	68[7]	489	391	394	876
351	255	277	176	69[2]	494	395	397	883
354	258	279	177	69[5]	498	398	401	891
357	260	282	178	70[1]	502	402	404	898

Table 15-4 continued

Hum. (mm)	Rad. (mm)	Ulna (mm)	Stature		Fem. (mm)	Tib. (mm)	Fib. (mm)	Fem. + Tib. (mm)
			(cm)	(in)[b]				
360	262	284	179	70[4]	506	405	407	905
363	264	286	180	70[7]	510	409	411	912
366	266	289	181	71[2]	514	412	414	919
369	268	291	182	71[5]	518	415	418	927
372	270	293	183	72	522	419	421	934
375	272	296	184	72[4]	526	422	425	941
			Black American Females					
245	186	195	140	55[1]	352	275	278	637
248	189	198	141	55[4]	356	279	282	645
251	191	201	142	55[7]	361	283	286	653
254	194	204	143	56[2]	365	287	290	661
258	197	207	144	56[6]	369	291	294	669
261	199	210	145	57[1]	374	295	298	677
264	202	213	146	57[4]	378	299	302	685
267	205	216	147	57[7]	383	303	306	693
271	208	219	148	58[2]	387	308	310	701
274	210	222	149	58[5]	391	312	314	709
277	213	225	150	59	396	316	318	717
280	216	228	151	59[4]	400	320	322	724
284	218	231	152	59[7]	405	324	326	732
287	221	235	153	60[2]	409	328	330	740
290	224	238	154	60[5]	413	332	334	748
293	227	241	155	61	418	336	338	756
297	229	244	156	61[3]	422	340	342	764
300	232	247	157	61[6]	426	344	346	772
303	235	250	158	62[2]	431	348	350	780
306	238	253	159	62[5]	435	352	354	788
310	240	256	160	63	440	357	358	796
313	243	259	161	63[3]	444	361	362	804
316	246	262	162	63[6]	448	365	366	812
319	249	265	163	64[1]	453	369	370	820
322	251	268	164	64[5]	457	373	374	828
326	254	271	165	65	462	377	378	836
329	257	274	166	65[3]	466	381	382	843
332	259	277	167	65[6]	470	385	386	851
335	262	280	168	66[1]	475	389	390	859
339	265	283	169	66[4]	479	393	394	867
342	268	286	170	66[7]	484	397	398	875
345	270	289	171	67[3]	488	401	402	883
348	273	292	172	67[6]	492	406	406	891

Table 15-4 continued

Hum. (mm)	Rad. (mm)	Ulna (mm)	Stature		Fem. (mm)	Tib. (mm)	Fib. (mm)	Fem. + Tib. (mm)
			(cm)	(in)[b]				
352	276	295	173	68[1]	497	410	410	899
355	279	298	174	68[4]	501	414	414	907
358	281	301	175	68[7]	505	418	418	915
361	284	304	176	69[2]	510	422	422	923
365	287	307	177	69[5]	514	426	426	931
368	289	310	178	70[1]	519	430	430	939
371	292	313	179	70[4]	523	434	434	947
374	295	316	180	70[7]	527	438	438	955
378	298	319	181	71[2]	532	442	442	963
381	300	322	182	71[5]	536	446	446	970
384	303	325	183	72	541	450	450	978
387	306	328	184	72[4]	545	454	454	986

a. The expected maximum stature should be reduced by 0.06 cm per year of age over 30 to obtain expected stature of individuals over 30 years of age.

b. The raised number indicates the numerator of a fraction of an inch expressed in eighths. Thus 59[7] should be read 59 7/8 inches.

16
TRAUMA
AND
DISEASE

Skeletal remains can preserve a record of events in the life of the individual, including traumas, which are any type of wound or injury, and disease. The effects of such events provide significant information about the past, both recent and distant, in which the individual lived. For example, a high frequency of healed fractures or wounds in males may suggest continual wars or raids, and a high frequency of pathologies in young children may suggest inadequate supplies of weaning foods.

BREAKAGE

Fractures are among the most common traumas that affect the bones. The response of living bone to fracture differs according to where the break is located, how severe the break is, and whether or not bone cell death occurs. In all cases, the first response of the bone is to mobilize osteoprogenitor cells to respond to the injury. These cells may come from one or more of five sources: the bone cells of the tissue itself or the marrow, the periosteum, the endosteum, the mesenchymal cells of the surrounding connective tissue, and the blood.

When the bone cells remain alive, they participate in healing injuries to the bone; when they die, usually because their blood supply has been interrupted by fracture or disease, the osteoprogenitor cells that respond are derived from the other four sources. In cases of bone cell death, the sequence of response differs according to the bone type, whether cancellous or compact.

When bone cell death occurs in coarse cancellous bone, healing occurs through a specific sequence of events. For example, when a fracture through the femoral neck interrupts the blood supply to the cancellous bone of the femoral head, first the vascular cells of the marrow die, and then the fat cells of the marrow die. The bone cells themselves die next—first the osteoprogenitor cells and osteoblasts, followed by the osteocytes and finally by the osteoclasts. Loose mesenchymal tissue, which is heavily vascularized, grows in from the point of fracture and begins filling in the spaces between the trabeculae. Some mesenchymal cells anchor themselves on the surfaces of the dead trabeculae, where they are transformed, mostly into osteoblasts and occasionally into osteoclasts.

The new osteoblasts begin laying down new, woven bone on top of the old, dead trabeculae. Since only a few of the mesenchymal cells turn into osteoclasts, the net effect of this new bone production is that the density of bone tissue in the area increases. That is, both the old, dead bone and the new, live bone are present, resulting in more bone tissue per unit volume than originally. Eventually, all of the dead trabeculae and the old marrow spaces are covered and filled with new woven bone, and bone density is high. At this point the number of osteoclasts increases, and they begin to resorb the dead bone. They also begin to remodel the new woven bone into lamellar bone. These responses proceed faster close to the fracture site and slower distant from the fracture site. Healing is complete when bone density and structure return to normal.

When bone cell death occurs in compact bone, there is little or no space in which new bone formation can occur. As in cancellous bone, the initial response is for loose mesenchymal tissue to grow from the fracture site. However, in compact bone, the initial transformation of the mesenchymal cells forms many osteoclasts and few osteoblasts. These osteoclasts burrow out spaces within the compact bone. The local regions of resorption show pointed hollows, called cutting cones, where old, dead, compact bone is being removed by osteoclasts. Once the osteoclasts have opened up spaces within the compact bone, other mesenchymal cells transform into osteoblasts, since there is now sufficient room for osteoid to be secreted and calcified. From this point on, healing proceeds as in cancellous tissue, with the production of new, woven bone followed by remodeling.

Linear defects are injuries, such as simple or incomplete fractures or stabbing wounds, in which the bone is damaged but little or no motion or displacement occurs at the site of injury. In such cases, bleeding usually occurs. A hematoma, or collection of blood, may be formed, but clotting proceeds normally at the fracture site. At the edge of the defect, bone cell death occurs. Osteoprogenitor cells from the marrow spaces, the periosteum, the endosteum, and the surrounding connective tissue respond in the sequence appropriate to the bone type, cancellous or compact.

The osteoprogenitor cells from these sources become osteoblasts and then begin to lay down new bone at a distance from the defect, working toward it, so as to span the defect with new, woven bone. At the same time, those cells within the bone tissue that remain alive and cells from the surrounding connective tissue proliferate into the defect. There, they form both fibrous connective tissue and woven bone to help fill the gap. The mass of new tissue from both sources is called the callus (Figure 16-1). In linear defects, the callus is primarily bony, but if there are greater amounts of movement at the fracture site than are common with linear defects, the callus becomes larger and more fibrous. Almost simultaneously with the new bone deposition, the osteoclasts start to resorb the new bone and remodel it into lamellar bone.

There are different ways to assess fracture healing. In one sense, healing has occurred when the fragments and pieces of the original bone are reunited by bony tissue. However, bony union occurs well before full functional strength is regained and remodeling is completed. In children especially, healing may occur so completely that it is impossible to detect any effects of a fracture, either in gross morphology or in microscopic architecture. In adults, functional healing may occur, but with the effects of the fracture remaining evident indefinitely. Clinical union, or the point at which the once-broken bone can bear stress without producing pain, precedes the regaining of full mechanical strength.

In studies of skeletal remains, a common problem is whether or not the injury was the cause of death and, if so, how long the individual lived after the injury occurred. Unfortunately, healing proceeds at different rates in different individuals. As a general rule, however, callus formation begins one to two weeks after the injury, at which time there may be some fine rounding and smoothing of the wound edges. After a month, callus formation is usually complete. Full healing, in which the remodeling has made the bone closely resemble its pretrauma condition, may take years to occur or may never occur. Untreated long bone fractures often heal functionally, but the muscles may pull the distal fragment upward, resulting in a permanent shortening or deformation of the bone. In well-nourished, otherwise healthy children, healing of fractures may occur astonishingly rapidly, leaving little or no evidence of fracture after one year.

Five factors govern the success of healing in a fracture: the amount and kind of motion of the fragments at the time of injury; the apposition, or degree of contact or separation, of the fragments from each other; the alignment of the fragments; the fixation or prevention of further movement of the fragments; and other individualized features, such as the age, health, and nutritional status of the person involved, the interposition of soft tissues between bone fragments, and the blood supply. The importance of these various factors depends upon their

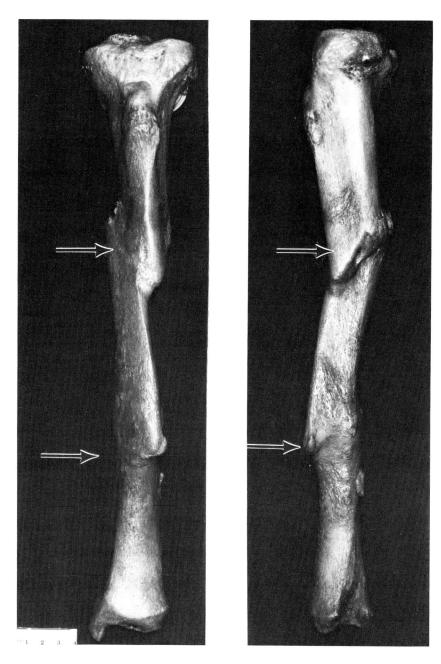

Figure 16-1

Bony callus *(arrows)* of an unset but fully healed fracture of the tibia in *(left)* anterior and *(right)* lateral view.

interaction. The results can range from successful healing to no healing. In all situations, healing is slowed or stopped if the individual is in poor health or poor nutritional condition.

Where there is little or no motion at the time of injury, close apposition, good alignment, and immobilization of the pieces after the injury, healing is likely to be highly successful. Good alignment includes a circumstance in which the two major pieces of the bone have their long axes aligned parallel to each other but one piece is slightly displaced to one side. In such a circumstance, the major response to the fracture comes from the osteoprogenitor cells within the bone itself, while a lesser response comes from the osteoprogenitor cells in the periosteum, endosteum, and surrounding connective tissues. The osteoblasts derived from these sources lay down new woven bone and little or no fibrous tissue. For healing to be highly successful, the individual must be in moderately good health and nutritional status and suffer no abnormalities of blood supply.

Where there is moderate motion, but no shear or rotation, and apposition, alignment, and fixation are good, the response from the osteoprogenitor cells of the periosteum and endosteum is intense. Starting at some distance from the fracture site, these osteoprogenitor cells give rise to osteoblasts that deposite woven bone. A lesser response comes from the surrounding connective tissue, but little or no response comes from the bone's own cells. Relatively little fibrous tissue is formed, and healing is good.

In cases with bad apposition and alignment and increased motion, including shear, the prognosis is not as good. The osteoprogenitor cells from the various sources tend to produce fibroblasts and chondroblasts rather than osteoblasts. These cells produce cartilage, much like that found in the cartilage models of bones in embryos, and fibrous tissue. Both types of cells undergo hypertrophy, calcification of the extracellular matrix, and degeneration, the end result being calcified cartilage. A callus is formed, made up of varying amounts of bone, fibrous tissue, cartilage, and calcified cartilage, which helps to immobilize the bone. If the callus prevents further significant motion, then osteoblasts can be formed and new woven bone laid down. The non-bony tissues may be resorbed in a manner similar to that found during cartilagenous ossification in the embryo. However, if immobilization through medical treatment or callus formation is not successful or does not occur rapidly enough, woven bone is not formed. Instead, the ends of the bone and the fragments are united by fibrocartilage in a condition known as nonunion. Nonunion is especially common in older patients whose fractures are not immobilized promptly.

Finally, if apposition and alignment are poor and shear or rotation is marked, healing cannot in any sense occur. The osteoprogenitor cells transform into chondroblasts and lay down cartilage similar to the hyaline cartilage found in joints. Other cells become synovial cells and give rise to synovial tissue, which in turn secretes synovial fluid. In the end, a pseudoarthrosis or false joint may be formed. This is an extreme case of nonunion.

Compressed fractures of the skull, in which an area of the cranial vault is pushed inward, are usually attributed to a blow with a blunt instrument. This kind of fracture has three distinguishing characteristics. First, cracks radiate from the depressed area. Second, within the depressed area the inner table of bone is beveled at the edges, because a larger segment of the inner table than of the outer is pushed inward. Third, the area surrounding the depressed region may be raised, having rebounded from the pressure that pushed the center inwards. If such damage occurred during life, then soft tissues will have cushioned the blow and held tiny fragments in place. However, compressed fractures may occur after death. For example, dry bones exposed on a surface or even buried by sediments and fossilized are frequently broken by nonhuman agencies. A classic confusion of natural, postmortem damage with intentional, antemortem damage occurred when some of the early hominid remains from South African caves were initially diagnosed as having received blows with blunt instruments, whereas they were actually damaged by roof-falls. Thus it is important to inspect compressed fractures of the cranium for their distinguishing characteristics before reaching conclusions about the cause of the injury.

Traumas other than fracture may also affect bones and teeth. These may include injuries produced deliberately by humans for reasons of health or fashion, incurred during fights or warfare, and caused by accident. These traumas leave characteristic marks, although distinguishing between intentional and accidental injuries may be impossible in many instances.

Cutting and piercing wounds have been well documented in skeletal remains. These wounds are often small and linear. Inspection of such marks reveals fine, parallel, microscopic striations oriented in the direction of the blow. These injuries may occur both in life and after death. Postmortem cutmarks may occur because some cultures engage in burial rites that involve defleshing or disarticulating of human remains prior to burial. In other instances, bones, especially skulls, may be decorated with elaborate, incised patterns that are obviously

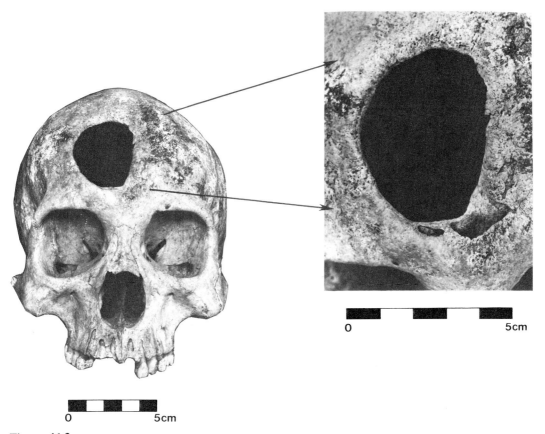

0   5cm

0   5cm

Figure 16-2

Cranium from a Mississipian Period site in Illinois, with a large, partially healed hole in the right frontal. Although deliberate trepination may have caused the hole, it was more likely caused by a blow to the forehead. Subsequent infection may have killed the bone tissue in the region, producing a hole. The large area of healed inflammation is shown in close-up.

made after death. Instances of sword, axe, or machete wounds have been found on skeletal remains, presumably attesting to wars or other battles. Occasionally an arrowhead or fragment of some other implement still remains in place in the bone.

Other types of trauma observed on bony remains include trephination, amputation, and the intentional deformation of body parts. Trephination involves cutting a hole in the skull of a living individual, often as a medical treatment, the results of which may resemble accidental injuries (Figure 16-2). The results of such practices have been observed on recent and prehistoric skulls from several continents. Amazingly,

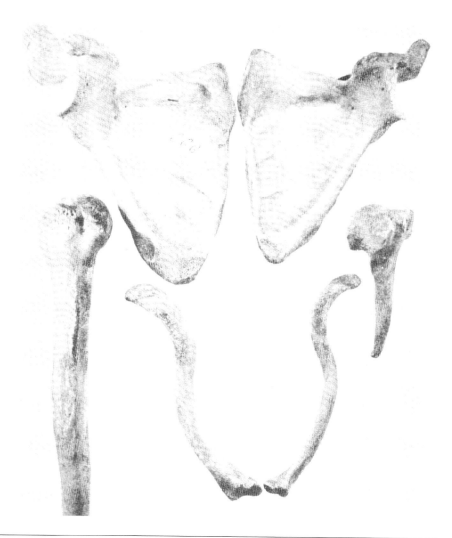

Figure 16-3

Effects of a healed left humeral amputation. The scapula, clavicle, and humeral stump have atrophied.

individuals frequently lived through the operation, as shown by partial or complete healing of the wound, and some skulls show several trephination holes. Several different techniques have been used for trephination, including making a rectangular hole via four linear incisions, drilling a large hole through the skull, and drilling many adjacent holes so that a plug of skull is separated.

Amputation, the severing of a part of the body, is another operation seen in skeletal remains that was presumably performed for medical reasons. The portion of the bone left on the body in amputations inevitably becomes smaller and less dense than the same bone on the intact side. The end of the amputated part in time becomes completely healed over. Once healed, its shaft smoothly diminishes in size to a blunt end (Figure 16-3).

Deliberate deformation of body parts, such as head-binding among various groups of American Indians or foot-binding in upper-class Chinese women before the twentieth century, often reveals itself as a consistent pattern within one or more skeletal populations. Such modifications can change the shape of the bones to an impressive extent, which often reflects the fact that the deforming procedures were initiated at or near birth (Figure 16-4).

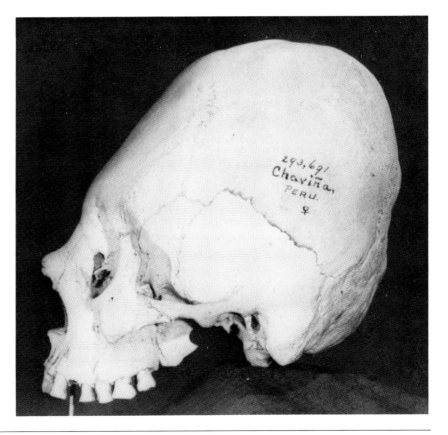

Figure 16-4

Effect of head-binding on the cranial shape. This practice, which was common among various aboriginal groups, resulted in a deliberate deformation.

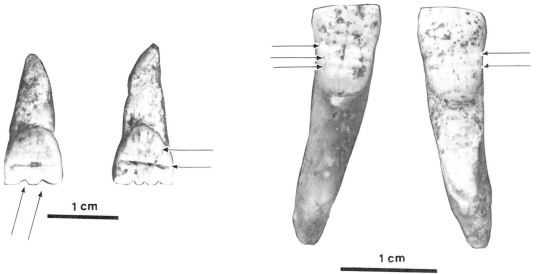

Figure 16-5

Dental abnormalities. *(Left)* Deliberate tooth-filing on central incisors creates a sinuous cutting edge and horizontal scratches *(arrows). (Right)* Enamel hypoplasia on lower canines results from nutritional stress during the formation of the enamel and produces indented horizontal bands *(arrows).*

Trauma to the teeth is also found on skeletal remains. For medical or ornamental reasons, a pattern of tooth removal, often of the lower incisors, or of tooth deformation through filing or incising may occur (Figure 16-5). When a consistent pattern of tooth loss is not observed in a skeletal population, individual instances can most probably be attributed to dental or periodontal disease rather than to human intervention. In any case, tooth loss during life is readily distinguished from postmortem tooth loss, which is extremely common, by the resorption of the alveolar bone and the growth of new bone over the socket.

DISEASE AND PATHOLOGIES

Many diseases can leave permanent effects on the skeleton. Three of the major or more common causes of bone pathology are malnutrition of various sorts, infection, and tumors. Each of these may alter bones sufficiently to permit diagnosis of the cause from skeletal remains.

The first class of pathologies, those caused by nutritional stress or deficiency, is divided into two groups: those that occur in utero or during the growth of an individual, and those that occur during adult life. A common result of nutritional stress in utero or early life is enamel hypoplasia, or arrested development (Figure 16-5). In this condition, one or more horizontal lines are visible across the surfaces of teeth; these lines represent the periods of time during which the enamel formation was defective, as a result of either dietary deficiency or disease. Because the timing of the formation of the crown of different teeth is known, the location of bands or pits of hypoplasia indicates the timing of the stress within the life of the individual.

The bones also show effects of stress by malnutrition or diet-related disease during the growing years. Dense horizontal lines, called transverse or Harris lines, are visible in radiographs of the long bones of such individuals (Figure 16-6). These lines reflect periods during which bone growth was arrested, because of stress, and then resumed once the stress was passed. The transverse line itself represents the first burst of osteoblast activity following the arrest. Such lines are most commonly found in the tibia, femur, radius, and metacarpals. Although lines laid down early in life may persist into adulthood, most are resorbed and remodeled within 10 years of their formation. Recurrent, regularly spaced transverse lines suggest that a population experienced periodic food shortage or, less probably, infection.

Nutritional stress alone is also responsible for such diseases as scurvy, rickets, hypervitaminosis A, and cribra orbitalia. Scurvy, which is due to a lack of vitamin C, inhibits the formation of collagen matrix and is therefore most evident in skeletons of infants under the age of one, since rapid bone growth is the norm during that period. The main skeletal symptom of scurvy is evidence of subperiosteal hemorrhage. These hemorrhages turn into fibrous clots that then become ossified or calcified and appear as areas of irregular bone deposited on long bone shafts. The cortical bone of scurvy victims is usually thin, and the metaphyses have a high frequency of fractures. Adult scurvy presents itself similarly, with the additional symptom of tooth loss.

Rickets, due to a lack of vitamin D or calcium in growing children, causes a deficit in the mineralization of bones. As a result, bones are weak, light-weight, and brittle. Bowing of the long bones is common in rickets, since the bones are unable to bear the weight of the individual or to resist normal stresses (Figure 16-7). Rickets may cause either thinning or thickening of the cranial vault. Thickening, which is most common in individuals 2–3 years of age, occurs primarily at the frontal eminence and the parietal bosses. Adult-onset rickets, known as osteomalacia, occurs because of deficient calcium, intestinal disease,

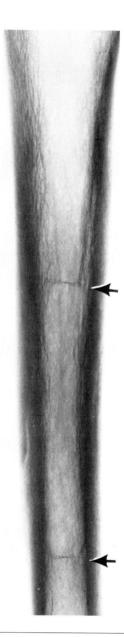

Figure 16-6

Transverse lines on the left tibial shaft, resulting from either nutritional stress or disease, which are visible on this radiograph as dark bands *(arrows)*.

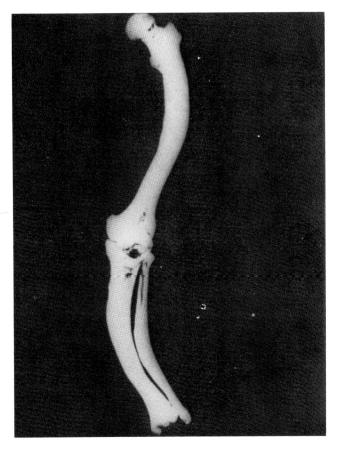

Figure 16-7

Effect of rickets on the left femur, tibia, and fibula. It causes a deficit in mineralization that results in a dramatic bowing of the bones.

or lack of sunlight and is intimately involved in vitamin D metabolism. One group especially vulnerable to osteomalacia are females who have had multiple pregnancies in rapid succession, since skeletal reserves of calcium and phosphorus can be severely depleted in such cases. Whereas rickets affects metaphyseal and cortical bone growth, in osteomalacia calcium and phosphorus are resorbed more generally from the skeleton. Softening, weakening, and deformation are particularly evident in the vertebral column, pelvis, femur, and tibia because these are the major weight-bearing bones of the skeleton. The vertebral column frequently shows either scoliosis, a lateral curvature, or kyphosis,

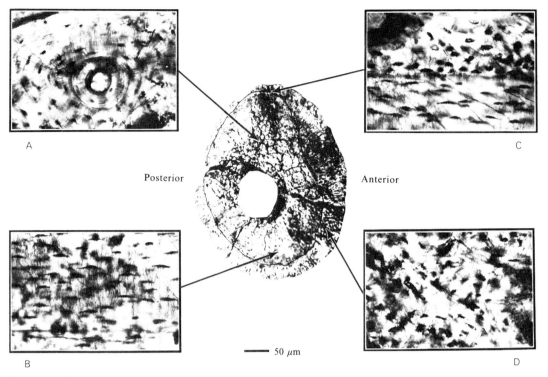

Figure 16-8

Effects of probable hypervitaminosis A on a *Homo erectus* femur. *(Center)* A cross-section through the shaft, showing the location of various micrographs *(arrows)*. The small marrow cavity is normal for this species, but the extra ring of bone surrounding the shaft is not. *(a)* Normal bone of the inner part of shaft, with an osteon that has concentric lamellae and darkly stained osteocyte lacunae and canaliculi. *(b)* Another area of normal concentric lamellae with regular arrays of osteocyte lacunae and canaliculi. *(c)* Interface of normal bone *(below)* and pathological bone *(above)*, where the organized normal tissue contrasts with the disorganized pathological tissue with its abnormal, rounded osteocyte lacunae. *(d)* The random orientation and distorted shapes of osteocyte lacunae farther out in the pathological bone.

an anteroposterior curvature also known as humpback. The skull is rarely involved in osteomalacia.

Hypervitaminosis A is a relatively rare condition brought on by an excessive dietary intake of vitamin A or by an enzyme deficiency. It results in massive, subperiosteal hemorrhage and subsequent ossification of irregular, disorganized spongy bone on the outer surface of various long bones. The skull may also be involved. Hypervitaminosis A

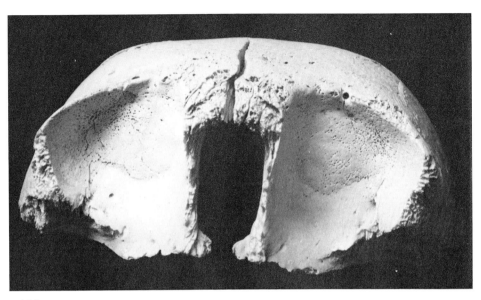

Figure 16-9

Effect of cribra orbitalia on the eye sockets. It produces the growth of extra, porous bone on the roofs of the orbits.

is best documented in individuals who have consumed quantities of carnivore liver, such as Arctic explorers trapped with limited food and equipment who eat raw seal or polar bear livers. A prehistoric case of hypervitaminosis A in *Homo erectus* has been found (Figure 16-8).

Cribra orbitalia, another disease tied to nutritional deficiencies, results in extra, spongy bone being deposited on the inferior surface of the roof of the bony orbits (Figure 16-9). The underlying cortical bone is also usually resorbed. Cribra orbitalia is more common in children than in adults. It may be related to iron deficiencies, especially during the weaning period, but its exact cause is unclear.

The second major class of bone diseases is caused by infection. Three of the more distinctive infectious diseases manifested in skeletal remains are tuberculosis, treponemal diseases, and leprosy. Tuberculosis osteitis is a classic bacterial disease, readily spread in crowded living quarters, and is often manifested in children's bones. Skeletal tuberculosis is considered a secondary infection, which arises from pulmonary tuberculosis in approximately 5–7 percent of all cases. Deformation of the vertebrae is a common symptom of skeletal tuberculosis (Figure 16-10). It starts as a resorption of the trabeculae of the central or anterior portions of the vertebral body, which leads to col-

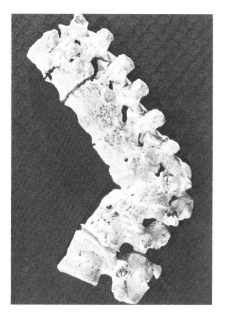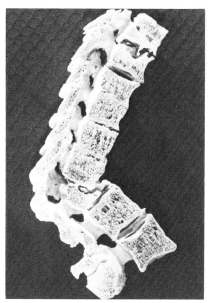

Figure 16-10

Effects of tuberculosis on the spinal column in *(left)* lateral view and *(right)* longitudinal section. The vertebrae have fused together and collapsed; the intervertebral disc between T7–8 is perforated.

lapse and fusion of that body with the adjacent one. The result is a pronounced kyphosis. The affected bone itself appears porous, irregular, and poorly organized. Other common sites of skeletal involvement are the hip and knee. In some or perhaps all parts of the world, early appearances of tuberculosis are associated with economic changes, such as the onset of pastoralism or agriculture, which permit or even require dense settlements.

Treponemal diseases are spread by various microorganisms called spirochetes, which result in yaws, bejel, and endemic or venereal syphilis. All three diseases may cause bone damage in the form of lesions, typically on either the long bones or the skull. All three are spread by close contact, such as occurs in crowded living quarters. Inflammation of the vault bones in these diseases begins with clusters of pits on the outer surface, which enlarge, coalesce into a larger pit, and then form radial scars (Figure 16-11). In severe cases the entire superior aspect of the cranium may be heavily pitted and scarred. In long bones, early involvement takes the form of subperiosteal pitting, striation, and deposition of clearly pathological extra bone. The cortical bone thickens

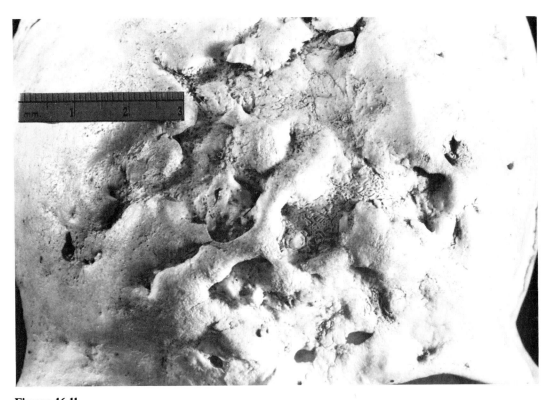

Figure 16-11

Effects of syphilis on the frontal. It produces scarring and pitting.

and takes on a swollen appearance. In later stages extreme bowing of long bones may occur, as in the condition known as sabre-shin tibia. It is difficult to differentiate between the various types of treponemal diseases in skeletal remains.

Leprosy is another infectious bacterial disease spread by close contact, although exposure must usually be prolonged. Leprosy has historically been a more common disease in the Old World than in the New. The most common type of bone lesion resulting from leprosy involves the hands and feet. The lower splanchnocranium is also often involved, with the nasal spine and maxillary alveoli atrophying, frequently causing loss of the upper incisors and resulting in porous, heavily pitted bone in the affected region. The palate is also often involved, through pitting, thinning, or perforation. In the hands and feet, the effects of leprosy appear first in the distal phalanges and then spread proximally. New bone is laid down in the medullary cavity, while the external surface of the bone is absorbed. Phalanges and metatarsals or metacarpals thin and dwindle to pointed stubs. Because leprotic changes in the hands and feet involve impaired nerve function during life, there is an increased rate of traumatic injury to those parts.

Finally, a wealth of tumors and tumor-like processes may permanently affect the bony skeleton. It is difficult to produce an exact diagnosis from skeletal remains, since biochemical and histological data are missing. Aside from the gross appearance of a tumor, its location may provide clues as to its origin, since different tumors occur characteristically in different regions of the skeleton. However, it is easy to confuse exostoses, or irregular outgrowths of bone, resulting from injuries — as when extensive hematomas ossify — with exostoses caused by cancer or similar disease processes. There is little information on the incidence of such pathologies in ancient populations.

A relatively common tumorous condition is an osteoma, which is observed as a lump or mound of compact bone, varying from a small button osteoma to a quite large growth. Osteomata are benign tumors formed in areas in which the bone normally ossifies intramembranously, for which reason they are common on the vault bones. It is not unusual for an individual to show several osteomata. They are often asymptomatic during life.

Malignant bone diseases include osteosarcomas and multiple myelomas. Osteosarcomas typically involve the production of malignant bone tissue, osteoid, or cartilage; the most common site is the distal femur. They usually occur in individuals between the ages of about 10 and 25. In contrast, multiple myelomas occur almost exclusively in individuals over 50 years of age. They involve a cancerous growth of plasma cells in the bone marrow and therefore are found predominantly in bones that contain a lot of marrow in adults: the vertebrae, ribs, pelvis, and cranial vault.

17
RECONSTRUCTION

Skeletal remains can reveal biological and historical information about the past. The specific aim of their study may vary from a simple question like, "Is this individual likely to be the one described on a recent missing persons report?" to a complex one like, "How did dietary changes affect the health, skeletal structure, and demography of populations in the New World?" Evidence gathered from estimating age or stature, determining race or sex, and detecting signs of stress, disease, or trauma is important in answering such questions. Additional information is provided by two very different but effective types of reconstruction based on bony remains: facial and dietary. Facial reconstruction focuses on detailed physical attributes of an individual, whereas dietary reconstruction yields information about an individual's behavior and habits during life.

FACIAL RECONSTRUCTION

Facial reconstruction involves visualizing the face of an individual from his or her skull. The technique has three important uses. It is used to help identify skeletal remains by comparing the facial reconstruction with photos of missing persons of the appropriate age and sex. It is used to assess skulls thought to be those of known individuals or to evaluate the accuracy of historic portraits. Finally, facial reconstruction is used to illustrate works on human evolution, in an attempt to give life and color to the "dry bones" of the past.

Facial reconstruction can take the form of a painting or drawing, but in many cases the most realistic and accurate reconstruction is produced by creating a clay sculpture directly on the skull or on a cast of the skull. The sculptural approach was pioneered in the late nineteenth century by scientists who measured the soft-tissue thickness at various points on the head of cadavers of different races. (Table 17-1, Figure 17-1). Because the thickness of skin, fat, muscle, and connective tissues differs between males and females and among different races, the accuracy of facial reconstruction must rely on the appropriateness of the population from which the data are collected.

Whatever its purpose, the technique of facial reconstruction is a skillful blend of statistics, anatomical knowledge, and artistry. Some people are more gifted than others at producing reconstructions that, when later identified, bear a striking resemblance to the living individuals whose skulls are in question (Figure 17-2).

Several problems plague the attempt to reconstruct facial features from skulls. These problems relate to the size, shape, and placement of soft tissue features that, when altered, can dramatically change facial appearance. These features include the placement of the eyeball within the bony orbit, the length and width of the nose, the width of the mouth,

Table 17-1 Average Tissue Depth at Eighteen Points on the Face in Male and Female Whites (mm)

Location of Point (Symbol)[a]		Study (Number of Subjects)[b]						
		W(13)	H(24)	K(21)	HK(45)	H(4)	K(4)	HK(8)
Midline of face			*Male*			*Female*		
Forehead: trichion	(A)	—	4.08	3.07	3.56	4.16	3.02	3.59
Forehead: middle	(B)	4.3	—	—	—	—	—	—
Forehead: glabella	(C)	—	5.17	4.29	4.69	4.75	3.9	4.32
Root of nose: nasion	(D)	5.9	5.45	4.31	4.93	5.0	4.1	4.55
Bridge of nose: middle of internasal suture	(E)	3.3	3.29	3.13	3.25	3.0	2.51	2.78
Bridge of nose: rhinion	(F)	2.2	—	2.12	2.12	—	2.07	2.07
Base of nasal septum: subnasale	(G)	—	11.25	11.65	11.59	9.75	10.1	9.92
Lower end of philtrum: prosthion	(I)	11.0	9.37	9.46	9.48	8.26	8.1	8.18
Mentolabial furrow	(J)	10.6	10.0	9.84	10.05	9.75	10.95	10.35
Chin: from in front	(L)	8.5	11.05	9.02	10.22	10.75	9.37	10.06
Chin: from below	(M)	—	6.16	5.98	6.08	6.5	5.85	6.18
Side of face								
Eyebrow: middle border	(N)	—	5.8	5.41	5.65	5.5	5.15	5.32
Orbit: middle of lower border	(O)	—	4.9	3.51	4.29	5.25	3.65	4.45
Cheekbone: prominence	(P)	—	—	6.62	6.62	—	7.73	7.73
Zygomatic arch: middle	(Q)	—	—	4.33	4.33	—	5.32	5.32
Zygomatic arch: near ear	(R)	—	6.05	7.42	6.74	6.75	7.1	6.92
Mandible: middle of ascending ramus	(S)	—	8.37	7.76	8.20	8.1	6.16	7.13
Mandible: corpus in front of masseter	(T)	—	17.55	17.01	17.53	17.0	14.83	15.91

a. See Figure 17.1.

b. W = Welcker, 1883; H = His, 1895; K = Kollmann, 1898; HK = His, 1895, and Kollmann, 1898, combined.

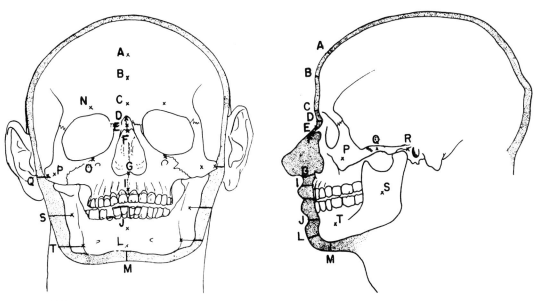

Figure 17-1

Location of tissue thickness measurements on the head in anterior and lateral view (see Table 17-1).

and the length of the ear. Guidelines have been developed by Gatliff and Snow for estimating the size or placement of each of these features.

In lateral view, the most anterior point of the curvature of the eyeball lies tangent to an imaginary line connecting the superior and inferior margins of the orbit. In anterior view, this same point, the apex of the cornea, lies at the intersection of two lines, one connecting the midpoint of the superior orbital margin with the midpoint of the inferior orbital margin and the other connecting the midpoints of the lateral and medial margins of the orbit. These two imaginary lines do not necessarily intersect at right angles.

In general, the width of the nasal aperture is approximately three-fifths that of the fleshy nose. The tip of the fleshy nose projects anteriorly from the base of the nasal aperture a distance that is about three times the length of the nasal spine. Unfortunately, nasal spines are frequently broken or damaged, in which case artistic talent and subjective judgment must be used.

The corners of the mouth, which determine its width, usually intersect an imaginary line drawn on each side between the midpoint of the inferior orbital margin and the widest point of the chin. The length of

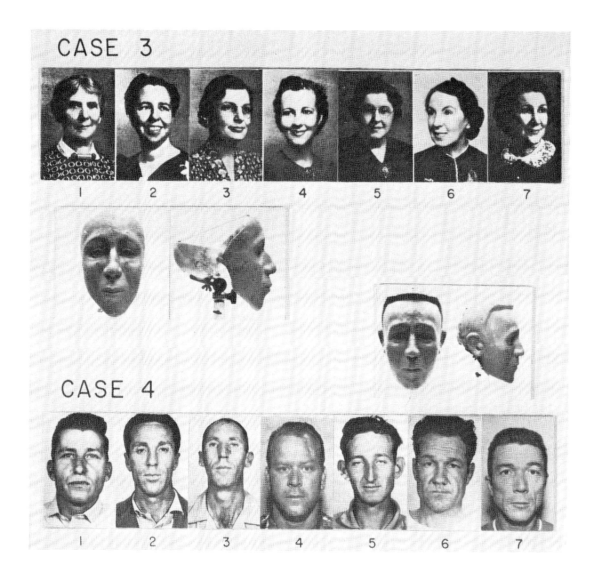

Figure 17-2

Poster used to test the usefulness of facial reconstruction in identifying individuals from cranial remains. In case 3, the reconstruction of a female cranium *(below left)* was compared with photos of seven women of similar age and ancestry; 26% of the observers correctly identified photo #2 as the individual in the reconstruction. In case 4, a similar test was performed on the reconstruction of a male cranium *(above right)*; 68% of the observers correctly identified photo #2.

the ear along a superoinferior axis is approximately equal to the total fleshy nose length, from bridge to tip.

Other features that may markedly affect appearance are less easily reconstructed. These include the color of skin, shape and width of lips, shape of ears, and hair style and color. Nevertheless, when Snow and his colleagues tested people's ability to match facial reconstructions made without recourse to photos with photos of a group of individuals of similar age and sex, the correct photos were chosen significantly more often than all others.

DIETARY RECONSTRUCTION

An entirely different set of aims motivates attempts at reconstructing the habitual diet of an individual or group. The concern is not to identify but rather to understand the lifestyle, ecology, and behavior of a past population or species. Simply put, diet is one of the most important biological facts about any species and thus is one of the most revealing points of information that can be gained from studying skeletal remains. Major questions in anthropology concern the causes and effects of changes in diet, modes of obtaining and processing food, and economic strategy in general.

There are eight principle modes of deducing diet from fossil or skeletal remains: interspecific comparisons of tooth morphology, biomechanical reconstruction, inspection of tooth microwear, isotope analysis, trace element analysis, application of ecological "rules", analysis of "food refuse" from archaeological sites, and diagnosis of metabolic diseases caused by diet (Walker, 1981:58). Another technique for reconstructing diet, which is only suitable within historic times, is reference to historic or ethnographic accounts of diet and food-procurement strategies.

Interspecific comparisons of tooth morphology often enable an extinct species to be grouped in a dietary category with known species that show similar dental adaptations. For example, grazing species tend to have tall (hypsodont) or evergrowing teeth with many plates or rods of enamel placed at right angles to the occlusal plane to form a masticatory system suitable for rasping or grinding. When human remains are at issue, however, this comparative approach is of little value, since all humans have morphologically similar teeth, despite the wide range of diets consumed by different human groups. This apparent uncoupling of form and function may be related in part to the human tendency to process food outside the mouth, such as using tools, water, and fire. However, it may also be true that human teeth are adapted for omnivory, so that they function equally well in processing foods of many types.

Similarly, biomechanical reconstructions of the muscles of mastication, their strength, and their lines of action may be useful in reconstructing the diet of extinct nonhuman species but is of little value in dealing with human remains. In fact, such reconstructions may in some cases be misleading. For example, female Eskimos living a traditional lifestyle have unusually large masticatory muscles and unusual wear on their incisors because they use these teeth to soften hides. Their masticatory muscle development thus has little to do with their diet per se but rather reflects other tasks performed with their jaws and teeth.

Tooth microwear studies make it possible to deduce the diet of extinct species or ancient populations. Walker and his co-workers have shown that food particles, extraneous material adhering to food, and even tooth-on-tooth wear produce distinctive patterns of microscopic wear on dentin and enamel. At the onset of tooth microwear study, qualitatively different patterns of dental microwear were compiled by inspecting the molars of species of a known diet. These patterns matched broad dietary categories, such as grazer, browser, frugivore, bone-crusher, and meat-eater, which made it possible to diagnose the diets of unknown groups if their microwear patterns matched those of a known dietary group.

A problem with this early methodology was that the comparison of different patterns was largely subjective. It provided no means of measuring resemblances or of evaluating the variation in dental microwear that might be expected between individuals eating essentially the same diet. Direct measurement of all microwear features, including pits, scratches, and grooves, occurring on photomosaics of the same facet on different individuals' teeth is possible, but it is extraordinarily time-consuming because each tooth facet bears thousands of microwear features. Teaford and Walker's more recent strategy for sampling areas within a facet and for using a computerized digitizing technique to quantify the size, shape, and frequency of microwear features permits a statistical comparison of the microwear observed on the unknown tooth with the microwear observed on a species of known diet (Figure 17-3). This technique allows much finer differences in diet to be detected than were possible with mere pattern recognition.

Isotope analysis is another useful technique for dietary reconstruction. It is based on the fact that the bones in the body incorporate different stable isotopes of carbon and nitrogen according to the iso-

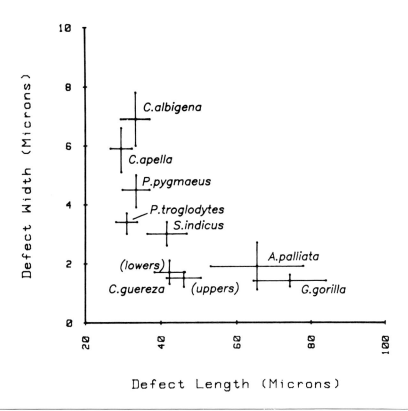

Figure 17-3

Diet and dental microwear features on M2's of living and fossilized primate species. The mean dimensions and 99.9% confidence limits of microwear defects separates the frugivores *(vertical axis)* from the folivores *(horizontal axis)* among the living species. The species with greater defect widths than lengths (mangabey, *Cercocebus albigena;* capuchin, *Cebus apella;* and orang-utan, *Pongo pygmaeus*) eat mostly fruits and nuts and form a gradient from harder to softer object feeders. The species with greater defect lengths than widths (colobus, *Colobus guereza;* howler monkey, *Alouatta palliata;* and gorilla, *Gorilla gorilla*) eat mostly leaves, stems, and flowers. The chimpanzee, *Pan troglodytes*, is intermediate in diet between these two groups, its microwear, and probably its diet, being statistically indistinguishable from that of the fossil species, *Sivapithecus indicus.*

topic composition of the diet that was being eaten while the bone was forming. Specifically, the different isotopes are found in the collagen fraction of bone. Isotope analysis can reveal whether a diet was based more heavily on meat or on one of several different categories of plants. It may also reveal whether the diet was derived from the marine or the terrestrial system.

In the case of carbon, different isotope ratios are found in various foods because two different chemical pathways, the C_3 and C_4, are used by plants during photosynthesis. The pathway used by a plant determines the ratios in the plant's tissue of two other carbon isotopes, ^{13}C and ^{12}C, that are available to be eaten by others. Thus, marine plants differ from terrestrial plants in the ratio of $^{13}C/^{12}C$ that they typically incorporate. In the case of nitrogen, different plant species obtain their nitrogen from different sources and therefore show different ratios of ^{15}N to ^{14}N. For this reason, marine and terrestial plants show different typical ratios of $^{15}N/^{14}N$. Within terrestrial plants, there is a further distinction between legumes, such as peas, and nonlegumes in the $^{15}N/^{14}N$ ratios in their tissues.

When a plant with its typical ratio of different carbon and nitrogen isotopes is eaten by an herbivore, the plant's isotopic ratio is transferred to the collagen in the herbivore's bones. The same transfer occurs when the herbivore's bones are eaten by a carnivore. Analyzing the ratios of carbon and nitrogen isotopes in bone collagen reveals the extent to which the different dietary items were consumed. Such analysis yields results in the δ notation, in which the measured isotopic ratios ($^{13}C/^{12}C$ or $^{15}N/^{14}N$) of the sample being analyzed are compared mathematically with those in known standards. The result is a $\delta^{13}C$ value or a $\delta^{15}N$ value that indicates how much the sample is altered relative to the standard.

A trophic level effect occurs in the nitrogen isotope system. That is, in the bones of animals of known diet, a small but significant enrichment of $\delta^{15}N$ values occurs at each step up the trophic pyramid from plant to herbivore to primary carnivore to secondary carnivore. A slightly greater enrichment occurs in the carbon isotope system in the step between plant and herbivore, but beyond this level the enrichment appears too small to be useful in dietary reconstruction.

The carbon isotope system is of particular interest in pinpointing the development and spread of agriculture in the New World. Most plants utilize the C_3 photosynthetic pathway, meaning that their tissues have lower $^{13}C/^{12}C$ ratios than tissues of plants that utilize the C_4 pathways. Although most C_4 plants are tropical grasses, one of the most important cultivated plants in the New World, maize, is also a C_4 plant. Therefore, the onset of major use of maize in a particular region will be reflected by a sudden increase in $\delta^{13}C$ values in the collagen of the maize-eating populations relative to the $\delta^{13}C$ values of their predecessors who did not eat maize.

A major difficulty with isotope analysis is that changes can occur in the collagen portion of bone after death due to processes known collectively as diagenesis. The preservation of organic matrix is highly variable in fossil and subfossil bones. If biochemically identifiable collagen cannot be isolated from a sample, that sample is not appropriate for isotope analysis. If only a trace of organic material can be isolated, the $\delta^{13}C$ and $\delta^{15}N$ values may have been altered from those existing in the original collagen.

Analysis of the trace element, strontium, in bones relies on a similar principle. Like isotope ratios, the ratio of strontium to the common element, calcium, in bone varies with trophic level. Different soils, waters, and plants contain different amounts of strontium. As animals feed upon the plants, the strontium is incorporated into their bones and flesh in proportions that reflect their dietary intake, giving a strontium/calcium ratio typical for their diet. Because the body discriminates against strontium in favor of calcium during bone deposition, herbivores contain less strontium, yielding lower strontium/calcium ratios than those of the plants upon which they feed. Omnivores that eat both plants and herbivores incorporate still less strontium into their bodies, which produces lower strontium/calcium ratios than in herbivores, and carnivores incorporate even less, so that they have the lowest strontium/calcium ratio of all. Because bone incorporates more strontium than does flesh, it is possible to distinguish between carnivores that consume mostly flesh, like cheetahs, and those that consume both bone and flesh, like hyenas. Cheetahs can be expected to have even lower strontium/calcium ratios than hyenas, although both are carnivores, because of the differences in their feeding habits.

Strontium analysis poses a number of problems. One is that the background levels of available strontium vary from place to place. It is necessary to normalize measured strontium levels so that these can be compared between sites. The usual approach is to make a ratio of the strontium values for carnivores and herbivores at each site. These ratios can then be compared without the interference of any extraneous effects produced by natural deviations in the level of strontium in the soil and groundwater from place to place. Although it is possible to avoid this problem by limiting analysis to the material from a single site, many questions about regional and temporal changes in diet cannot be answered without intrasite comparisons.

Another problem with strontium analysis derives from the metabolic differences between tissues. Since strontium is incorporated into the skeleton as a substitute for calcium, poorly mineralized tissues contain less strontium than well-mineralized ones. For this reason the values of both strontium and calcium are measured, and a ratio of the two values is used rather than the measured strontium level alone. A further metabolic difference that may confound strontium analysis involves teeth that were formed in utero or during breast feeding. In these cases neither the strontium/calcium ratios nor the strontium levels per se accurately reflect the adult dietary consumption of strontium. This distortion occurs because both the placenta and the breast discriminate strongly against strontium; therefore, very little of the mother's intake of strontium is available to the fetus or infant for incorporation into its body. Abnormally low strontium values also appear in the bones of newborn infants, whereas the bones of older children and adults accurately reflect the dietary intake of strontium. This distinction occurs because bones remodel but teeth do not, with the result that teeth retain the strontium levels that were incorporated during amelogenesis and odontogenesis. In species with evergrowing teeth, new dentin and enamel are produced continually and the strontium/calcium ratios in all teeth thus reflect dietary intake. Finally, if calcium intake was deficient in the population under study, then strontium will have been incorporated in the bones at a much higher rate than would have occurred had the calcium intake been normal.

The final problem with strontium analysis concerns possible diagenetic changes in the inorganic matrix. As with isotope analysis, trace element analysis may yield misleading results if the bone mineral composition has been changed postmortem. X-ray diffraction studies, which yield information about the crystalline structure of substances, can show whether the biological hydroxyapatite has been replaced by the geological mineral apatite during diagenesis. Samples that show the x-ray diffraction pattern typical of biological hydroxyapatite can be assumed to have an unaltered strontium/calcium ratio. Comparison of these ratios in herbivores, carnivores, and humans within a single site also reveals diagenesis. When the strontium/calcium values for herbivores and carnivores do not separate well, all of the skeletal materials from the site are probably diagenetically altered. However, the mammals classified as carnivores differ widely in the amount of meat, bone, and vegetable food in their diet. Thus, if the only carnivores present are omnivorous-feeders, like foxes and striped hyenas, a failure to separate carnivores and herbivores may not indicate that diagenesis has occurred. Finally, spurious strontium/calcium ratios may be obtained in some cases because the cracks, Haversian canals, and osteocyte lacunae of bones have been filled with contaminants during fossilization. In such cases, careful preparation of the samples, either mechanically or chemically, is needed to exclude the contaminating material.

Other trace elements less commonly analyzed include zinc and lead. Lead analysis is of particular interest because techniques commonly used in the past to make pewter and pottery create utensils that contaminate food or drink with lead. Measured lead levels in some prehistoric populations indicate the occurrence of chronic lead poisoning.

Ecological rules or generalizations are useful in eliminating diets that cannot be successfully maintained by species of a given body size. For example, small-bodied species cannot digest cellulose rapidly enough to live on leaves, and large-bodied species cannot obtain sufficient insects to be insectivores, unless they eat social insects occurring in large colonies. Such rules are based on the attributes of the food item in terms of its nutritional yield, its distribution in space and time, and its necessary processing in order to yield usable food substances. Humans, like all other species, selectively utilize the foods theoretically available in their habitats. Thus, their choices, whether conscious or not, are probably affected strongly by the energetic costs of obtaining or processing a given food item, by the size of the units in which it can be acquired, and by the reliability with which the food item can be located.

Analysis of archaeological food refuse, such as bones or shells, may be a valuable source of information about diet. The difficulty with this approach lies in distinguishing food refuse from items that are only accidentally present at the site. For example, animal bones are often found spatially associated with stone tools, traces of dwellings, or other signs of human activity and yet do not reflect dietary intake. Such bones may have been accumulated before or after the human activities and may bear no causal relationship to them. Alternatively, bones may be present at a site because of human activities and yet not represent food items. For example, pets or work animals not regarded as edible may be buried or disposed of in a refuse pit.

Several techniques can be applied to archaeological assemblages in order to establish a causal link between humans or their ancestors and animal bones that may represent food refuse. Cutmarks made by stone, bone, or metal tools can be distinguished microscopically from similar marks made by carnivore chewing, sedimentary abrasion, trampling, weathering, and other such events (Figure 17-4). The presence of verified cutmarks on bones establishes a firm, causal connec-

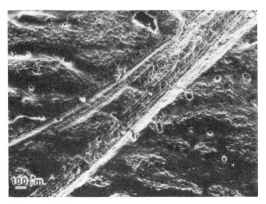 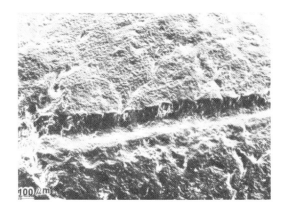

Figure 17-4

Microscopic morphology as a means of identifying linear grooves on bones. *(Left)* A cutmark made by a stone tool. Cutmarks typically are elongate grooves with many fine, parallel striations within the main groove. *(Right)* A toothmark made by a hyena. Toothmarks typically are smooth on the bottom or else show chatter-marks oriented perpendicular to the long axis of the groove.

tion between the tool-user and the bone, although cutmarks alone do not indicate that the flesh from the bone was eaten. Cutmarks are also left by skinning and dismembering procedures, which are not neces-sarily accompanied by the consumption of flesh.

Butchery, in the sense of a systematic processing of carcasses for the removal of flesh, leaves a highly patterned distribution of cut-marks. Most species of animals are butchered similarly, by disarticu-lating the major joints to separate convenient units of meat and bone. As a result, butchered animals show a heavy concentration of cut-marks around the major joints, sometimes accompanied by regular patterns of breakage where tough or difficult-to-reach tendons and joint capsules are found. These facts can be used to evaluate patterns of cutmarks and breakage statistically and thereby determine whether the observed damage represents butchery.

The burning of skeletal remains can also be detected microscopi-cally. Since controlled fires produce substantially higher tempera-tures for a longer period of time than natural fires, the temperature reached by a bone may indicate whether it was heated in a man-made fire. Again, although burning does not invariably indicate meat con-sumption, a regular pattern of burning on particular elements of par-ticular species provides strong circumstantial evidence of dietary practices.

Similarly, plant material that does not represent food refuse may also accrue on archaeological sites. The presence of large quantities of particular plant remains strongly suggests that they were eaten, as does the existence of cultivated, rather than wild, types. Human groups that rely heavily on plant foods usually leave indirect evidence as well, in the form of storage containers and processing tools.

The diagnosis of metabolic diseases caused by diet is possible when bone pathologies are found. In most cases, serious dietary deficiencies alter bones and teeth in ways that can be detected even if the individual lived for several years afterward on a sufficient diet. However, there are few skeletal signs that point to a specific dietary problem. Many pathologies indicate only that some stress, whether caused by diet or disease, occurred at a particular point in an individual's life.

Exploration of all these lines of evidence, where appropriate, usually provides a broad picture of the diet of a population or species. Generally, only the major components of a diet are well represented in skeletal remains, and occasional or minor parts of the diet remain archaeologically invisible. This loss of fine detail is inevitable, reflecting the current level of precision of the techniques of dietary reconstruction. However, in terms of the major demands and concerns of the daily life of a population, such reconstruction probably reflects accurately the past. With new research and refined techniques, dietary reconstruction promises to be one of the most powerful tools available for transforming skeletal remains back into living organisms.

GLOSSARY

abduction: the action of moving a limb or limb segment laterally, away from the body's midline

adduction: the action of moving a limb or limb segment medially, toward the body's midline

alignment: the orientation of bone fragments following a fracture

amelogenesis: the process of making enamel

anterior: of or toward the front of the body

appendicular: pertaining to the bones of the limbs

apposition: the degree of contact or separation of bone fragments following a fracture

appositional growth: increase in width, due to the recruitment of new chondroblasts from the periochondrium

articular cartilage (also called hyaline cartilage): a special type of cartilage that covers the surfaces of bones where they participate in joints

articulation: the point at which any two bones meet and participate in a joint

axial: of or pertaining to the bones of the trunk and thorax, including the vertebrae, sacrum, ribs, innominates, and sternum

balancing side: in mastication, the side of the mouth where there is little or no food but where the resultant force is taken

bilaminar embryonic disc: the two-layer mass of cells, including both ectoderm and endoderm, found at about the eighth or ninth day after fertilization

blastocyst: a morula, or 16-cell ball, that has developed a central cavity

boundary lubrication: reduction of friction due to the presence of mutually repellant, opposing surfaces during movement

browser: a herbivorous species that habitually eats leaves

buccal: of or toward the cheek

calcification: the deposition of hydroxyapatite onto osteoid to form new bone tissue

calcitonin: the hormone secreted by the thyroid gland that decreases the circulating levels of calcium and phosphate ions by blocking bone resorption and fostering calcification, antagonistic to parathyroid hormone

callus: the mass of woven bone and fibrocartilaginous tissue that forms during the initial stages of fracture healing

calvaria (*pl.* calvariae): the superior portion of the skull where it roofs the cranial vault, covering the superior surface of the brain

canaliculus (*pl.* canaliculi): a microscopic tunnel in bone tissue, which houses a dendritic projection used by osteocytes to communicate with each other and with the blood stream

cancellous bone (also called spongy bone): bone tissue that characteristically has many grossly visible pores and openings, typically found in the ends of long bones or in the bodies of vertebrae

carnivore: a species, such as a lion, that habitually eats other animals

carpus: the wrist

cartilaginous ossification. *See* ossification

cervical: of or pertaining to the neck region

chondroblast: the cell that secretes the organic matrix of cartilage

chondroclast: the large, multinucleate cell responsible for resorbing cartilage

chondrocyte: a transformed chondroblast that is trapped in cartilage matrix

circumduction: the action whereby a limb or limb segment is pivoted around a joint, causing the distal end to describe the base of a cone with its apex at the joint

collagen: the primary component of the organic matrix of bone, occurring as fibers made up of many tropocollagen molecules that typically show a light and dark banding pattern with 64nm repeats

compact bone (also called cortical bone): bone tissue that is relatively dense, having few spaces or canals, typically found in the shafts of long bones

compass gait: a hypothetical form of bipedal locomotion involving a fixed ankle and knee

compression: a force that tends to move the atoms or molecules of a substance closer to each other

coronal: a midline plane or section that divides the body in anterior and posterior halves

cortical bone. *See* compact bone

costal: of or pertaining to the ribs

cranium: the part of the skull that includes the bony face, upper jaw, and the various bones that surround the brain

dental microwear: microscopic alterations of dentin and enamel caused by use

dentin: the yellowish substance that makes up the root and interior part of the crown of teeth

dentinoenamel junction (DEJ): the interface between the dentin and enamel within a tooth

diaphysis: the shaft of a long bone

digit: a toe or finger

dimorphism: the condition of having two different morphs, or shapes, as in sexual dimorphism

distal: in the limbs, away from the trunk or toward the terminal part of the limb; in the mouth or dentition, toward the back of the tooth row, where the molars are located

dorsiflexion: the action of flexing the ankle, so that the dorsum of the foot is moved closer to the anterior tibia

dorsum: the back, especially the posterior surface of the thorax or the superior surface of the foot ectoderm: the embryonic tissue that gives rise to the superficial skin layers, hair, nails, some glands, and the central nervous system

elasticity. *See* Young's modulus of elasticity

enamel: the hard, white substance that covers the outer surface of the tooth crown

endoderm: the embryonic tissue that gives rise both to the lining of the pulmonary and digestive systems and to the tonsils, pharynx, and thyroid gland

endoplasmic reticulum: an organelle that synthesizes many cell products and contains many cisternae or compartments for the temporary storage of cell products; rough endoplasmic reticulum is studded with ribosomes containing RNA-encoded directions for protein synthesis

endosteum: a membrane that lines the medullary or marrow cavity of bones

energy: the capacity for doing work, as in moving a given load over a given distance, measured as foot-pounds or joules

epiphyseal plate (also called epiphyseal growth plate or physis): in immature bones, the remnant of the original cartilaginous model that persists between the primary center of ossification in the shaft and the epiphyses, which is replaced by bone in a mature skeleton

epiphysis: a secondary center of ossification of a bone, found especially at the articular ends of long bones, which in immature bones is separated from the primary center of ossification, in the shaft, by a cartilaginous growth plate

extension: the action that increases, or straightens, the angle at a joint

fine cancellous bone: rapidly deposited, finely porous bone laid down in response to unusual, transient stress

fixation: the immobilization or prevention of further movement of fragments following a fracture, often by medical intervention

flat foot: in walking, a position in which the foot of the stance leg is placed flat on the ground

flexion: the action that decreases, or makes more acute, the angle at a joint

fontanelle: in immature crania, an expanse of dense connective tissue that lies between the growing cranial bones

foramen (*pl.* foramina): a hole or small, rounded opening in a bone

fracture: one type of trauma, involving breakage of a bone

Golgi apparatus (also called Golgi complex): an organelle found within cells, which is responsible for processing cell products and packaging them in membranes or for removing cell membranes from vesicles bringing substances into the cell

grazer: a herbivorous species that habitually eats grass

hallux: the big or first toe

Haversian canal: the bony tube surrounding a blood vessel and oriented longitudinally within a bone, which nourishes bone tissue as part of the Haversian system

heel strike: in walking, the placing of the heel on the ground and starting to transfer weight to that heel, at the onset of a new step

hemopoietic (also called hematopoietic): producing blood cells

herbivore: a species, such as a deer, that habitually eats plant food

hyaline cartilage. *See* articular cartilage

hydrodynamic lubrication: reduction of friction due to the presence of a fluid film that is drawn between two opposing surfaces by their movements

hydrostatic lubrication: reduction of friction due to the presence of a fluid film that is pumped between two opposing surfaces during movement

hydroxyapatite: the crystalline compound of calcium and phosphorus that is the inorganic component of bone

inferior: of or toward the bottom or lower part of the body

inner cell mass: the cells of the blastocyst that give rise to the tissues of the new individual

interstitial growth: increase in length, due to the multiplication of chondroblasts

intramembranous ossification. *See* ossification

isotope: an alternative form of an element

joint capsule: the connective tissue structure that completely encloses a joint

joule: a measure of energy equal to 0.74 foot-pounds or 1 newton per meter

kyphosis: an exaggerated thoracic curvature of the vertebral column or hunchback

labial: of or toward the lips

lamellar bone: mature bone tissue organized into concentric rings or lamellae of bone, with 15–20 lamellae surrounding a Haversian canal through which a blood vessel runs, produced by remodeling some type of immature bone tissue

laminar bone: an immature bone tissue typical of young, rapidly growing animals, having sheets or laminae of bone tissue separated by networks of canals for blood vessels, which is usually remodeled into mature lamellar bone

lateral: away from the body's midline

lingual: of or toward the tongue

lumbar: of or pertaining to the lower back

lysosome: an organelle consisting of digestive enzymes bound by a membrane

medial: toward the body's midline

medullary cavity: the marrow cavity inside long bones

mesenchyme: a loose connective tissue that is a source of osteoprogenitor cells and gives rise to the mesoderm, the last embryonic tissue to appear

mesoderm: the embryonic tissue that gives rise to the muscles, bones, urogenital system, digestive system, and all connective tissues

metaphysis: the region at either end of an immature long bone at which growth occurs, adjacent to the epiphyseal plate

micron: a unit of measurement equal to 1/1000 of a millimeter

mitochondrion: the organelle that produces energy for the cell

morula: the 16-cell ball that appears in early embryonic life

nanometer: a unit of measure equal to 1/1,000,000 of a millimeter

neurocranium: the bony housing of the brain

newton: a unit of force equal to 0.225 pounds or 0.102 kilograms

nucleation: the process of forming a nucleus or initial aggregation of substances, especially molecules, which then aggregate to form larger crystals or other structures. Homogeneous nucleation occurs spontaneously, by precipitation caused by concentration fluctuations; heterogeneous nucleation is triggered by the addition of some foreign substance

odontogenesis: the process of making dentin

omnivore: a species that habitually eats both plant and animal food

opposition: the movement of the thumb that involves simultaneous rotation about its long axis and flexion of the carpometacarpal joint, so that the fleshy ball of the thumb faces the balls of the other fingers

ossification: the formation of new bones by the replacement of pre-existing tissues. Cartilaginous ossification is typical of long bones that are formed by the replacement of a cartilage model; intramembranous ossification is typical of cranial vault bones that are formed within a membrane

osteoblast: the cell responsible for secreting osteoid, the organic component of bone, and forming new bone tissue

osteoclast: the large, multinucleate cell responsible for resorbing bone tissue and initiating remodeling of bone tissue

osteocyte: a transformed osteoblast cell trapped in calcifying osteoid, which communicates with other bone cells via a network of dendritic processes housed in canaliculi and is capable of digesting bone tissue in rapid response to the body's needs for calcium and phosphorus

osteogenesis: the process of making bone tissue

osteoid: the organic component of bone, most of which is collagen

osteolysis: the cellular process of digesting bone to free calcium and phosphate ions

osteon: the basic unit of mature bone, consisting of a blood vessel in a bony canal comprised of concentric lamellae or rings of bone

osteonectin: a protein in the osteoid that may facilitate calcification by binding to collagen on one site and to calcium and phosphate ions or hydroxyapatite on other sites

osteoprogenitor: the pluripotent cell that gives rise to both osteoblasts and osteocytes, typically found in mesenchyme, the periosteum, or the marrow cavity

palmar: of or pertaining to the anterior surface of the hand

parathyroid hormone: the hormone secreted by the parathyroid gland that increases the circulating levels of calcium and phosphate ions by inducing osteolysis and suppressing calcification, antagonistic to calcitonin

pelvic inlet: the superior aperture of the pelvis, defined by the pubic symphysis anteriorly, the superior pubic ramus and linea terminalis medially, and the sacral promotory posteriorly. Pelvic inlet shape is the basis of a gynecological classification

pelvic outlet: the inferior aperture of the pelvis, defined by the pubic symphysis anteriorly, the ischiopubic ramus and ischial tuberosity medially, and the sacrotuberous ligaments and coccyx posteriorly

perichondrium: the membrane that surrounds the cartilagenous model of a bone during its initial formation, which is transformed into periosteum when invaded by capillaries

periosteum: a tough, highly vascularized membrane that covers the outer surfaces of bones

physis. *See* epiphyseal plate

piezoelectric: producing an electrical current when deformed, characteristic of both whole bones and collagen

plantar: of or pertaining to the sole of the foot

plantarflexion: the action of straightening the ankle

pollex: the thumb or first finger

postcranial: of or pertaining to the region of the skeleton that includes all parts except the skull

posterior: of or toward the back of the body

procollagen: the precursor of collagen, similar in structure to tropocollagen but including extra peptide chains that prevent the formation of fibrils

pronation: the action of the forearm that results in the standard anatomical position of the upper limb with palm facing anteriorly and the long axes of the radius and ulna lying parallel to each other

proximal: toward the trunk or superior part of the limb

pseudoarthrosis: a false joint, including a synovial joint capsule, that results from poor healing of a fracture due to excessive, continued movement of the fragments

sagittal: a midline plane or section that divides the body into symmetrical right and left halves

scoliosis: an abnormal, lateral curvature of the vertebral column

sesamoid: a bone that grows within a tendon, such as the patella

skull: the cranium, including the bony face, upper jaw, cranial vault, and mandible or lower jaw

splanchnocranium: the bony face

spongy bone. *See* cancellous bone

stance phase: in walking, the segment of a stride involving weight-bearing by a leg

strain: the change in dimension, often in length, produced by a force

streaming potential: production of electricity during the movement of a fluid through a solid, due to the preferential attraction of one type of ion, either positive or negative, to the solid

strength: the amount of force required to induce failure of a substance, often measured as tensile strength

stress: the strength of tension or compression, typically measured in pounds per square inch, kilograms per square centimeter, or meganewtons per square meter (1 newton = 0.225 pounds or 0.102 kilograms of force)

stride: in walking, the unit of the cycle that begins with heel strike on one side and ends with the initiation of another heel strike on that side

subchondral bone: highly vascular bone tissue that underlies articular cartilage at joint surfaces

supination: the action of the forearm that results in the palm facing posteriorly and the shaft of the radius crossing anterior to the ulnar shaft, so that the distal radius lies medial to the ulna while the proximal radius lies lateral to the ulna

suture: a specialized type of fibrous joint at which little movement is permitted, as in the interdigitating sutures between various cranial bones

swing phase: in walking, the segment of a stride in which a leg is not weight-bearing but swings around to initiate heel strike

synovia: the thick, slimy fluid found in the capsule of synovial or freely moving joints, which is important in lubricating joints and thus reducing friction during movement

tarsus: the ankle

tension: a force that tends to separate the atoms or molecules of a substance

thoracic: of or pertaining to the thorax or chest

toe off: in walking, the movement of pushing off with a foot as weight is transferred from that foot to the other

torsion: a twisting force

trabecula (*pl.* trabeculae): a small bony spicule or strut typical of cancellous bone

transverse: a horizontal plane or section that divides the body into superior and inferior portions

trauma: any wound or injury

trophic level: the place in the food web that reflects a species' most common energy source or food

trophoblast: the cell type that gives rise to the placenta

volar: of or pertaining to the back or posterior surface of the hand

Volkmann's canal: a bony tube surrounding a blood vessel that runs obliquely or transversely within a bone, which is part of the Haversian system that nourishes bone

working side: in mastication, the side of the mouth where the food resides and is deformed by the bite force

Young's modulus of elasticity (E): the stiffness or flexibility characteristic of a substance, equal to the stress divided by the strain and typically expressed in pounds per square inch, kilograms per square centimeter, or meganewtons per square meter

zygote: the fertilized egg

BIBLIOGRAPHY

PART ONE. THE NATURE OF BONE

Bloom, W., and D. W. Fawcett. 1975. *A Textbook of Histology.* W. B. Saunders, Philadelphia.

Currey, J. D. 1970. *Animal Skeletons.* Edward Arnold, London.

Halstead, L. B. 1974. *Vertebrate Hard Tissues.* Wykeham Publications, London.

Hopkins, C. R. 1978. *Structure and Function of Cells.* W. B. Saunders, London.

Jee, W. S. S. 1983. "The skeletal tissues." In L. Weiss, ed., *Histology: Cell and Tissue Biology.* Elsevier, New York: 200–255.

Thompson, C. W. 1973. *Manual of Structural Kinesiology.* C. V. Mosby, St. Louis.

Williams, P., and R. Warwick, ed. 1980. *Gray's Anatomy.* 36th ed. W. B. Saunders, Philadelphia.

1. Basic Concepts

Livingston, R. B., D. W. Woodbury, and J. L. Patterson, Jr. 1965. "Fluid compartments of the brain: Cerebral circulation." In T. C. Ruch and H. D. Patton, ed., *Physiology and Biophysics.* W. B. Saunders, Philadelphia: 935–958.

Shea, B. 1977. "Eskimo craniofacial morphology, cold stress and the maxillary sinus." *Am. J. Phys. Anthrop.* 47 (2): 289–300.

2. Bone Structure

Friedenstein, A. J. 1976. "Precursor cells of mechanocytes." *Int. Rev. of Cytol.* 47: 327–359.

Galliard, P. J. 1952. "Parathyroid gland and bone in vitro." *Develop. Biol.* 1: 152–171.

Goldhaber, P. 1960. "Behavior of bones in tissue culture." In R. F. Soggnaes, ed., *Calcification in Biological Systems.* Am. Assoc. Adv. Sci. Pub. #64, Washington, D.C.: 349–372.

Hall, B. K. 1978. *Developmental and Cellular Skeletal Biology.* Academic Press, New York.

Jande, S. S., and L. F. Bélanger. 1973. "The life cycle of the osteocyte." *Clin. Orthop.* 94: 281–305.

Jee, W. S. S., and P. N. Nolan. 1963. "Origin of osteoclasts from fusion of phagocytes." *Nature* 200: 255–257.

Kahn, A. J., M. D. Fallon, and S. L. Teitelbaum. 1984. "Structure-function relationships in bone: An examination of events at the cellular level." In W. A. Peck, ed., *Bone and Mineral Research: Annual 2.* Excerpta Medica, Amsterdam: 125–170.

Kember, N. F. 1960. "Cell division in endochondral ossification: A study of cell proliferation in rat bones by the method of tritiated thymidine autoradiography." *J. Bone Jt. Surg.* 42B: 824–839.

Owen, M. 1963. "Cell population kinetics of an osteogenic tissue." *J. Cell Biol.* 19: 19–32.

———. 1978. "Histogenesis of bone cells." *Calcif. Tiss. Res.* 25: 205–207.

Patt, H. M., and M. A. Maloney. 1975. "Bone marrow regeneration after local injury: A review." *Exp. Hemat.* (Copenhagen) 3: 135–146.

Posner, A. S. 1978. "The chemistry of bone mineral." *Bull. Hosp. Joint. Cis.* 39: 126–144.

Prockup, D. J., K. I. Kivirikko, L. Tuderman, and N. A. Guzman. 1979. "The biosynthesis of collagen and its disorders." *New Eng. J. Med.* 301: 13–23, 77–85.

Young, R. W. 1964. "Specialization of bone cells." In H. M. Frost, ed., *Bone Biodynamics.* Little Brown, Boston: 117–137.

3. Collagen and Calcification

Bourne, G. H., ed. 1972. *The Biochemistry and Physiology of Bone,* vols. I–IV. Academic Press, London.

Fleisch, H. 1964. "Role of nucleation and inhibition in calcification." *Clin. Orthop.* 32: 170–180.

Glimcher, M. J. 1976. "Composition, structure, and organization of bone and other mineralized tissues and the mechanism of calcification." In R. O. Greep and E. B. Astwoods, ed., *Handbook of Physiology, 7: Endocrinology VII.* Williams and Wilkins, Baltimore: 25–116.

———. 1984. "Recent studies of the mineral phase in bone and its possible linkage to the organic matrix by protein-bound phosphate bonds." *Phil. Trans. Roy. Soc. Lond.* ser. B 304: 479–508.

Hodge, A. J., J. A. Petruska, and A. J. Bailey. 1965. "The subunit structure of the tropocollagen macromolecule and its relation to various ordered aggregation states." In S. Fitton Jackson, R. D. Harkness, S. M. Partridge, and G. R. Tristam, ed., *Structure and Function of Connective and Skeletal Tissue.* Butterworth, London: 31–41.

McLean, F. C., and M. R. Urist. 1968. *Bone: An Introduction to the Physiology of Skeletal Tissues.* University of Chicago Press, Chicago.

Miller, A. 1984. "Collagen: The organic matrix of bone." *Phil. Trans. Roy. Soc. Lond.* ser. B 304: 455–477.

Russell, R. G. E., and H. Fleisch. 1970. "Inorganic pyrophosphate and pyrophosphatases in calcification and calcium homeostasis." *Clin. Orthop.* 69: 101–117.

Talmage, R. V., and P. L. Munson, ed. 1972. *Calcium, Parathyroid Hormone and the Calcitonins.* Intl. Cong. Series no. 243, Excerpta Medica, Amsterdam.

Termine, J. D. 1983. "Osteonectin and other newly described proteins of developing bone." In W. A. Peck., ed., *Bone and Mineral Research: Annual 1.* Excerpta Medica, Amsterdam: 144–156.

Termine, J. D., and A. S. Posner. 1966. "Infrared analysis of rat bone: Age dependency of amorphous and crystalline mineral fractions." *Science* 153: 1523–1525.

Termine, J. D., H. K. Kleinman, S. W. Whitson, K. M. Conn, M. L. McGarvey, and G. R. Martin. 1981. "Osteonectin, a bone-specific protein linking mineral to collagen." *Cell* 26 (Part 1): 89–105.

4. Bone Growth

Aiello, L. 1981. "The allometry of primate body proportions. *Symp. Zool. Soc. Lond.* 48: 331–358.

Alexander, R. M., A. S. Jayes, G. M. O. Maloiy, and E. M. Wathuta. 1979. "Allometry of the limb bones of mammals from shrews *(Sorex)* to elephant *(Loxodonta)*." *J. Zool. Lond.* 189: 305–314.

Fitzgerald, M. J. T. 1978. *Human Embryology: A Regional Approach*. Harper and Row: Hagerstown.

Langman, J. 1981. *Medical Embryology*. Williams and Wilkins, Baltimore.

McMahon, T. 1973. "Size and shape in biology." *Science* 179: 1201–1204.

———. 1975. "Using body size to understand the structural design of animals: Quadrupedal locomotion." *J. Appl. Physiol.* 39: 619–627.

Radin, E. L., H. G. Parker, J. W. Pugh, R. S. Steinberg, I. L. Pauk, and P. M. Rose. 1973. "Response of joints to impact loading—III; Relationship between trabecular microfractures and cartilage degeneration." *J. Biomech.* 6: 51–57.

Ruff, C. B. 1984. "Allometry between length and cross-sectional dimensions of the femur and tibia in *Homo sapiens sapiens.*" *Am. J. Phys. Anthrop.* 65: 347–358.

Simon, S. R., E. L. Radin, I. L. Paul, and R. M. Rose. 1972. "The response of joints to impact loading—II; In vivo behavior of subchondral bone." *J. Biomech.* 5: 267–272.

5. Bone as a Material

Bassett, C. A. L. 1965. "Electrical effects in bone." *Sci. Am.* 213 (4): 18–25.

Bassett, C. A. L., and R. O. Becker. 1962. "Generation of electric potentials by bone in response to mechanical stress." *Science* 137: 1063–1064.

Bassett, C. A. L., R. J. Pawluk, and R. O. Becker. 1964. "Effects of electric currents on bone in vivo." *Nature* 204: 652–654.

Bonnucci, E., and G. Graziani. 1975. "Comparative thermogravimetric, x-ray diffraction and electron microscope investigations of burnt bones from recent, ancient and prehistoric age." *Atti Della Accademia Nazionale dei Lincei. Sci. Fis. Matem. Natur.* ser. 8, 59: 517–534.

Currey, J. D. 1964. "Three analogies to explain the mechanical properties of bone of different histological types." *J. Anat.* 93 (1): 87–95.

———. 1968. "The adaptation of bones to stress." *J. Theoret. Biol.* 20: 91–106.

———. 1984a. "Effects of differences in mineralization on the mechanical properties of bone." *Phil. Trans. Roy. Soc. Lond.* ser. B 304: 509–518.

———. 1984b. *The Mechanical Adaptations of Bones*. Princeton University Press, Princeton.

Evans, F. G. 1973. *Mechanical Properties of Bone*. Charles C Thomas, Springfield.

Frankel, V. H., and A. H. Burstein. 1970. *Orthopedic Biomechanics*. Lea and Febiger, Philadelphia.

Frankel, V. H., and M. Nordin. 1980. *Basic Biomechanics of the Skeletal System*. Lea and Febiger, Philadelphia.

Fung, Y.-C. 1981. *Biomechanics: Mechanical Properties of Living Tissues.* Springer-Verlag, New York.

Gross, D., and W. S. Williams. 1982. "Streaming potential and the electromechanical response of physiologically-moist bone." *J. Biomech.* 15 (4): 277–295.

Gordon, J. E. 1978. *Structures, or Why Things Don't Fall Down.* Penguin Books, Middlesex.

———. 1968. *The New Science of Strong Materials, or Why You Don't Fall Through the Floor.* Penguin Books, Middlesex.

Mack, R. W. 1964. "Bone — a natural two-phase material." Technical memorandum, Biomechanics Lab, University of California, San Francisco–Berkeley.

Shipman, P., G. Foster, and M. J. Schoeninger. 1984. "Burnt bones and teeth: An experimental study of color, morphology, crystal structure and shrinkage." *J. Arch. Sci.* 11: 307–325.

Williams, W. 1982. "Piezoelectric effects on biological materials." *Ferroelectrics* 41: 225–246.

Yamada, H. 1970. *Strength of Biological Materials.* Williams and Wilkins, Baltimore.

6. Joints and Lubrication

Dowson, D. 1967. "Modes of lubrication in human joints." Paper no. 12, *Lubrication and Wear in Living and Artificial Human Joints.* Proc. Instn. mech. Engrs. 181, part 3J: 45–67.

Dowson, D., A. Unsworth, and V. Wright. 1970. "Analysis of 'boosted lubrication' in human joints." *J. Mech. Eng. Sci.* 12(5): 364–369.

———. 1971. "The cracking of human joints — A study of 'cavitation' in the metacarpo-phalangeal joint." *Instn. mech. Engrs.* 9: 120–127.

Hildebrand, M. 1974. *Analysis of Vertebrate Structure.* John Wiley, New York.

Linn, F. C., and E. L. Radin. 1968. "Lubrication of animal joints, III. The effect of certain chemical alterations of the cartilage and lubricant." *Arth. and Rheum.* 11 (5): 674–682.

McCutcheon, C. W. 1959. "Sponge-hydrostatic and weeping bearings." *Nature* 184: 1284–1285.

———. 1962. "The frictional properties of animal joints." *Wear* 5: 1–17.

———. 1969. "Why did nature make synovial joints slimy?" *Clin. Orthop.* 64: 18.

Mow, V. C., V. Roth, and C. G. Armstrong. 1980. "Biomechanics of joint cartilage." In V. H. Frankel and M. Nordin, ed., *Basic Biomechanics of the Skeletal System.* Lea and Febiger, Philadelphia: 61–86.

Radin, E. L. 1968. "Synovial fluid as a lubricant." *Arth. and Rheum.* 11 (5): 693–695.

Radin, E. L., I. L. Paul, D. A. Swann, and E. S. Schottstaedt. 1970. "Lubrication of synovial membrane." *Ann. Rheum. Dis.* 30: 322–324.

PART TWO. THE FUNCTION OF BONES

Basmajian, J. V. 1979. *Muscles Alive: Their Function Revealed by Electromyography.* Williams and Wilkins, Baltimore.

Bass, W. 1971. *Human Osteology: A Laboratory and Field Manual.* Missouri Archaeological Society, Columbia.

Breathnach, A. S., ed. 1965. *Frazer's Anatomy of the Human Skeleton*. J. and A. Churchill, London.

Brothwell, D. R. 1981. *Digging Up Bones*. Cornell University Press, Ithaca.

Joseph, J. 1963. *Aids to Osteology*. Ballière, Tindall and Cassell, London.

7. The Axial Skeleton

Lindh, M. 1980. "Biomechanics of the lumbar spine." In V. H. Frankel and M. Nordin, ed., *Basic Biomechanics of the Skeletal System*. Lea and Febiger, Philadelphia: 255–290.

8. Breathing

Hildebrandt, J., and A. C. Young. 1965. "Respiration." In T. C. Ruch and H. D. Patton, ed., *Physiology and Biophysics*. W. B. Saunders, Philadelphia: 733–760.

9. The Upper Limb

Napier, J. 1961. "Prehensility and opposability in the hands of primates." *Symp. Zool. Soc. Lond.* 5: 115–132.

10. Manipulation

Matsen, F. A., III. 1980. "Biomechanics of the shoulder." In V. H. Frankel and M. Nordin, ed., *Basic Biomechanics of the Skeletal System*. Lea and Febiger, Philadelphia: 221–242.

———. 1980. "Biomechanics of the elbow." In V. H. Frankel and M. Nordin, ed., *Basic Biomechanics of the Skeletal System*. Lea and Febiger, Philadelphia: 243–254.

11. The Lower Limb

Ruff, C. B., C. S. Larsen, and W. C. Hayes. 1984. "Structural changes in the femur with the transition to agriculture on the Georgia coast." *Am. J. Phys. Anthrop.* 64: 125–136.

12. Walking

Eberhart, H. O., V. T. Inman, and B. Bresler. 1954. "The principal elements in human locomotion." In P. E. Klopsteg and P. D. Wilson, ed., *Human Limbs and Their Substitutes*. McGraw-Hill, New York: 437–471.

Frankel, V. H., and M. Nordin. 1980. "Biomechanics of the ankle." In V. H. Frankel and M. Nordin, ed., *Basic Biomechanics of the Skeletal System*. Lea and Febiger, Philadelphia: 179–192.

———. 1980. "Biomechanics of the foot." In V. H. Frankel and M. Nordin, ed., *Basic Biomechanics of the Skeletal System*. Lea and Febiger, Philadelphia: 192–220.

Inman, V. T., H. J. Ralston, and F. Todd. 1981. *Human Walking*. Williams and Wilkins, Baltimore.

Napier, J. 1967. "Antiquity of human walking." *Sci. Am.* 216: 56–66.

Nordin, M., and V. H. Frankel. 1980. "Biomechanics of the hip." In V. H. Frankel and M. Nordin, ed., *Basic Biomechanics of the Skeletal System*. Lea and Febiger, Philadelphia: 149–178.

———. 1980. "Biomechanics of the knee." In V. H. Frankel and M. Nordin, ed.,

Basic Biomechanics of the Skeletal System. Lea and Febiger, Philadelphia: 113–148.

Saunders, J. B. de C. M., V. T. Inman, and B. Bresler. 1953. "The major determinants in normal and pathological gait." *J. Bone & Jt. Surg.* 35A: 543–558.

13. The Skull

Dahlberg, A., ed. 1975. *Dental Morphology and Evolution.* University of Chicago Press, Chicago.

Hiatt, J., and L. Gartner. 1982. *Textbook of Head Anatomy.* Appleton-Century Crofts, Baltimore.

14. Chewing

Rowe, N. H., ed. 1976. *Occlusion: Research in Form and Function.* University of Michigan School of Dentistry, Ann Arbor.

Sicher, H., and E. L. DuBrul. 1975. *Oral Anatomy.* C. V. Mosby, St. Louis.

Walker, A. C. 1978. "Functional anatomy of the oral tissues: Mastication and deglutition." In J. H. Shaw, E. A. Sweeney, C. C. Cappucino, and S. M. Meller, ed., *Textbook of Oral Biology.* W. B. Saunders, Philadelphia: 277–296.

PART THREE. INTERPRETING BONES

Krogman, W. M. 1962. *The Human Skeleton in Forensic Medicine.* Charles C Thomas, Springfield.

Rathbun, T. A., and J. E. Buikstra. 1984. *Human Identification: Case Studies in Forensic Anthropology.* Charles C Thomas, Springfield.

Stewart, T. D. 1970. *Personal Identification in Mass Disasters.* National Museum of Natural History, Smithsonian Institution, Washington, D.C.

———. 1979. *Essentials of Forensic Anthropology.* Charles C Thomas, Springfield.

Ubelaker, D. H. 1978. *Human Skeletal Remains: Excavation, Analysis, Interpretation.* Aldine, Chicago.

15. Age, Sex, Race, and Stature

Ahlqvist, J., and O. Damsten. 1969. "Modification of Kerley's method for the microscopic determination of age in human bone." *J. Forensic Sci.* 14: 205–214.

Buikstra, J. E., and J. H. Miekle. 1984. "Demography, diet, and health." In R. I. Gilbert and J. H. Mielke, ed., *Techniques for the Analysis of Prehistoric Diet.* Academic Press, New York: 360–422.

DiBennardo, R., and J. V. Taylor. 1979. "Sex assessment of the femur: A test of a new method." *Am. J. Phys. Anthrop.* 50: 635–638.

Genovés, S. 1967. "Proportionality of the long bones and their relation to stature among Mesoamericans." *Am. J. Phys. Anthrop.* 26: 67–77.

Giles, E., and O. Elliot. 1962. "Race identification from cranial measurements." *J. Forensic Sci.* 7: 147–157.

———. 1963. "Sex determination by discriminant analysis." *Am. J. Phys. Anthrop.* 21: 53–68.

Gustafson, G. 1950. "Age determinations of teeth." *J. Am. Dent. Assoc.* 41: 45–54.

Hanihara, G. 1958a. "Sex diagnosis of Japanese skulls and scapulae by means of discriminant function." *J. Anthropol. Soc. Nippon* 67: 191–197.

———. 1958b. "Sexual diagnosis of Japanese long bones by means of discriminant function." *J. Anthropol. Soc. Nippon* 66: 187–196.

Howell, N. 1982. "Village composition implied by a paleodemographic life table: The Libben Site." *Am. J. Phys. Anthrop.* 53: 263–270.

Howells, W. W. 1973. *Cranial Variation in Man.* Paper of Peabody Mus. Arch. and Ethn. #67, Harvard University Press, Cambridge.

Keen, J. A. 1965. "A study of the differences between male and female skulls." *Am. J. Phys. Anthrop.* 8: 65–79.

Kelley, M. A. 1978. "Phenice's visual sexing technique for the os pubis: A critique." *Am. J. Phys. Anthropol.* 48: 121–122.

Kerley, E. R. 1965. "The microscopic determination of age in human beings." *Am. J. Phys. Anthrop.* 23: 149–163.

Lovejoy, C. O., R. S. Meindl, R. P. Mensforth, and T. J. Barton. 1985. "Multifactorial determination of skeletal age at death." *Am. J. Phys. Anthr.* 68: 1–14.

Lovejoy, C. O., R. S. Meindl, T. R. Pryzbeck, T. S. Barton, K. G. Heiple, and D. Kotting. 1977. "Paleodemography of the Libben Site, Ottawa County, Ohio." *Science* 198: 291–293.

Maples, W. R. 1978. "An improved technique using dental histology for estimation of adult age." *J. Forensic Sci.* 23: 747–770.

McKern, T. W., and T. D. Stewart. 1957. "Skeletal age changes in young American males." Technical Report EP-45, Quartermaster Research and Development Command, Natick, Mass.

Meindl, R. S., and C. O. Lovejoy. 1985. "Ectocranial suture closure." *Am. J. Phys. Anthrop.* 68: 57–66.

Meindl, R.S., C.O. Lovejoy, R.P. Mensforth, and R.A. Walker. 1985. "A revised method of age determination using the os pubis." *Am. J. Phys. Anthr.* 68: 29–46.

Olivier, G., and H. Pineau. 1958. "Determination de l'age foetale et de l'embryon." *Arch. Anat. (La Semaine des Hôpitales)* 6: 21–28.

———. 1960. "Nouvelle determination de la taille foetale d'apres les longeurs diaphysaires des os longs." *Ann. Med. Leg.* 40: 141–144.

Owsley, D. W., and R. S. Webb. 1983. "Misclassification probability of dental discriminant functions for sex determination." *J. Forensic Sci.* 28: 181–185.

Parson, F. G. 1916. "On the proportions and characteristics of the modern English clavicle." *J. Anat. Lond.* 51: 71–93.

Phenice, T. W. 1969. "A newly developed visual method of sexing the os pubis." *Am. J. Phys. Anthrop.* 30: 297–302.

Pons, J. 1955. "The sexual diagnosis of isolated bones of the skeleton." *Hum. Biol.* 37: 12–21.

Richman, E. A., M. E. Michel, F. P. Schulter-Ellis, and R. S. Corrucini. 1979. "Determination of sex by discriminant function analysis of postcranial skeletal remains." *J. Forensic Sci.* 24: 159–167.

Schulter-Ellis, F. P., D. J. Schimdt, L. A. Hayek, and J. Craig. 1983. "Determination of sex with a discriminant analysis of new pelvic bone measurements: Pat I." *J. Forensic Sci.* 24: 159–167.

Singh, I. J., and D. L. Gunberg. 1970. "Estimation of age at death in human males from quantitative histology of bone fragments." *Am. J. Phys. Anthrop.* 33: 373–381.

Snow, C. C., S. Hartman, E. Giles, and F. A. Young. 1979. "Sex and age determination of crania by calipers and computer: A test of the Giles and Elliot functions in 52 forensic science cases." *J. Forensic Sci.* 24: 448–460.

Steel, L. D. 1976. "Further observations on the osteometric discriminant function: The human clavicle." *Am. J. Phys. Anthrop.* 25: 319–322.

Stewart, T. D. 1948. "Medico-legal aspects of the skeleton. I. Sex, age, race, and stature." *Am. J. Phys. Anthrop.* 6: 315–322.

——. 1951. "What the bones tell." *FBI Law Enf. Bull.* 20 (2): 2–5.

Swedlund, A., and G. Armelagos. 1976. *Demographic Anthropology.* Brown, Dubuque.

Thieme, F. P., and W. J. Schull. 1957. "Sex determination from the skeleton." *Hum. Biol.* 29: 242–273.

Trotter, M., and G. C. Gleser. 1952. "Estimation of stature from long bones of American Whites and Negroes." *Am. J. Phys. Anthrop.* 10: 463–514.

——. 1958. "A re-evaluation of stature based on measurements taken during life and of long bones after death." *Am. J. Phys. Anthrop.* 16: 79–123.

Ubelaker, D. H. 1974. *Reconstruction of Demographic Profiles from Ossuary Skeletal Samples: A Case Study from the Tidewater Potomac.* Smithsonian Contrib. Anthrop. no. 18, Smithsonian Institution Press, Washington, D.C.

Washburn, S. 1948. "Sex differences in the pubic bone." *Am. J. Phys. Anthrop.* 6: 199–207.

Weiss, K. M. 1973. *Demographic Models for Anthropology.* Mem. Soc. Am. Arch. #27. *Am. Antiq.* 38(2), Part II.

16. Trauma and Disease

Brothwell, D. R., and A. T. Sandeson, ed. 1963. *Diseases in Antiquity.* Charles C Thomas, Springfield.

Ortner, D. J., and W. G. J. Putschar. 1981. *Identification of Pathological Conditions in Human Skeletal Remains.* Smithsonian Contrib. Anthrop. no. 28, Smithsonian Institution Press, Washington, D.C.

Steinbock, R. T. 1976. *Paleopathological Diagnosis and Interpretation.* Charles C Thomas, Springfield.

Tyson, R. A., and E. S. Dyer Alcauskas, ed. 1980. *Catalogue of the Hrdlicka Paleopathology Collection.* San Diego Museum of Man, San Diego.

Walker, A. C., M. R. Zimmerman, and R. E. Leakey. 1981. "A possible case of hypervitaminosis A in *Homo erectus.*" *Nature* 296: 248–250.

17. Reconstruction

Bender, M. M. 1971. "Variations in the $^{13}C/^{12}C$ ratio of plants in relation to the pathway of photosynthetic carbon dioxide." *Phytochem.* 10: 1239–1244.

Gatliff, B. P. 1979. "Facial reconstruction in forensic medicine." Videotape, Department of Biomedical Communications, University of Texas Health Science Center, Dallas.

Gatliff, B. P., and C. C. Snow. 1979. "From skull to visage." *J. Biocommunication* 6(2): 27–30.

His, W. 1895. "Anatomische Forschungen ueber Johann Sebastian Bach's Gebeine und Antlitz' nebst Bemerkungen ueber dessen Bilder." *Abhandl d k sächs Gesellsch d Wissensch zu Leipz* 22 (whole ser. 37): 379–420.

Kollman, J., and W. Büchly. 1898. "Die Persistenz der Rassen und die Reconstruction der Physiognomie prähistorischer Schädel." *Arch. Anthrop.* 25: 329–359.

Rhine, J. S., and H. R. Campbell. 1980. "Thickness of facial tissues in American blacks." *J. Forensic Sci.* 25: 847–858.

Rhine, J. S., and C. E. Moore. 1982. "Facial reproduction tables of facial tissue thicknesses of American Caucasoids in forensic anthropology." Maxwell Museum Technical Series no. 1, Albuquerque.

Schoeninger, M. J. 1979. "Diet and status at Chalcatzingo: Some empirical and technical aspects of strontium analysis." *Am. J. Phys. Anthrop.* 51: 295–310.

Schoeninger, M. J., and M. DeNiro. 1982. "Carbon isotope ratios of apatite from fossil bone cannot be used to reconstruct diets of animals." *Nature* 297: 577–578.

———. 1984. "Nitrogen and carbon isotopic composition of bone collagen in marine and terrestrial vertebrates." *Geochim. Cosmochim. Acta* 48: 625–639.

Schoeninger, M. J., M. DeNiro, and H. Tauber. 1983. "^{15}N/^{14}N ratios of bone collagen reflect marine and terrestrial components of prehistoric diet." *Science* 220: 1381–1383.

Shipman, P. 1981. "Applications of scanning electron microscopy to taphonomic problems." In A.-M. Cantwell, J. B. Griffin, and N. Rothschild, ed., *The Research Potential of Anthropological Museum Collections.* Ann. N.Y. Acad. Sci. 276: 357–385.

———. 1983. "Early hominid lifestyle: Hunting and gathering or foraging and scavenging?" In J. Clutton-Brock and C. Grigson, ed., *Animals and Archaeology,* vol I. *Hunters and Their Prey.* B. A. R., London: 31–50.

Sillen, A., and M. Kavanaugh. 1982. "Strontium and paleodietary research." *Yrbk. Phys. Anthrop.* 25: 67–90.

Snow, C. C., B. P. Gatliff, and K. R. McWilliams. 1970. "Reconstruction of facial features from the skull: An evaluation of its usefulness in forensic anthropology." *Am. J. Phys. Anthrop.* 33: 221–227.

Teaford, M. F., and A. C. Walker. 1984. "Quantitative differences in dental microwear between primate species with different diets and a comment on the presumed diet of *Sivapithecus*." *Am. J. Phys. Anthrop.* 64: 191–200.

Toots, H., and M. R. Voorhies. 1965. "Strontium in fossil bones and the reconstruction of food chains." *Science* 149: 849–855.

van der Merwe, N., and J. C. Vogel. 1978. "^{13}C content of human collagen as a measure of prehistoric diet in Woodland North America." *Nature* 276: 815–816.

Vogel, J. C., and N. van der Merwe. 1977. "Isotopic evidence for early maize cultivation in New York state." *Am. Antiq.* 42: 238–242.

Walker, A. C. 1981. "Dietary hypotheses and human evolution." *Phil. Trans. Roy. Soc. Lond.* ser. B, 292 (1057): 57–63.

Walker, A. C., H. N. Hoeck, and L. M. Perez. 1978. "Microwear on mammalian teeth as an indicator of diet." *Science* 201: 908–910.

Welcker, H. 1883. *Schiller's Schädel und Todenmaske, nebst Mittheilungen über Schädel und Todenmaske Kants.* Braunschweig.

CREDITS

Figures

12-19 Based on data from Eberhart et al., 1954. David Bichell.
12-20 Based on Saunders et al., 1953. David Bichell.
13-1 – 21 David Bichell.
14-1 – 20 David Bichell.
15-1 From G. Olivier and H. Pineau, 1960. *Ann. Med. Leg.* 40: 143.
15-2 – 6 David Bichell.
15-7 – 8 Reprinted from D. R. Brothwell, 1981. *Digging Up Bones.* By permission of the author, Cornell University Press, and the British Museum (Natural History).
15-9 Reprinted from R. A. Tyson and E. S. Alcauskas, ed., 1980. *Catalogue of the Hdrlicka Paleopathology Collection,* with permission of the San Diego Museum of Man.
15-10 David Bichell.
15-11 Based on Washburn 1948. David Bichell.
15-12 – 13 David Bichell.
16-1 Photo by Pat Shipman and Tom Urquhart.
16-2 Photos by Jeff Abrams. Reprinted from G. Milner, 1984. *Paleopathology Newsletter* 45: 11 – 12, by permission of the author and publisher.
16-3 Reprinted from W. M. Krogman, 1962. *The Human Skeleton in Forensic Medicine.* Courtesy of Charles C Thomas, Publisher, Springfield, Illinois.
16-4 By permission of the Smithsonian Institution Press, from *Identification of Pathological Conditions in Human Skeletal Remains,* Smithsonian Contributions to Anthropology Number 28, by Donald J. Ortner and Walter G. J. Putschar. Fig. 106, p. 91. Smithsonian Institution, Washington, D.C. 1981.
16-5 Photo by Jeff Abrams. Reprinted from G. Milner, 1984, in C. J. Bareis and J. W. Porter, ed., *American Bottom Archaeology,* with permission of the authors, editors, and the University of Illinois Press, Urbana. Copyright 1984 University of Illinois Press.
16-6 Photo courtesy of George Milner.
16-7 By permission of the Smithsonian Institution Press, from *Identification of Pathological Conditions in Human Skeletal Remains,* Smithsonian Contributions to Anthropology Number 28, by Donald J. Ortner and Walter G. J. Putschar. Fig. 427, p. 278. Smithsonian Institution, Washington, D.C. 1981.
16-8 Reprinted from Walker et al., 1981. *Nature* 296: 249. Copyright © 1984 Macmillan Journals Limited.
16-9 Reprinted from R. A. Tyson and E. S. Alcauskas, ed., 1980. *Catalogue of the Hrdlicka Paleopathology Collection,* with permission of the San Diego Museum of Man.
16-10 By permission of the Smithsonian Institution Press, from *Identification of Pathological Conditions in Human Skeletal Remains,* Smithsonian Contributions to Anthropology Number 28, by Donald J. Ortner and Walter G. J. Putschar. Fig. 427, p. 278. Smithsonian Institution, Washington, D.C. 1981.
16-11 Reprinted from R. A. Tyson and E. S. Alcauskas, ed., 1980. *Cata-*

logue of the Hrdlicka Paleopathology Collection, with permission of the San Diego Museum of Man.

17-1   Based on Kollman and Büchly, 1889. Reprinted from T. D. Stewart, 1979. *Essentials of Forensic Anthropology.* Courtesy of Charles C Thomas, Publisher, Springfield, Illinois.

17-2   Reprinted from Snow et al., 1970. *American Journal of Physical Anthropology.* By permission of the authors and publisher.

17-3   Reprinted from M. F. Teaford and A. C. Walker, 1984. *American Journal of Physical Anthropology.* By permission of the authors and publisher.

17-4   Reprinted from P. Shipman, 1981. *Life History of a Fossil.* Harvard University Press, Cambridge, by permission of the author and publisher.

Tables

5-1   Data from Mack, 1964, cited in Evans, 1973.

15-1   Data from Stewart, 1979.

15-2   Reprinted from McKern and Stewart, 1957, by permission from the Headquarters, Quartermaster Research and Development Center, U.S. Army, Natick, Mass.

15-3   Data from J. E. Buikstra and J. H. Miekle in R. I. Gilbert and J. H. Miekle, ed., 1984. *Techniques for the Analysis of Prehistoric Diet.* New York: Academic Press.

15-4   Reprinted from M. Trotter, in T. D. Stewart, ed., 1970. *Personal Identification in Mass Disasters.* National Museum of Natural History, Washington, D.C., by permission of the editor. Corrections proposed in Trotter (1977) are incorporated.

17-1   Reprinted from T. D. Stewart, 1979. *Essentials of Forensic Anthropology.* Courtesy of Charles C Thomas, Publisher, Springfield, Illinois.

Index

Foramina: vertebral, 83; cecum, 203; infraorbital, 207, 208; incisive, 209; zygomaticofacial, 209; mandibular, 212; mental, 212; sphenopalatine, 216; rotundum, 220, 221; ovale, 220–221; spinosum, 221; parietal, 224; mastoid, 225; lacerum, 226; jugular, 226, 230; stylomastoid, 226–227; condyloid, 229. *See also* Obturator foramen; Optic foramen

Forearm, 101, 108–111, 130, 134, 139

Fossae: infraspinous, 105; supraspinous, 105; coronoid, 107; acetabular, 143; condyloid, 148, 229; iliac, 177; cranial, 199, 201, 220; canine, 207; incisive, 207, 209; digastric, 212, 226; sublingual, 212; submandibular, 212; pterygoid, 221; parietal, 223; jugular, 226–227, 230; for brain, 229. *See also* Glenoid fossa

Fractures, 57, 63, 285–294

Frankfurt horizontal, 234, 236

Frontal, 196, 197, 199, 202–205, 207–208; and sphenoid, 209, 221; and temporalis muscle, 239

Gatliff, B. P., 305

Genovés, S., 279

Giles, E., 274

Glenoid fossa: and scapula, 13, 104, 120, 123, 127; and elbow, 128; of temporal bone, 212, 225, 237, 243, 245

Gleser, G. C., 279

Gliding, 17. *See also* Bones: movements of

Gluteus maximus, 173–174, 178

Gluteus medius, 174, 192, 194

Gluteus minimus, 175, 192, 194

Golgi apparatus, 23–24, 26, 31

Gonial angle, 212, 236, 240

Gordon, J. E., 53

Gustafson, G., 270

Hallux, 14; phalanges of, 153, 162, 163; muscles of, 156, 158, 161, 186, 187, 188, 189; in walking, 183, 192

Hamate, 3, 113, 115

Hamstrings, 173, 181, 194

Hand, 3, 5, 101, 111–117, 139; extrinsic muscles of, 130–135; intrinsic muscles of, 135–138; phalanges of, 162–163

Harris lines, 295

Haversian system, 21, 22, 48, 49; Volkmann's canals in, 22; Haversian canals in, 22, 24, 269, 312

Hearing, 196, 226, 232

Heel. *See* Calcaneus

Heel strike, 190, 191, 192, 194

Hip: joint of, 14; in walking, 145, 148, 164–165, 190, 192, 194, 195; movements of, 165, 171, 176–177; muscles of, 173–181; fusion of, 264; and tuberculosis, 300

Hodge, A. J., 30

Hormone, parathyroid, 36, 37

Howship's lacunae, 25, 26

Humerus, 9, 13, 101, 105–107, 108, 139; joints of, 14; fusion of, 40, 263; movement of, 120, 123, 124–127, 128–130, 134; in interpreting bones, 277

Hunchback. *See* Kyphosis

Hyaluronic acid, 67, 72

Hydroxyapatite, 53, 54–55, 56, 59, 312; formation of, 31, 33, 34

Hyoid, 9, 12, 196, 202, 227, 233–234; ossification of, 233–234; and digastric muscle, 242

Hypervitaminosis A, 295, 298–299

Hypoglossal canal, 230

Hypophysis (pituitary gland), 201

Ilium, 14, 89, 126, 141, 143, 164, 177; in interpreting bones, 275

Incus, 13, 196, 230, 231, 232

Indians, American, 251, 254, 293

Infection, 299

Inferior concha, 213, 214, 216

Infratemporal crest, 221

Innominate, 11–12, 14, 42, 89, 126, 275; fusion of, 139; three major regions of, 141, 143–146; and interpreting bones, 275. *See also* Pelvic girdle

Ischium, 141, 143–144, 164, 275, 276. *See also* Pelvic girdle

Isotope analysis, 307, 308–310, 312

Joints, 11, 13–14, 64–77; fibrous, 64; basic types of, 64–65; cartilaginous, 64–65; synovial, 65, 67, 68, 71, 75, 84, 89, 101, 164, 237; lubrication of, 65–72; sternoclavicular, 67; temporomandibular (TMJ), 67, 225, 237–238; and muscles, 68, 118; cracking, 72–73; as levers, 73–75; multiaxial, 75, 76; biaxial, 75, 76, 77; uniaxial, 75–76; shapes of, 76–77; humeroulnar, 76, 108, 120; planar, 76–77; condylar, 77; ellipsoidal, 77; pivotal, 77; sellar, 77; spheroidal, 77; radiocarpal, 77, 118; hinge, 77, 123, 171, 172; manubrioster-